ANNALS OF
THE NEW YORK ACADEMY
OF SCIENCES

Volume 895

EDITORIAL STAFF

Executive Editor
BARBARA M. GOLDMAN

Managing Editor
JUSTINE CULLINAN

Associate Editors
JOHN W. KENNEDY
RICHARD STIEFEL

The New York Academy of Sciences
2 East 63rd Street
New York, New York 10021

THE NEW YORK ACADEMY OF SCIENCES
(Founded in 1817)

BOARD OF GOVERNORS, September 15, 1999–September 15, 2000

BILL GREEN, *Chairman of the Board*
TORSTEN WIESEL, *Vice Chairman of the Board*
RODNEY W. NICHOLS, *President and CEO* [ex officio]

Honorary Life Governors
WILLIAM T. GOLDEN   JOSHUA LEDERBERG

JOHN T. MORGAN, *Treasurer*

Governors

D. ALLAN BROMLEY	LAWRENCE B. BUTTENWIESER	PRAVEEN CHAUDHARI
JOHN H. GIBBONS	RONALD L. GRAHAM	HENRY M. GREENBERG
ROBERT G. LAHITA	MARTIN L. LEIBOWITZ	JACQUELINE LEO
WILLIAM J. McDONOUGH	KATHLEEN P. MULLINIX	JOHN F. NIBLACK
SANDRA PANEM	RICHARD RAVITCH	RICHARD A. RIFKIND
	SARA LEE SCHUPF	JAMES H. SIMONS

ELEANOR BAUM, *Past Chairman of the Board*

HELENE L. KAPLAN, *Counsel* [ex officio]   PETER H. KOHN, *V.P. & Secretary* [ex officio]

UNCERTAINTY IN THE RISK ASSESSMENT OF ENVIRONMENTAL AND OCCUPATIONAL HAZARDS

AN INTERNATIONAL WORKSHOP

ANNALS OF THE NEW YORK ACADEMY OF SCIENCES
Volume 895

UNCERTAINTY IN THE RISK ASSESSMENT OF ENVIRONMENTAL AND OCCUPATIONAL HAZARDS

AN INTERNATIONAL WORKSHOP

Edited by A. John Bailer, Cesare Maltoni,
John C. Bailar III, Fiorella Belpoggi,
Jill V. Brazier, and Morando Soffritti

The New York Academy of Sciences
New York, New York
1999

Copyright © 1999 by the New York Academy of Sciences. All rights reserved. Under the provisions of the United States Copyright Act of 1976, individual readers of the Annals *are permitted to make fair use of the material in them for teaching and research. Permission is granted to quote from the* Annals *provided that the customary acknowledgment is made of the source. Material in the* Annals *may be republished only by permission of the Academy. Address inquiries to the Executive Editor at the New York Academy of Sciences.*

Copying fees: *For each copy of an article made beyond the free copying permitted under Section 107 or 108 of the 1976 Copyright Act, a fee should be paid through the Copyright Clearance Center, Inc., 222 Rosewood Drive, Danvers, MA 01923. The fee for copying an article is $3.00 for nonacademic use; for use in the classroom it is $0.07 per page.*

∞ *The paper used in this publication meets the minimum requirements of American National Standard for Information Sciences—Permanence of Paper for Printed Library Materials. ANSI Z39.48-1984.*

Library of Congress Cataloging-in-Publication Data

[applied for]

K-M Research/PCP
Printed in the United States of America
ISBN 1-57331-236-3 (cloth)
ISBN 1-57331-237-1 (paper)
ISSN 0077-8923

ANNALS OF THE NEW YORK ACADEMY OF SCIENCES

Volume 895

UNCERTAINTY IN THE RISK ASSESSMENT OF ENVIRONMENTAL AND OCCUPATIONAL HAZARDS

AN INTERNATIONAL WORKSHOP[a]

Editors
A. JOHN BAILER, CESARE MALTONI, JOHN C. BAILAR III,
FIORELLA BELPOGGI, JILL V. BRAZIER, AND MORANDO SOFFRITTI

Conference Organizers
JOHN C. BAILAR III, A. JOHN BAILER,
CESARE MALTONI, AND MARCEL VAN DEN BROECKE

CONTENTS

Foreword. *By* JOHN C. BAILAR III ix

Introductory Remarks. *By* CESARE MALTONI x

Uncertainty in Risk Assessment. *By* MARCEL VAN DEN BROECKE xii

Part I. Introduction

Risk Assessment for Children and Other Sensitive Populations.
  By PHILIP J. LANDRIGAN 1

Part II. Uncertainty in Hazard Identification

The Scientific and Methodological Bases of Experimental Studies for Detecting and Quantifying Carcinogenic Risks. *By* CESARE MALTONI, MORANDO SOFFRITTI, AND FIORELLA BELPOGGI 10

A Bayesian Approach to Hazard Identification: the Case of Electromagnetic Fields and Cancer. *By* ANDERS AHLBOM AND MARIA FEYCHTING 27

Mega-experiments to Identify and Assess Diffuse Carcinogenic Risks.
  By MORANDO SOFFRITTI, FIORELLA BELPOGGI, FRANCO MINARDI, LUCIANO BUA, AND CESARE MALTONI 34

Long-Term Chemical Carcinogenesis Bioassays Predict Human Cancer Hazards: Issues, Controversies, and Uncertainties. *By* JAMES HUFF 56

[a]This volume is the result of an international workshop entitled **Uncertainty in the Risk Assessment of Environmental and Occupational Hazards**, which was organized by the European Foundation of Oncology and Environmental Sciences B. Ramazzini, the International Statistical Institute, the University of Chicago, and Miami University and was held on September 24–26, 1998 in the Council Chamber of the Town Hall of Bologna, Italy.

Part III. Uncertainty in Exposure Assessment

Uncertainty in Biomonitoring and Kinetic Modeling. *By* LUTZ EDLER 80

Using Molecular Epidemiology in Assessing Exposure for Risk Assessment.
By P.A. SCHULTE AND M. WATERS 101

Kaplan-Meier Tumor Probability as a Starting Point for Dose-Response Modeling Provides Accurate Lifetime Risk Estimates from Rodent Carcinogenicity Studies. *By* WIL F. TEN BERGE................................. 112

Uncertainty in Estimating Exposure Using a Toxicokinetic Model: the Example of 2,3,7,8-Tetrachlorodibenzo-*p*-Dioxin. *By* ALBERTO SALVAN, KARL THOMASETH, PAOLA BORTOT, AND NICOLA SARTORI................. 125

Uncertainty in the Relation between Exposure to Magnetic Fields and Brain Cancer due to Assessment and Assignment of Exposure and Analytical Methods in Dose-Response Modeling. *By* HANS KROMHOUT, DANA P. LOOMIS, AND ROBERT C. KLECKNER 141

Measures of Exposure to Environmental Tobacco Smoke: Validity, Precision, and Relevance. *By* ALISTAIR WOODWARD AND WAEL AL-DELAIMY 156

The Contribution of Environmental Monitoring in the Epidemiological Assessment of Exogenous Risk: the Experience of ARPA in the Emilia-Romagna Region of Italy. *By* A. ZAVATTI AND P. LAURIOLA............. 173

Part IV. Uncertainty in Dose-Response Modeling

Combining Uncertainty Factors in Deriving Human Exposure Levels of Noncarcinogenic Toxicants. *By* RALPH L. KODELL AND DAVID W. GAYLOR   188

Statistical Methods for Developmental Toxicity: Analysis of Clustered Multivariate Binary Data. *By* LOUISE RYAN AND GEERT MOLENBERGHS ... 196

Sources of Uncertainty in Dose-Response Modeling of Epidemiological Data for Cancer Risk Assessment. *By* LESLIE STAYNER, A. JOHN BAILER, RANDALL SMITH, STEPHEN GILBERT, FAYE RICE, AND EILEEN KUEMPEL.......... 212

Nonparametric Analysis of Dose-Response Relationships. *By* K. ULM........ 223

Estimates of the Proportions of Carcinogens and Anticarcinogens in Bioassays Conducted by the U.S. National Toxicology Program: Application of a New Meta-analytic Approach. *By* KENNY S. CRUMP, DANIEL KREWSKI, AND CYNTHIA VAN LANDINGHAM................................ 232

Characterization of Uncertainty and Variability in Residential Radon Cancer Risks. *By* D. KREWSKI, S.N. RAI, J.M. ZIELINSKI, AND P.K. HOPKE 245

Part V. Uncertainty in Risk Characterization and Communication

Risk Assessment—the Mother of All Uncertainties: Disciplinary Perspectives on Uncertainty in Risk Assessment. *By* JOHN C. BAILAR III AND A. JOHN BAILER 273

Foreword

JOHN C. BAILAR III

Department of Health Studies and Harris School of Public Policy, University of Chicago, 5841 South Maryland Avenue, MC 2007, Chicago, Illinois 60637, USA

It is a pleasure to introduce this volume of the *Annals of the New York Academy of Sciences*, which grew from a workshop on Uncertainty in the Risk Assessment of Environmental and Occupational Hazards. The workshop was sponsored jointly by the European Ramazzini Foundation and the International Statistical Institute. Many other organizations also provided financial support and these are identified at the end of the table of contents. The volume includes papers by authors from many different parts of the world. This is welcome, because the problems of uncertainty in risk assessment are universal, and require the dedicated attention of leading scientists everywhere.

We are particularly grateful to the city of Bologna for allowing us to use its Council Chambers for the workshop. These Chambers combine the most modern audio-visual tools with an appearance and ambiance that has remained unchanged over centuries, and I understand that the building has never needed to be restored because it has been continually maintained to the highest standards.

Risk assessment is fundamental to protection of the public health from environmental and occupational hazards, but any estimate of risk is subject to numerous and large uncertainties. These uncertainties can go far beyond the uncertainty expressed by the usual statistical confidence bounds. Thus, risk assessments of the same hazard commonly differ by factors of that exceed 1,000. We do not believe that the public is well served by ignoring or sweeping away these differences, nor is it well served by an exclusive focus on either the high end or the low end of what may seem to be a plausible range. This volume deals with many aspects of uncertainty, including its origins, its general magnitude, and its implications for public policy. For the most part, the authors present real examples with real data.

The Scientific Committee did a fine job of including papers from world experts that discuss uncertainty in risk assessment. It is also a pleasure to acknowledge the constant and vigorous support of Dr. Jill Brazier in arranging for the workshop from which this volume resulted. He would also like to thank the Editorial Department of the New York Academy of Sciences, and particularly Dr. John W. Kennedy, for their professional adeptness in seeing this volume through the press.

Introductory Remarks

CESARE MALTONI[a]

European Ramazzini Foundation for Oncology and Environmental Sciences, Bologna, Italy

Cancer is quite clearly mankind's major disease, in our day and for the future. Cancer incidence and mortality have risen dramatically over the last century, chiefly as a result of two factors: the ageing of the population and an increase in pollution from carcinogens present in, and released into the environment at work and at large as a result of our industrial consumer pattern of development.

The elimination or reduction of environmental carcinogens by primary prevention strategies could cause a dramatic fall in cancer incidence over the coming years—no mean feat if one reflects on the limitations to our clinical control over the disease.

From this perspective, identification of hazards and assessment of their risk are of decisive importance as we embark on strategies of primary prevention and set our priorities among them. Yet, for the time being, there is a dearth of studies on the identification of cancer hazards. Only a fraction of what pollutes the work and wider environment has undergone experimental and epidemiologic carcinogenicity trials or risk assessment. The methods used in such studies show built-in limitations; and often these methods are improperly used. What is called for is an intensification of research in this branch of toxicology and oncology, together with a critical reappraisal and rethinking of study methodology.

Hazard identification and risk assessment stand in equal need of solid basic laboratory, epidemiologic, and clinicopathologic data, of exposure assessment, and of adequate techniques for statistical analysis. In other words, cancer risk identification and assessment is based upon statistical significance and (or) biological plausibility and relevance. I wish to stress that the basic data form a necessary prerequisite that, if lacking, cannot be remedied by any amount of statistical elaboration. Rather, it is true that the value of statistical elaboration and the interpretation of data mirror the quality of the basic data themselves. All too often our analysts, laboratory researchers, epidemiologists, and biostatisticians continue to work in isolation. A tight-knit concerted effort would ease and improve the planning of research and the use made of its results. Hence, it is most gratifying to see this volume resulting from a gathering of laboratory researchers, epidemiologists, and biostatisticians working together to uncover the roots of uncertainty in risk assessment and to devise new ways of curtailing it.

I am grateful to John C. Bailar for having the idea for a workshop on Uncertainty in the Risk Assessment of Environmental and Occupational Hazards; to John Bailer and Marcel Van Den Broecke for assisting John Bailar so valiantly to make it possi-

---

[a]Address for correspondence: Cancer Research Center, European Ramazzini Foundation for Oncology and Environmental Sciences, Bentivoglio Castle, 40010 Bentivoglio (BO), Italy.
e-mail: crcfr@tin.it

Distributions of Individual Susceptibility among Humans for Toxic Effects: How Much Protection Does the Traditional Tenfold Factor Provide for What Fraction of Which Kinds of Chemicals and Effects? *By* DALE HATTIS, PRERNA BANATI, AND ROBERT GOBLE 286

Analysis of PBPK Models for Risk Characterization. *By* FRÉDÉRIC YVES BOIS . 317

Uncertainty in Risk Characterization of Weak Carcinogens.
By NAOHITO YAMAGUCHI 338

Reducing Uncertainty in the Derivation and Application of Health Guidance Values in Public Health Practice: Dioxin as a Case Study.
By CHRISTOPHER T. DE ROSA, HANA R. POHL, HUGH HANSEN, ROBIN C. LEONARD, JAMES HOLLER, AND DENNIS JONES 348

Uncertainty in Risk Characterization and Communication: Discussion. *By* ALISTAIR WOODWARD.. 365

Part VI. Conclusions

Uncertainty in Risk Assessment: Current Efforts and Future Hopes.
By A. JOHN BAILER... 367

Common Themes at the Workshop on Uncertainty in the Risk Assessment of Environmental and Occupational Hazards. *By* JOHN C. BAILAR III AND A. JOHN BAILER 373

Index of Contributors 377

Financial assistance was received from:

Sponsors
- AKZO NOBEL NV
- REGIONAL AGENCY FOR PREVENTION AND ENVIRONMENT (EMILIA-ROMAGNA REGION)
- AGENCY FOR TOXIC SUBSTANCES AND DISEASE REGISTRY
- COLLEGIUM RAMAZZINI
- DSM
- EUROPEAN FOUNDATION OF ONCOLOGY AND ENVIRONMENTAL SCIENCES B. RAMAZZINI
- INTERNATIONAL STATISTICAL INSTITUTE
- MIAMI UNIVERSITY
- NATIONAL CENTER FOR TOXICOLOGICAL RESEARCH
- NATIONAL INSTITUTE OF ENVIRONMENTAL HEALTH SCIENCES
- NATIONAL INSTITUTE FOR OCCUPATIONAL SAFETY AND HEALTH
- UNIVERSITY OF CHICAGO

Contributors
- ASSOCIAZIONE COOPERATIVE DI CONSUMATORI DEL DISTRETTO ADRIATICO
- CAAB MERCATI S.R.L.
- CANALI & C. S.P.A.
- COCA-COLA COMPANY
- EVC ITALIA
- GRANAROLO FELSINEO S.P.A.
- INTERPORTO BOLOGNA S.P.A.
- ISAGRO S.P.A.
- LEGA DELLE COOPERATIVE DI BOLOGNA
- SEABO S.P.A.

The New York Academy of Sciences believes it has a responsibility to provide an open forum for discussion of scientific questions. The positions taken by the participants in the reported conferences are their own and not necessarily those of the Academy. The Academy has no intent to influence legislation by providing such forums.

ble; to the Italian Ministry of Health; to those agencies, institutions, organizations, and industries who contributed their support; and to the Mayor of Bologna for providing an illustrious setting for the gathering.

Uncertainty in Risk Assessment

MARCEL VAN DEN BROECKE[a]

International Statistical Institute, Prinses Beatrixlaan 428, Voorburg, The Netherlands

The meeting from which this volume results, grew from an initiative of John C. Bailar and the International Statistical Institute to organize a cutting edge workshop on risk assessment. We were pleasantly surprised by the positive response received from industry, from academic circles, and from government agencies in Italy and elsewhere.

Why is it that a volume on risk assessment within the context of environmental and occupational safety fulfils such a clear need and has attracted papers from authors in Western Europe, the USA, Canada, Japan, and New Zealand? Because we all recognize the need to improve our understanding of the sources and nature of uncertainty in the risk assessment process, to reduce this uncertainty, and to develop policy measures accordingly.

Risk in a statistical context was defined by Bullock *et al.,* as those circumstances where the different outcomes and their probabilities are known objectively or subjectively. In the latter case, we are talking about perceived risks, and we all know how deceptive perceptions can be. Marriot is more straightforward, with the definition in his Dictionary of Statistical Terms (incidentally an ISI publication): "*risk* in statistics is a word used in its ordinary sense."

Risk, then, is the probability that something unpleasant may happen. In this volume, we focus on the necessity to assess unpleasant risks as they occur in the environment and in the work place. It is well recognized by statisticians in industry, academia, and governmental agencies that policies to assess risks and to minimize risks require a better understanding of their nature and causes than we presently have available. This is a more mature approach than to require that the probability of running risks should be zero. Desirable as that may be, we all know that there is no such thing as life without risks. I am confident that this volume will help us to understand the nature of risks so that we can manage them—if we cannot exclude them.

I want to conclude by congratulating the organizers of the workshop, specifically John C. Bailar, A. John Bailer, and Cesare Maltoni, for their excellent preparations.

---

[a]Address for correspondence: Marcel van den Broecke, Director of the International Statistical Institute, Prinses Beatrixlaan 428, 2273X2 Voorburg, the Netherlands. 31-70-3375737 (voice); 31-70-3860025 (fax).

e-mail: isi@cbs.nl

Risk Assessment for Children and Other Sensitive Populations

PHILIP J. LANDRIGAN

Department of Community and Preventive Medicine, Mount Sinai School of Medicine, One Gustave L. Levy Place, New York, NY 10029, USA

ABSTRACT: Children form a unique subgroup within the population who require special consideration in risk assessment. Children are not little adults. Their tissues and organs grow rapidly, developing and differentiating. These development processes create windows of great vulnerability to environmental toxicants. Furthermore, the exposure patterns of children to environmental chemicals are very different from those of adults. Traditional risk assessment has generally failed to consider the special exposures and the unique susceptibilities of infants and children. Adoption of a new child-centered agenda for research and risk assessment is necessary if disease in children of toxic environmental origin is to be identified, understood, controlled, and prevented. This agenda needs to be multidisciplinary. Specific requirements within the agenda include: (1) exploration and quantification of unique patterns of exposure for children; (2) adoption of new, more sensitive approaches to testing chemicals that can recognize the consequences of exposure during early development; (3) identification, through clinical and epidemiologic studies, of etiologic associations between environmental exposures and pediatric diseases; and (4) elucidation, at the cellular and molecular levels, of the pathogenetic mechanisms of pediatric environmental illness. In the United States, an important start toward adoption of this new agenda has occurred since passage of the Food Quality Protection Act in 1996. A Presidential Executive Order on Children's Health and the Environment has been promulgated. This Order requires all federal agencies to make protecting the health of children against environmental hazards a high priority. A new Office of Children's Health Protection has been established at the U.S. Environmental Protection Agency. Programs in children's environmental health have been created at the Centers for Disease Control and Prevention, the Agency for Toxic Substances and Disease Registry, and the National Institute of Environmental Health Sciences. A national network of eight new Children's Environmental Health Research and Disease Prevention Centers has been formed. These developments will enhance research on previously understudied issues in the environmental health of children and will provide a scientific basis for child-centered risk assessment.

INTRODUCTION

Children form a unique subgroup within the population. They have unusual patterns of exposure to environmental chemicals. They also have vulnerabilities to chemicals that are quite distinct from those of adults. Children constitute a classic example of a population subgroup who should receive special consideration in risk assessment.[1]

Traditionally, risk assessment has not examined the special vulnerabilities or particular patterns of exposure of infants and children. Neither has it considered other vulnerable subgroups, such as the elderly and individuals with chronic disease. Traditional risk assessment has for the most part considered only exposures of adults (usually adult white males) and has evaluated risks according to the exposure and disease outcomes of this one group.[2]

The central thesis of this essay is that children, and perhaps other vulnerable subgroups, need to receive appropriate consideration in risk assessment. Specifically, this consideration needs to examine the unusual exposures and unique vulnerabilities of children. If high-risk groups, such as children, do not receive appropriate consideration, then risk assessment and the regulatory decisions that follow from it will, in many cases, fail to adequately protect these most vulnerable members of society from environmentally induced disease and dysfunction.[3]

ENVIRONMENTAL HAZARDS FOR CHILDREN

Children today live in an environment that is vastly different from that of two or three generations ago. Thanks to vaccines, antibiotics, and improved nutrition, many once lethal pediatric diseases are now largely under control. The predicted lifespan of an infant born today is substantially greater than that of a child born in the early years of the 20th century.[4]

However, children today face hazards that were neither known nor imagined decades ago. Most notably, children today are exposed to thousands of synthetic chemicals that have been newly developed since world war II and that are disseminated widely in the environment.[5] More than 75,000 unique chemical substances are registered with the U.S. Environmental Protection Agency (EPA), and these materials are combined into more than ten million mixtures, formulations, and blends.[6] The toxicity of the majority of these chemicals has not been tested.[7,8] Gaps in our knowledge are especially great concerning the toxicity of chemicals to development. By default, we are conducting a massive toxicologic experiment, and our children are the experimental subjects.[5]

The rest of this section highlights some of the more noteworthy environmental hazards—both old and new—to which children today are exposed.[5]

The Old Hazards

Lead. Although lead levels in the United States have been reduced by more than 90% by the removal of lead from gasoline, nearly one million preschool children continue to have blood lead levels of 10 µg/dL and higher.[9] Epidemiologic studies have shown that blood lead levels in this range are associated with diminished levels of neurologic and behavioral function.[10] Lead-based paint remains the major source of child exposure to lead, but lead in drinking water is also an important source. Other less widely distributed sources include lead in folk medicines and cosmetics, lead transported home from industry on the shoes and clothing of workers, and lead exposure through home hobbies.[9]

Asbestos. Asbestos is a proven carcinogen that can cause lung cancer, malignant mesothelioma, certain gastrointestinal cancers, and laryngeal cancer.[11] Asbestos was used widely in the construction of schools and public buildings in the United States and, to a lesser extent, in home construction. In place and intact, asbestos poses no hazard to children. However, when asbestos in buildings becomes cracked and broken, it may liberate microscope sized fibers into the air. Inhalation of these fibers by children increases their future risk of lung cancer and mesothelioma.[12]

Cigarette Smoke. Secondhand cigarette smoke has been shown to increase the frequency of developing upper respiratory infections, bronchitis, and pneumonia in children. Moreover, epidemiologic studies indicate that exposure to secondhand smoke increases their future risk of cancer.[13]

The New Hazards

Pesticides. Children are exposed to pesticides on a daily basis.[14] The majority of fruits and vegetables contain residues of pesticides that are applied in agriculture; it is not uncommon to find multiple pesticides on a single fruit.[14] Pesticides are applied also on lawns, to gardens, in schools, and in homes.

An analysis by the National Academy of Sciences found that, prior to 1996, risk assessment and regulations in the United States for pesticides in food crops permitted children to be exposed to unsafe levels of many pesticides.[2] Passage, in 1996, of the Food Quality Protection Act put in place a new approach to risk assessment, an approach that is specifically intended to protect the health of children.[15] (see TABLE 1).

Air Pollution. Outdoor air pollution is a pervasive problem in the United States and in other industrially developed nations, particularly in urban areas where automotive emissions are the principal source.[16] The major components are ozone, oxides of nitrogen, carbon monoxide, and fine particles (less than 2.5 µg in diameter). Children exposed to air pollution have been shown to have a higher frequency of acute asthmatic exposure and respiratory infections than unexposed children.[17] Ambient air pollution in combination with exposure to passive cigarette smoke and contaminated, mold-laden air inside inadequately ventilated buildings is thought to be a major contributor to increasing rates of childhood asthma.[18]

TABLE 1. Major provisions of the Food Quality Protection Act of 1996[15]

Requires that standards for pesticide residues in food be health-based. Standards must be set at levels that ensure a "reasonable certainty of no harm."

Exposure and vulnerabilities of infants and children must be specifically considered in establishing pesticide residue standards.

When insufficient data exist to assess the special exposures and/or vulnerabilities of infants and children, an additional tenfold safety factor must be considered in setting standards.

Consideration of the potential benefits of pesticides must be limited.

All pesticide standards must be reviewed every ten years.

Endocrine effects of pesticides must be systematically evaluated in toxicity testing.

Diseases in Children Associated with Environmental Exposures

During the past 50 years a range of chronic diseases have replaced infectious illnesses as major causes of morbidity and mortality among children in the developed world. These new diseases have been termed the *new pediatric morbidity.*[4] Some may be caused, at least in part, by toxic hazards in the environment. Research to identify possible etiologic associations is sorely needed. Examples include:

1. Lead Poisoning. Nearly one million children have elevated blood lead levels and suffer chronic neuropsychologic impairment as a consequence of lead exposure.[9]

2. Asthma. The incidence of childhood asthma has doubled in the past decade from this cause, and mortality is also increasing.[18]

3. Childhood Cancer. The reported incidence rates of childhood leukemia and brain cancer are increasing;[19,20] the causes of these increases are not known, but possibly include environmental factors.[20] Improved diagnostic detection does not appear to be an adequate explanation for the observed rates of increase.

4. Male Reproductive Dysfunction. Among young adults, sperm counts are decreasing and the incidence of testicular cancer has increased by 70%.[19] Incidence of hypospadias has doubled in baby boys.[21] These trends may be interrelated and may reflect intrauterine exposures to environmental chemicals that disrupt endocrine function.[22]

Vulnerability of Children to Toxins in the Environment

Children are uniquely vulnerable to environmental toxins. Their heightened susceptibility stems from several sources.

1. Children have greater exposures to environmental toxins than adults.[2] Kilogram per kilogram of body weight, children drink more water, eat more food, and breathe more air than adults. For example, in the first six months of life infants consume seven times as much water (in total) per kilogram than does the average adult. Children aged one through five years eat three to four times more food per kilogram. Furthermore, children have unique food preferences. For example, the average one-year-old drinks 21 times more apple juice, 11 times more grape juice, and eats two to seven times more grapes, bananas, pears, carrots, and broccoli than does the average adult.[14] The air intake of a resting infant is twice that of an adult. These patterns of increased consumption reflect the rapid metabolism of children as well as their growth and development. The implication for health is that children have substantially greater exposure per kilogram to any toxic materials that are present in water, food, or air. Two additional characteristics of children further magnify their exposures to toxins in the environment: (1) their hand-to-mouth behavior, which increases their ingestion of any toxins in dust or soil, and (2) they play close to the ground, which increases their exposure to toxins in dust, soil, and carpets as well as to toxins that form low-lying layers in the air, such as certain pesticide vapors.

2. The metabolic pathways of children, especially in the first months after birth, are immature compared with those of adults.[24] As a consequence of this biochemical immaturity, the ability of a child to detoxify and excrete certain toxins is different from that of adults. In some instances, children are actually better able than adults to deal with environmental toxins. More commonly, however, they are less

TABLE 2. Examples of developmental vulnerability to environmental toxicants

Increased risk of cancer following intrauterine exposure to nitrosamines.[34]
Increased susceptibility to the neurotoxic effects of lead.[10]
Increased susceptibility to alcohol (fetal alcohol syndrome).
Thalidomide and phocomelia.
DES and adenocarcinoma of vagina.

able than adults to deal with toxic chemicals and, thus, are more vulnerable to them.[2]

3. Children undergo rapid growth and development, and their delicate developmental processes are easily disrupted.[2] Many organ systems in young children, such as the nervous system, the reproductive organs, and the immune system, undergo very rapid growth, development, and differentiation during the first months and years of life. During this period, structures are developed and vital connections are established. These developmental processes create windows of great vulnerability to environmental toxicants, in which even minute exposures can produce devastating results (see TABLE 2). The nervous system, for example, is not well able to repair any structural damage that is caused by environmental toxins. If cells in the developing brain are destroyed by chemicals such as lead, mercury, or solvents; or if formation of vital connections between nerve cells is blocked; then there is high risk that the resulting neurobehavioral dysfunction will be permanent and irreversible. The consequences can be loss of intelligence and alteration of normal behavior.[5] Similar considerations pertain in the reproductive, immune, endocrine, and cardiovascular systems.

Approaches to Prevention

Despite extensive exposures and heightened vulnerability to environmental toxins that children experience, until very recently there has been no coherent research or policy agenda to ensure that children will grow up in a safe environment.[3] Most previous regulatory efforts have not been health-based, but instead have represented attempts to balance health issues against economic factors; issues pertaining to the health of children have been largely ignored.[5] New toxins are introduced into the environment because they are seen as useful in their own right, or as byproducts of processes considered useful. Too often the toxicity of these materials is untested and the potential hazards that they may pose to children have not been examined.[7,8] Finally, there is little information available concerning the patterns or extent of children's exposures to chemicals in the environment.

Prerequisites for Child-Centered Risk Assessment

Carlson[1] has written eloquently on the need to formulate a new paradigm for environmental research and risk assessment that is centered on the needs and exposures of children. She states,

> The essence of this paradigm is to place the child, not the chemical or hazard, at the center of the analysis. The analysis would then begin with the child, his or her biology, exposure patterns, and developmental stage. This paradigm calls for a new way of thinking, and a retooling of the risk assessment process so that it takes into account not only the increased vulnerability of children but also the effects of multiple and cumulative exposures over the course of a lifetime.[1]

Specific tasks that need to be accomplished to develop and implement this new child-centered paradigm for research and risk assessment include the following:

1. Exploration and quantification of the unique patterns of exposure of children.[14,21] Studies are needed that specifically examine patterns of exposure for infants and children and that quantify these exposures. It may be useful in such studies to incorporate biological markers for exposure.

2. Creation of new approaches to chemical toxicity testing that are reliably able to detect the unanticipated developmental consequences of exposures during windows of early developmental vulnerability.[26] Extensive past experience has demonstrated that infants and young children are uniquely vulnerable to certain chemicals that are relatively innocuous to adults (TABLE 2). To detect such unanticipated consequences, it is necessary to undertake studies in which chemicals are administered either *in utero,* or shortly after birth and the subjects then followed over their entire lifespan in order to detect delayed effects. Moreover, such studies must incorporate sophisticated tests for function including neurological, immunological, and reproductive function. It is not sufficient to rely solely on observational test batteries.

3. Identification and elucidation through clinical, toxicologic, and epidemiologic studies, of etiologic associations between environmental exposures and pediatric disease.[10,27] A strong case can be made here for the need to establish a major prospective study of children's health in relation to toxic environmental exposures—a *pediatric Framingham study.*

4. Elucidation at organ, cellular, and molecular levels of the pathogenic mechanisms of environmentally-induced disease in children.[28,29] These studies could be undertaken either conjunction with toxicologic testing of chemicals in newborn infant animals or in the context of epidermiologic studies.

5. Overcome problems with traditional risk assessment methods, especially failure to consider simultaneous exposures to multiple chemicals, often with potential for synergistic interaction.[28,29] Until these problems with traditional risk assessment can successfully be overcome, it is necessary to incorporate additional safety factors in the risk assessment paradigm, as was specifically mandated by the Food Quality Protection Act of 1996.[15]

Recent Developments in the United States Toward Development of a Child-Centered Agenda

There have been a series of developments in the United States in the past three years that bode well for establishment of a new child-centered agenda in research, risk assessment, and regulation. The major developments are as follows:

- Publication in 1993 of the National Academy of Sciences Report, *Pesticides in the Diets of Infants and Children.*[2] This report established the scientific basis for the unique patterns of exposure and the specific biologic vulnerabilities of children. It provided an intellectual basis for the Food Quality Protection Act.

- Passage of the Food Quality Protection Act in 1996, by unanimous vote of both Houses of Congress.[15] (TABLE 1).

- Promulgation, in April 1997, of the Presidential Executive Order on Protection of Children from Environmental Health Risks and Safety Risks.[31] This order established the protection of health of children from environmental factors as paramount priority of all agencies of the U.S. federal government under the Clinton/Gore Administration. Under this executive order, a task force was established under the joint leadership of the EPA and HHS. Heads of all federal agencies now meet quarterly under the aegis of this task force to review progress towards the protection of children's health.

- Development by the U.S. Environmental Protection Agency of a child-centered agenda for research, risk assessment of regulation, and creation by the EPA of a new Office of Children's Health Protection.[6] These developments extend the themes and directives of the Presidential Executive Order to all of the operating arms and regional offices of the U.S. Environmental Protection Agency.

- Development of child-centered programs for research and prevention in the Agencies of the Department of Health and Human Services including the Centers for Disease Control and Prevention (CDC), the Agency for Toxic Substances and Disease Registry (ATSDR),[32] and the National Institute of Environmental Health Sciences (NIEHS).

- Establishment of a new national network of eight Children's Environmental Health Disease and Disease Prevention Centers in universities across the United States. This network undertakes wide ranging research to analyze the preventable causes of environmental disease in American children. Centers focus variously on asthma, early childhood development, and neurological development.

- Promulgation, by the environmental leaders of the eight leading world economies (the G-8), of an international declaration on the environmental health of children.[33] Through this declaration, the leaders of these eight major nations commit to the protection of children's health from environmental toxins. Specifically, this declaration included a resolution to remove lead from gasoline in nations around the world.

CONCLUSION

The protection of children against environmental toxins is a major challenge to modern society.[3] Hundreds of new chemicals are developed every year and are released into the environment. The majority of these chemicals are untested for their toxic effects on children.[7,8] The challenge, in this context, is to design policies that specifically protect children against environmental toxins and that allow children to grow, develop, and reach maturity without incurring neurologic impairment, immune dysfunction, reproductive damage, or increased risks of cancer as a consequence of toxic environmental exposures.[1]

To meet this challenge, a new paradigm for environmental health policy needs to be developed that is centered on the needs and exposures of children.[30] The essence of this paradigm is to place the child, not the chemical or hazard, at the center of the analysis. The analysis then begins with the child, his or her biology, exposure patterns, and developmental stage. This paradigm calls for a new way of thinking and a retooling of the risk assessment process so that it takes into account, not only the increased vulnerability of children, but also the effects of multiple and cumulative exposures over the course of a lifetime.

As we move toward the 21st century, the issue of environmental exposure and degradation looms large not only in the United States, but globally. It is imperative that we develop policies that will protect the health of our children now and in the future.

REFERENCES

1. LANDRIGAN, P.J. & J.E. CARLSON. 1995. Environmental policy and children's health. The Future of Children **5**: 34–52.
2. NATIONAL ACADEMY OF SCIENCES. 1993. Pesticides in the Diets of Infants and Children. National Academy Press, Washington.
3. SCHAFFER, M. 1998. Children and toxic substances: confronting major public health challenge. Environ. Health Perspect. **102**(Suppl. 2): 155–156.
4. HAGGERTY, R., J. ROTHMAN & I.B. PRESS. 1975. Child Health and the Community. John Wiley & Sons, New York.
5. WARGO, J. 1996. Our Children's Toxic Legacy. Yale University Press, New Haven.
6. BROWNER, C. 1996. Environmental Health Threats to Children. U.S. Environmental Protection Agency, Washington.
7. NATIONAL ACADEMY OF SCIENCES. 1984. Toxicity Testing: Needs and Priorities. National Academy Press, Washington.
8. ENVIRONMENTAL DEFENSE FUND. 1997. Toxic Ignorance: The Continuing Absence of Basic Health Testing for Top-Selling Toxic Chemicals in the United States. Environmental Defense Fund, Washington.
9. CENTERS FOR DISEASE CONTROL AND PREVENTION. Update—blood lead levels—United States, 1991–1994. MMWR **46**: 141–146.
10. NEEDLEMAN, H.L., C. GUNNOE & A. LEVIRON. 1979. Deficits in psychological and classroom performance of children with elevated dentine lead levels. N. Engl. J. Med. **300**: 689–695.
11. SELIKOFF, U., J. CHURG & E.C. HAMMOND. 1964. Asbestos exposure and neoplasia. J.A.M.A. **188**: 22–26.
12. AMERICAN ACADEMY OF PEDIATRICS. COMMITTEE ON ENVIRONMENTAL HEALTH. 1987. Asbestos in schools. Pediatrics **79**: 301–305.
13. AMERICAN ACADEMY OF PEDIATRICS. 1997. Environmental tobacco smoke: a hazard to children. Pediatrics **999**: 639–642.
14. WILES, R. & C. CAMPBELL. 1993. Pesticides in children's food. Environmental Working Group, Washington.
15. U.S. CONGRESS. 1996. Food Quality Protection Act.
16. AMERICAN ACADEMY OF PEDIATRICS. 1993. Ambient air pollution: respiratory hazards to children. Pediatrics **91**: 1210–1214.
17. DOCKERY, W. & C.A. POPE. 1994. Acute respiratory effects of particulate air pollution. Ann. Rev. Public Health **15**: 107–132.

18. CENTERS FOR DISEASE CONTROL AND PREVENTION. 1996. Asthma mortality and hospitalization among children and young children and young adults—United States, 1980–1993. MMWR **45:** 350–353.
19. FRAUMENI, J.F., JR. 1995. Recent cancer trends in the United States. J. Natl. Cancer Inst. **87:** 175–182.
20. ROBISON, L.L., J.D. BUCKLEY & G. BUNIN. 1995. Assessment of environmental and genetic factors in the etiology of childhood cancers: the Children's Cancer Group Epidemiology Program. Environ. Health Perspect. **103**(Suppl. 6): 111–116.
21. PAULOZZI, L.L.J., J.D. ERICKSON & R.J. JACKSON. 1997. Hypospadias, trends in two American surveillance systems. Pediatrics **100:** 831–834.
22. LONGNECKER, M.P., W.J. ROGAN & G. LUCIER. 1997. The human health effects of DDT (dichlorodiphenyltrichloroethane) and PCBs (polychlorinated biphenyls) and an overview of organochlorines in public health. Ann. Rev. Public Health **18:** 211–244.
23. COLBORN, T., D. DUMANOSKI & T.P. MYERS. 1996. Our Stolen Future. Dutton, New York.
24. SPIELBERG, S.P. 1992. Anticonvulsant adverse drug reactions: age dependent and age independent. *In* Similarities and Differences Between Children and Adults; Implications for Risk Assessment. P.S. Guzelian, C.J. Henry & S.S. Olin, Eds.: 104–106. International Life Sciences Institute Press, Washington.
25. GURUNATHAN, S., M. ROBSON, N. FREEMAN, B. BUCKLEY, R. MEYERS, J. BUKOWSKI & P.J. LIOY. 1998. Accumulation of chloropyrifos on residential surfaces of toys accessible to children. Environ. Health Perspec. **106:** 96–99,
26. TILSON, H.A. 1998. Developmental toxicology of endocrine disrupters and pesticides: identification of information groups and research needs. Environ. Health Perspec. **106**(Suppl. 3): 807–812.
27. JACOBSON, J.L. & S.W. JACOBSON. 1996. Intellectual impairment in children exposed to polychlorinated biphenyls *in utero*. N. Engl. J. Med. **335:** 783–789.
28. WHITNEY, K.D., F.J. SEIDLER & T.A. SLOTKIN. 1995. Developmental neurotoxicity of chloropyrifos: cellular mechanisms. Toxicology and Applied Pharmacology **134:** 53–62.
29. CAMPBELL, C.G., F.J. SEIDLER & T.A. SLOTKIN. 1997. Chlorpyrifos interferes with cell development in rat brain regions. Brain Research Bulletin **43**(2): 179–189.
30. LANDRIGAN, P.J., J.E. CARLSON, C.F. BEARER, J.S. CRAMMER, R.D. BULLARD, R.A. ETZEL, J. GROOPMAN, J.A. MCLACHLAN, F.P. PERERA, J.R. REIGART, L. ROBISON, L. SHELL & W.A. SUK. 1998. Children's health and the environment: a new agenda for prevention research. Environ. Health Perspect. **106**(Suppl. 3): 787–794.
31. CLINTON, W.J. & A. GORE. 1997. Executive Order on Protection of Children from Environmental Health Risks and Safety Risk. The White House, Washington.
32. AGENCY FOR TOXIC SUBSTANCES AND DISEASE REGISTRY. 1997. Healthy Children--Toxic Environments. Acting on the Unique Vulnerability of Children who Dwell Near Hazardous Waste Sites. ATSDR, Atlanta.
33. ENVIRONMENTAL LEADERS SUMMIT. 1997. Declaration of the Environment Leaders of the Eight on Children's Environmental Health. Miami, Florida, May 6, 1997.
34. GRAY, R., R. PETO, P. BRANTON & P. GRASSO. 1991. Chronic nitrosamine ingestion in 1040 rodents: the effect of choice of nitrosamines, the species studied, and the age of starting exposure. Cancer Research **51:** 6470–6490.

The Scientific and Methodological Bases of Experimental Studies for Detecting and Quantifying Carcinogenic Risks

CESARE MALTONI,[a] MORANDO SOFFRITTI, AND FIORELLA BELPOGGI

European Ramazzini Foundation for Oncology and Environmental Sciences, Bologna, Italy

ABSTRACT: This paper outlines the aims and potential scope of experimental research for risk identification and assessment in industrial carcinogenesis (environmental and occupational). It then reviews the basic, general, and specific requisites of a rigorously scientific nature that are required to render experiments to be more appropriate and better geared to the information they seek. A range of experimental approaches to risk assessment are illustrated by results achieved in the Cancer Research Centre of the Ramazzini Foundation (CRC/RF). The paper ends with a call for closer relations and integration among experimental, epidemiologic, and biostatistical studies.

INTRODUCTION TO THE ROLE OF EXPERIMENTAL CARCINOGENICITY STUDIES (BIOASSAYS)

The risks of cancer can be identified, characterized, and quantified by means of two basic methodologies, epidemiologic research on man and experimental research on animals.

Epidemiology studies would theoretically be the most direct method. However, this method grows less and less viable, in that it presupposes prolonged exposure of a human population. It is also complicated by a series of factors: (1) the need for extremely long observation periods, according to the length of latency time; (2) the large number of confounding situations; (3) the ensuing need to find sufficiently broad and relatively homogeneous exposed populations as well as proper control groups; (4) the complex web of political interference. Such factors explain why far too few epidemiology studies are being performed, why they often give ambiguous or borderline results, and why, if they are to give any useful result, their duration tends to outstrip that of the industrial compounds they refer to and the market for these compounds.

Experimental studies on animals, if conducted in keeping with certain binding scientific requirements, may provide information that leads not only to identification of cancer risk factors, but also to the quantification of those cancer risks according to the dose (dose-response ratio), duration, and chronology of exposure. This applies both to characterization of specific risks (i.e., the type of tumor produced), and to

---

[a]Address for correspondence: Cancer Research Center, European Ramazzimi Foundation for Oncology and Environmental Sciences, Bentivoglio Castle, 40010 Bentivoglio (BO), Italy.
e-mail:crcfr@tin.it

correlating the biological risk factors with exposed individual/population characteristics. Such information may be extrapolated to man and form a basis for preventive norms and strategies. The experimental trial run by our laboratories on vinyl chloride, the largest trial ever published on a single chemical agent, stands as a paradigm.[1] To date, bioassays have been performed on some 200 industrial agents[2,3] by the CRC/RF. Many of the agents studied have involved trials that are comparable with that for vinyl chloride. Such studies concern, for example, gamma radiation, vitamins, and aldehydes. Many of these studies have been published, some are being written up, some are still in progress. It has been claimed that experimental research is unduly expensive, especially when run on adequate groups and using a sufficiently large number of animals with the trials protracted throughout their life. Such a fallacy cannot be too forcibly rebutted. It is without substance, serving as an excuse to justify limiting the number of adequate bioassays conducted on environmental carcinogens, especially of an industrial kind. The real cost of such studies, as with our mega-experiment on vinyl chloride, is meager in comparison with the economic impact of the agents being studied, and damage to health and environment that they may cause. Accordingly, we should persevere with the experimental studies. They can: (1) make a decisive contribution to risk assessment, which forms the kernel of primary tumor prevention in the case of agents that are already at large in the environment; and (2) offer viable prospects for predicting the existence of potential cancer risks from agents that result from mass production and commercialization.

To date, attention has been limited, almost exclusively, to cancer risks from exposure to individual agents. However, humans are exposed, at the same or at different times, to a whole range of carcinogens, whereas a body of data in the literature suggests that exposure to multiple carcinogens may give rise to additional/multiplicative effects (syncarcinogenesis). The time has come to promote syncarcinogenesis research and to deal with multiple carcinogen exposure and mixtures of various agents. The data and arguments that follow concern both single and multiple exposures.

BASIC KNOWLEDGE OF CARCINOGENESIS TO BE CONSIDERED IN EXPERIMENTAL CARCINOGENICITY BIOASSAYS

Physical or chemical carcinogens occur with a range of carcinogenetic power. In general highly potent agents are found to give rise to a high incidence of tumors, with a relatively short latency time (high potency carcinogen). Others have a low tumor incidence and a long latency (low potency carcinogen). Between these extremes lie agents with various degrees of carcinogenetic power. Chemical carcinogens may act directly on the tissues (direct carcinogens), or may achieve their effect by metabolic biotransformation in the organism (procarcinogens).

The type of tumor produced partly depends on the physicochemical properties of the agents involved, how they spread and are metabolized by the organisms exposed, how they are administered (since this may affect both absorption and diffusion/metabolism), and how toxic they are. The latter may in turn affect the weight and survival of the animal. Such factors are known to play an important part in the neoplastic response. A wide range of data show the connection between exposure level (dose/agent concentration multiplied by duration of treatment) and neoplastic response.

The type of animal experiment is all important. According to the species, strain and sex of the animals, large differences are to be found in their tendency for spontaneous general or specific tumor formation (basic tumorigram). Under the effect of carcinogens, various experimental animal types tend to preferentially develop, with a greater incidence and/or shorter latency time, those tumors that they are prone to generate spontaneously. There are, therefore, both qualitative and quantitative parallelisms between the basic tumorigram and the type of neoplastic response to be expected from exposure to carcinogens. This emerges clearly in the case of agents that, by virtue of their properties, are able to reach the various anatomical regions of an organism.[4] The choice of animal, therefore, has a decisive influence on the results of experimental carcinogenicity trials, both in assessing the general carcinogenicity of an agent, and in defining the precise oncological action for the site and type of tumor produced. The age of animals at the start of exposure also affects the neoplastic response. Biological targets may react differently at various ages.

Many carcinogens have been shown to be multipotent; that is, to cause various kinds of tumor in various tissues and organs of various kinds of animals. This effect depends on the ability of the agent to reach targets in various organs and tissues, and on the specific tissue/organ responsiveness of the animals studied. From the evidence we possess and basic assumptions from biology, we may conclude that, if appropriately tested, all carcinogens are presumably multipotent. The possibility that an agent may cause various kinds of tumor leads to a sort of tumor competition. More specifically, depending on the experimental conditions, animals treated with a carcinogen die mainly of high-incidence/short-latency tumors, thus curtailing the chance for other neoplasias to develop.

The neoplastic response depends not only on the kind of agent, its physicochemical and toxicologic properties, the mode of exposure, and the type of animal, but also to a great extent, on the length of the biophase in relation to the latency time of the tumor being caused, which varies and may be very long. The experimental findings concur that the latent neoplastic potential for causing a tumor increases with the length of the biophase (i.e., observation time or age). That is why we are convinced that experimental carcinogenicity trials should continue until spontaneous animal death and not be cut short before. Cutting short an experiment after two years of biophase may mask a possible carcinogenic response. Beginning exposure in the embryo or neonate may have a positive effect on the neoplastic response, not only through the greater responsiveness of some organs at that age, but also because it prolongs the experimental biophase. For experiments to be planned correctly these basic notions of carcinogenesis must on no account be ignored.

GENERAL PLANNING AND METHODOLOGY PREREQUISITES FOR OPTIMIZING EXPERIMENTAL CARCINOGENICITY BIOASSAYS

There are several prerequisites that must be fulfilled if experimental carcinogenicity trials are to be optimized. Some of them are general in nature, others concern specific points of information that the bioassays are designed to provide.

The following general prerequisites are imperative, in our view, for protecting this branch of research from the amateur or anecdotal approach:

1. Use of animal species and strains whose basic tumorigram and kind of response to cancer stimuli is not too remote from the human counterpart. For example, one should avoid strains of mouse or rat that are peculiarly prone to certain kinds of tumor that may shorten their life-span, compete with other potential neoplastic latencies and, hence, cramp the onset of other kinds of tumor, and may potentially giving rise to metabolic alterations in the organism that confuse the picture of neoplastic response.

2. Continuing bioassays until the end of the life of an animal. Truncation of experiments is an artificial departure from the human model for the principal reason that, in humans, tumors tend to appear mainly in later life. According to the data of the Nominal Mortality Registry, for all causes of death, especially tumors, in Bologna Province, more than 85% of all deaths from cancer occur after age 60. Sacrificing mice or rats after about two years is like carrying out epidemiologic studies on man excluding the "third age" that is only taking subjects younger than 45–55 (in reference to the lifespan of the rodents most often used in bioassays).

3. Following the rules of Good Laboratory Practice as a minimum standard in experiment management. Those practices may of course themselves be improved.

4. Choosing precise parameters to assess neoplastic response. In our opinion, such parameters are: total number and percentage of animals carrying benign and malignant tumors and the various kinds of tumor; total number of benign and malignant tumors, and number of the various kinds per 100 animals (in view of the fact that one and the same animal may develop multiple tumors of various kinds at various sites); latency time for all specific benign and malignant tumors; and incidence of malignancy precursors.

5. Standardizing the experimental conditions for conducting experiments, parameter assessment, and data presentation. Thus, the results of various experiments may be compared and used, say, in assessing the relative cancer risk of various agents — an important factor in industrial decisions and prevention strategy.

All too frequently the failure to adopt such minimal standards leads, on one hand, to a spate of inadequate data and, on the other, to spawning nonintegrable, usually discordant, information that no amount of systematic revision will ever bring into line (and that obviously brings discredit on the whole experimental approach).

Planning experimental bioassays and setting the specific methodological prerequisites depends on the type and extent of the information the research is required to provide. The bioassay plan must, therefore, make it quite clear just what kind of information is desired.

WHAT INFORMATION MAY BE OBTAINED FROM BIOASSAYS

Potentially, bioassays may provide a whole range of scientific information. This may consist of:
1. Exposure of the carcinogenic potential of an agent in general terms, whatever the experimental conditions used, but always observing the rules outlined in the previous section.

2. Information on the effect of exposure routes and chronology with special regard to those features that link with human scenarios.
3. Information on the neoplastic response at various doses of the risk agents under test; that is, information on dose-response.
4. Indicating the organs that form the main targets, the types of tumor and precursors that are found with the agent under study.
5. Detection of any correlated or cancer-associated pathologies.
6. Information on the relative carcinogenic potency among agents.
7. Exposing weak/diffuse cancer risks, including those due to multiple exposure or mixtures of agents.

As previously mentioned, in planning a proper carcinogenicity bioassay one must clearly establish what information one wishes to know about, so that a targeted experiment protocol may be drawn up. As a general rule, it is not professional to make assumptions, or ask questions, about a bioassay beyond the scope for which it was specifically designed.

PLANNING BIOASSAYS IN RELATION TO THE INFORMATION FOR WHICH THEY ARE BEING PERFORMED

It follows from the aforegoing argument that bioassays must take account of the list of general requisites common to all bioassays, as well as specific requisites that vary from experiment to experiment, and yet are absolutely essential to the rationale of the study in question.

Identifying Potential Carcinogens

In this case any type of responsive animal may be used (except for those overly prone to developing certain kinds of tumor), and any exposure route (even widely divergent from the routes encountered by humans), employing high doses, although not so high as to markedly shorten the life-span through toxic effects. Such experiments are obviously most limited. In particular, should the data prove negative, one cannot be sure that by varying the dose, exposure route, and, hence, the target organ one might not find them positive. In any case, the result is always to be interpreted within the context of the test conditions.

Information on the Effect of the Administration Route and the Exposure Chronology

The route of administration may affect distribution of the test agents and hence the tissue/organ dose of the agent or its biotransformation products, thereby conditioning the neoplastic response in qualitative or quantitative terms. The tissue or organ dose can likewise be affected by varying the exposure schedule. The administration route may again influence the neoplastic response with direct or topical action agents, depending on the responsiveness of the tissues they are brought into contact with. Hence, if one is seeking information on the effects of a dose and administration schedule that may be extrapolated to man, the experiment needs to test various forms of administration and various schedule, with close reference to the human scenario and its characteristics.

Information on the Dose and its Effect

It has long been known that the carcinogenic effect, however expressed, increases as the dose increases. Quantifying the risk in relation to the dose is of vital importance and is a *sine qua non* in deciding the compatibility or otherwise of an agent in the environment and *socially acceptable* exposure standards (although let it be stressed, once and for all, there are no biologically safe dose levels in carcinogensis). The doses tested must, at least, include the highest tolerable dose, a dose of the order of those that humans are exposed to, and a midlevel dose. Naturally, the higher the number of doses studied, the better the information for quantitative assessment. In our bioassay project on vinyl chloride, 14 concentrations were tested by inhalatory exposure. Having those data available accelerated the implementation of international norms to establish an acceptable exposure level in the workplace.[1,2]

Information on the Site and Type of Tumors and Their Precursors

In experimental conditions, various kinds of animal are prone to develop tumors and their precursors of various kinds. Thus, there is a range of neoplastic responses to carcinogen exposure in qualitative and quantitative terms. If we wish to acquire knowledge leading to a forecast for which human organs will be targeted by exposure to a given carcinogen, we must choose experimental animals with the closest possible tumorigram to that of man (or, at least, one that is not too dissimilar).

Information on Pathologies in some way Related to Carcinogens

As well as tumors and their precursors, carcinogens may produce pathological alterations of a phlogistic and degenerative kind in the main tumor site organs and tissues, or at other sites, and these may relate in some way to, or be associated with, the neoplastic process. In any case, they may act as short- or medium term markers, or may throw light on the cancer mechanisms specifically triggered by the agent in question. To acquire information on such lesions, the clinical, necropsy, histopathology, and laboratory investigations must include systematic observation of all lesion types.

Information on the Relative Cancer Potential of Various Agents

Such information bears heavily on production and marketing decisions, as well as on setting priorities for preventive action. It may be obtained by comparing the data from carcinogenicity tests on a range of agents, provided the tests have been carried out under comparable experimental conditions.

Weak or Diffuse Cancer Risk Exposure

One of the main problems with industrial carcinogensis today is the weak cancer risk connected with exposure to single, multiple, or mixed cancer agents, often involving broad segments of the population, and, at times, the whole human race. These risk situations are due to low- or extremely-low doses of high- or medium-power carcinogens, or to weak or very-weak carcinogens at various doses (even small doses) and combinations of these factors.

By their very nature, traditional epidemiologic investigations are unsuited to detecting the tiny variations in cancer effects produced by such kinds of exposure.

Experimental trials offer a clear advantage in that they are conducted in strictly controlled conditions. For bioassays to be effective, their protocols must step up their power to reveal the effects of risks. In this case, not only must one make sure all the previously described general and specific requisites are met, but we must also have available a large animal population so as to reduce chance fluctuations and, as far as is possible, prolong the observation times, anticipating exposure to the prenatal period, and thus managing to cause a sufficient number of pathological events. The CRC/RF has wide experience here[5] and has reported on it in another paper in this volume.[6]

EXAMPLES OF VARIOUS TYPES OF EXPERIMENT GEARED TO PROVIDING CLEARLY DEFINED PLANNED INFORMATION

Paradigm examples of data that provide information for risk identification and assessment are reported here. All derive from lifespan experiments performed at the CRC/RF laboratories.

Experiments to Identify Potential Carcinogens

Such experiments may be rather simple, the number of animals being limited and the exposure route easy. Subcutaneous injection or insertion is a speedy way of treatment for agents predicted to act topically or directly (direct carcinogen).

A clear example of this type of bioassay is provided by a series of experiments performed on the carcinogenicity of inorganic pigments. The test compounds were injected *one-off* in the subcutaneous tissues of 8–13-week-old, male and female Sprague-Dawley rats (a type of animal known to respond to this type of testing). The animals were kept under observation until spontaneous death. The carcinogenicity of these compounds was evaluated by the onset of sarcomas at the point of injection. The experimental plan and carcinogenicity results are presented in TABLE 1.

Experiments to Provide Information on the Effects of the Route and Site of Administration of Carcinogens

Experiments on the carcinogenic effects (production of local mesotheliomas) of crocidolite and erionite, by injection in the pleural and peritoneal cavities of male and female Sprague-Dawley rats held under observation until spontaneous death, have shown clear differences in carcinogenic potency depending on the site of injection. Furthermore, such experiments have shown that the capacity of crocidolite to produce mesothelioma is higher when the fibers are injected in the peritoneum, the opposite being true for erionite (see TABLE 2).

Experiments to Provide Information on the Effects of the Carcinogen Dose Administered (Dose-Response Relationship)

An example is provided by the carcinogenicity of ceramic fibers. The test compound was delivered one-off at various doses by intraperitoneal injection to male and female Sprague-Dawley rats kept under observation until spontaneous death. The onset of topical peritoneal mesotheliomas directly parallel the dose delivered (see TABLE 3).

TABLE 1. Carcinogenicity bioassays on inorganic pigments indicative of the carcinogenic potential (see Refs. 7 and 8)

Test compound[a]	Animals N			Animals with local sarcomas					
	M	F	M+F	M		F		M+F	
				N	%	N	%	N	%
Chromium yellow (lead chromate)	20	20	40	10	50.0	16	80.0	26	65.0
Chromium orange (basic lead chromate)	20	20	40	14	70.0	13	65.0	27	67.5
Chromium red (lead chromate, sulphate, molybdate)	20	20	40	19	95.0	17	85.0	36	90.0
Zinc chromate (C2O3: 20%)	20	20	40	3	15.0	3	15.0	6	15.0
Zinc chromate (C2O3: 40%)	20	20	40	9	45.0	8	40.0	17	42.5
Silica coated chromium-yellow	20	20	40	10	50.0	15	75.0	25	62.5
Cadmium yellow (cadmium sulphide)	20	20	40	9	45.0	7	35.0	16	40.0
Iron Yellow (iron oxide)	20	20	40	0	–	0	–	0	–
Iron Red (iron oxide)	20	20	40	1	5.0	0	–	1	2.5
Titanium oxide	60	60	120	0	–	0	–	0	–
None	20	20	40	0	–	0	–	0	–

[a] Administered by subcutaneous injection of 30 mg, one-off, to 8–13-week-old male (M) and female (F) Sprague-Dawley rats (Exp. BO 12 and BT 2007).

TABLE 2. Effect of route/site of exposure from carcinogenicity bioassays of crocidolite and erionite (see Ref. 9)

Test compound[a]	Site of injection	Animals N.			Animals with local mesotheliomas					
					M		F		M + F	
		M	F	M + F	N	%	N	%	N	%
Crocidolite	Peritoneum	20	20	40	19	95.0	20	100.0	39	97.5
	Pleura	20	20	40	13	65.0	5	25.0	18	45.0
Erionite	Peritoneum	20	20	40	9	45.0	11	55.0	20	50.0
	Pleura	20	20	40	18	90.0	17	85.0	35	87.5
None	Peritoneum	20	20	40	0	—	0	—	0	—
	Pleura	20	20	40	0	—	0	—	0	—

[a]Administered by intraperitoneal and intrapleural injection of 25 mg, one-off, to eight week-old male (M) and female (F) Sprague-Dawley rats (Exp. BT 2101 and BT 2103).

TABLE 3. Effect of exposure doses from carcinogenicity bioassays on ceramic fibers (see Ref. 10)

Dose of ceramic fibers (mg)[a]	Animals N.			Animals with peritoneal mesotheliomas						
	M	F	M+F	M		F		M+F	
				N	%	N	%	N	%
10	20	20	40	7	35.0	6	30.0	13	32.5
5	20	20	40	1	5.0	3	15.0	4	10.0
1	20	20	40	1	5.0	0	—	1	2.5
0	50	50	100	0	—	0	—	0	—

[a]Administered by intraperitoneal injection one-off, to eight week-old male (M) and female (F) Sprague-Dawley rats (Exp. BT 2111).

TABLE 4. Effects of the concentration/dose on carcinogenicity bioassays for vinyl chloride (VC) (see Refs. 1 and 11)

Dose of VC (ppm)[a]	Animals N.			Animals bearing liver angiosarcomas (%)			Total number of malignant tumors per 100 animals (%)		
	M	F	M+F	M	F	M+F	M	F	M+F
30,000	30	30	60	16.6	43.3	30.0	76.7	123.3	100.0
10,000	30	30	60	10.0	13.3	11.7	80.0	83.3	81.7
6,000	30	30	60	10.3	33.3	22.0	46.7	73.3	60.0
2,500	30	30	60	20.0	23.3	21.7	53.3	73.3	63.3
500	30	30	60	–	20.0	10.0	23.3	80.0	51.7
250	30	30	60	3.4	6.7	5.1	23.3	36.7	30.0
50	30	30	60	3.3	–	1.7	6.7	23.3	15.0
0	30	30	60	–	–	–	–	26.7	13.3

[a]Administered by inhalation, four hours daily, five days weekly, for 52 weeks, to 13–17 week-old male (M) and female (F) Sprague-Dawley rats (Exp. BT 6).

Another clear example of this type of bioassay is provided by experiments performed on the carcinogenicity of vinyl chloride (VC). The test compound was delivered by repeated exposure through inhalation, at different concentrations, to male and female Sprague-Dawley rats, kept under observation until spontaneous death. Since VC is a multipotential carcinogen and, therefore, there may be competition for the onset of various different tumors, the dose-response relationship was more consistently revealed by plotting the total malignant tumors per 100 animals, rather than the percentage of animals bearing a specific tumor, even when the tumor type acts as a *sentinel* event, as does liver angiosarcoma in the case of VC (see TABLE 4).

Experiments to Provide Information on the Site and Type of Tumors (and Possibly Their Precursors)

The type of neoplastic response is greatly affected by the type of the animal tested. Thus, in order to assess the extent of multipotential carcinogenic effects of the test agent it is necessary to use animals that are prone to respond with a variety of tumors, and to use various types of animals with differing kinds of responsiveness. Under these experimental conditions we were able to show that VC and benzene are typical multipotential carcinogens, producing a large spectrum of tumors of different types or at different sites (see TABLES 5 and 6). Were bioassays to have been conducted on a more limited number of animal types, important information would be missed.

Experiments to Provide Information on Pathologies Related to Carcinogenesis

Such information may help throw light on risk assessment and carcinogenesis mechanisms. A classic case of this type is the lesions (necrosis) to the renal tubules of rodents exposed to vinylidene chloride. The incidence and intensity of these in Sprague-Dawley rats and male and female Swiss mice parallel the induction of renal tumors (see TABLE 7).

Experiments to Provide Information on the Relative Cancer Risk of Various Agents

Two sets of experiments show paradigmatically that experimental bioassays may contribute to relative quantitative risk assessment: the first deals with different types of asbestos (see TABLE 8), and the other deals with benzene and several zelated compounds (see TABLE 9).

For instance, the data on various different types of asbestos provide support for the assumption that there are no major differences in the carcinogenic potency of the different type of asbestos, when the results are evaluated as incidence of mesotheliomas.

Experiments to Assess Weak or Diffuse Cancer Risks

This is a highly important field in our opinion.[5,6] For years the CRC/RF has been engaged in this type of experiment, the role of which continues to be mysteriously underestimated. Five mega-experiments have been, or are being, conducted or planned in our laboratories. Initial results point to their importance and also show

TABLE 5. Effects of the type of test animals on tumor response from carcinogenicity bioassays on vinyl chloride (VC) (see Refs. 1 and 10)[a]

Animal Type		Tumor response[b]												
Species	Strain	Angiosarcomas of liver	Angiosarcomas and angiomas of other sites	Nephroblastomas	Hepatomas/ hepatocarcinomas	Tumors of brain	Tumors of lung	Lymphomas and leukemias	Zymbal gland (sebaceous carcinomas)	Ear duct epithelial tumors	Cutaneous epithelial tumors	Mammary carcinomas	Forestomach papillomas and acanthomas	Melanomas
Rat	Sprague-Dawley	+	+	+	+	+	(+)		+		(+)	+	+	
	Wistar	+	+	+	(+)	+			+	+	(+)	+		
Mouse	Swiss	+					+				(+)	+	(+)	
Hamster	Syrian golden	+	(+)					(+)					+	(+)

[a] Administered by inhalation (Exp. BT1, BT4, BT6, BT7, and BT4001).
[b] +, clear evidence; (+), borderline evidence.

TABLE 6. Effects of the type of test animals on tumor response from carcinogenicity bioassays on benzene (see Ref. 12)[a]

Animal Type		Tumor response[b]									
Species	Strain	Zymbal gland (sebaceous carcinoma)	Carcinomas of oral cavity	Carcinomas of nasal cavity	Carcinomas of the skin	Carcinomas of the forestomach	Carcinomas of the mammary gland	Hepatomas	Angiosarcomas of the liver	Hemolymphoreticular neoplasias	Tumors of the lung
Rat	Sprague-Dawley	+	+		+	+	(+)	(+)	+	(+)	
	Wistar	+	+	+				(+)			
Mouse	Swiss					+	+		+	+	+
	RFJ						+			+	+

[a] Administered by ingestion and by inhalation (Exp. BT 901, BT 902, BT 907, BT 908, BT 909, and BT 4004).
[b] +, clear evidence; (+), borderline evidence.

TABLE 7. The correlation between tubular kidney necrosis and onset of kidney adenocarcinomas in male (M) and female (F) Sprague-Dawley rats and Swiss mice, exposed to vinylidene chloride (see Ref. 13)[a]

Animal type	Sex	Kidney tubular necrosis	Kidney carcinogenesis (incidence of adenocarcinomas)
Sprague-Dawley rats	M	(+)	–
	F	–	–
Swiss mice	M	+++	+++
	F	(+)	(+)

[a]Adminstered by inhalation (Exp. BT 401, BT 402, BT 403, and BT 404).

that they are the most suitable instrument nowadays to assess such risks. The plans of the five projects and preliminary data are presented in this volume.[5]

CONCLUSION

When planned for precise purposes with attention to the key, general, and specific requisites, and when conducted by standardized methods (throughout the biophase, in processing and examining the pathological specimens, and in data elaboration and presentation), experimental studies form an important instrument capable of providing adequate information and reducing the uncertainties of risk assessment. The need for adequacy in these data cannot be overlooked: such data cannot be upstaged by other kinds of information, or by sophisticated biostatistical analysis on improper

TABLE 8. Relative quantitative risk assessment from carcinogenicity bioassays of several types of asbestos (see Ref. 14)

Test compound[a]	Animals with peritoneal mesotheliomas		
	N.	%	Average latency time (weeks)
Crocidolite (UICC)	39	97.5	59.5
Amosite (UICC)	36	90.0	66.7
Anthophyllite (UICC)	35	82.5	73.3
Chrysotile (Canada, UICC)	32	80.0	92.2
Chrysotile (Rhodesia, UICC)	33	82.5	89.7
Chrysotile (California)	29	72.5	85.3
None	0	–	–

[a]Injected at the dose of 25 mg, one-off, in the peritoneal cavity, to groups of 40 eight-week-old Sprague-Dawley rats (20 males and 20 females) (Exp. BT 2101).

Table 9. Relative quantitative risk assessment from carcinogenicity bioassays on benzene, toluene, xylenes, and ethylbenzene (see Ref. 15)

Test compound[a]	Number of total malignant tumors per 100 animals
Benzene	161
Toluene	69
Xylenes	56
Ethylbenzene	40
Olive oil	24

[a]Administered by ingestion, at a daily dose of 500 mg/kg b.w., 4–5 days weekly for 104 weeks, to 80 seven-week-old Sprague-Dawley rats (40 male and 40 female) (Exp. BT 902, BT 903, BT 904 and BT 905).

data. On the other hand, in planning and performing their experiments, researchers must strive to produce consistent data, fit for statistical analysis.

It is high time for a get together on risk assessment, concerted group action linking experimental researchers, epidemiologists, and biostatisticians, in order to decide how their efforts can best be integrated. The present forum certainly stands as an attempt, let us hope successful, to pursue this line.

REFERENCES

1. MALTONI, C., G. LEFEMINE, A. CILIBERTI, G. COTTI & D. CARRETTI. 1981. Carcinogenicity bioassays of vinyl chloride monomer: a model of risk assessment on experimental basis. Environ. Health Perspect. **41:** 3–29.
2. MALTONI, C. 1995. The contribution of experimental (animal) studies to the control of industrial carcinogenesis (1995 Herbert Stokinger Lecture). Appl. Occup. Environ. Hyg. **10:** 749–760.
3. MALTONI, C., M. SOFFRITTI, F. BELPOGGI, F. MINARDI & A. PALAZZINI. 1999. La ricerca primaria in oncologia con particolare riguardo agli studi sperimentali. Gli Ospedali della Vita **25:** 19–37.
4. TANNENBAUM, A. & C. MALTONI. 1962. Neoplastic response of various tissues to the administration of urethan. Cancer Research **22:** 1105–1112.
5. MALTONI, C., M. SOFFRITTI & F. BELPOGGI. 1998. Mega-experiments enhancing the evaluation of diffuse exogenous carcinogenic risks. Eur. J. Oncol. **3:** 5–10
6. SOFFRITTI M., F. BELPOGGI, F. MINARDI, L. BUA & C. MALTONI. 1999. Mega-experiments to identify and assess diffuse carcinogenic risks. Ann. N.Y. Acad. Sci. **895:** this volume.
7. MALTONI, C., L. MORISI & P. CHIECO. 1982. Experimental approach to the assessment of the carcinogenic risk of industrial inorganic pigments. In Advances in Modern Environmental Toxicology. Occupational Health Hazards of Solvents, Vol II. A. Englund, K. Ringen & M. Mehlman, Eds.: 77–92. Princeton Scientific Publishers, Princeton.
8. MALTONI, C., F. MINARDI, L. MORISI & F. BELPOGGI. 1982. Early results of long-term carcinogenicity bioassays of silica-coated lead chromate pigment, by subcutaneour injection on Sprague-Dawley rats. Acta Oncol. **3:** 89–94.
9. MALTONI, C. & F. MINARDI. 1989. Recent results of carcinogenicity bioassays of fibers and other particulate materials. In Non-Occupational Exposure to Mineral fibres. J. Bignon, J. Peto & R. Saracci, Eds.: 46–53. IARC Scientific Publications N. 90, Lyon.

10. MINARDI, F. & C. MALTONI. 1998. Results of long-term carcinogenicity bioassays of ceramic fibres ("Fiberfrax") on Sprague-Dawley rats. Eur. J. Oncol. **3:** 241–249.
11. MALTONI, C., G. LEFEMINE, A. CILIBERTI, G. COTTI & D. CARRETTI. 1984. Experimental research on vinyl chloride carcinogenesis. *In* Archives of Research on Industrial Carcinogenesis, Vol. II. C. Maltoni & M.A. Mehlman, Eds.: Princeton Scientific Publishers, Princeton.
12. MALTONI, C., A. CILIBERTI, G. COTTI, B. CONTI & F. BELPOGGI. 1989. Benzene, an experimental multipotential carcinogen: results of the long-term bioassays performed at the Bentivoglio Institute of Oncology. Environ. Health Perspect. **82:** 109–124.
13. MALTONI, C., G. LEFEMINE, G. COTTI & V. PATELLA. 1985. Experimental research on vinylidene chloride carcinogenesis. *In* Archives of Research on Industrial Carcinogenesis, Vol III. C. Maltoni & M.A. Mehlman, Eds.: Princeton Scientific Publishers, Princeton.
14. MALTONI, C., M. SOFFRITTI, C. PINTO, P. CARMENTANO, A. PALAZZINI & F. MINARDI. 1990. Models of development, environmental and cancer. In Update in Oncology. F. Pannuti & G. Robustelli della Cuna, Eds.: 107–158. Edizioni Medico-Scientifiche, Pavia.
15. Maltoni, C., A. Ciliberti, C. Pinto, M. Soffritti, F. Belpoggi & L. Menarini. 1997. Results of long-term experimental carcinogenicity studies of the effects of gasoline, correlated fuels, and major gasoline aromatics on rats. *In* Preventive Strategies for Living in a Chemical World. E. Bingham & D.P. Rall, Eds. Ann. N.Y. Acad. Sci. **837:** 15–52.

A Bayesian Approach to Hazard Identification

The Case of Electromagnetic Fields and Cancer

ANDERS AHLBOM[a] AND MARIA FEYCHTING

Karolinska Institute, S 171 77 Stockholm, Sweden

ABSTRACT: This paper discusses certain issues related to uncertainty in hazard identification. Research on the hypothesis that exposure to 50–60-Hz magnetic and electric fields (EMF) increases the risk of cancer has been ongoing for two decades. Epidemiological studies provide a somewhat consistent pattern indicating an increased risk for childhood leukemia and adult chronic lymphatic leukemia and possibly also for other leukemias and brain cancer. However, there is still no good candidate for a mechanism. Epidemiological studies have throughout the two decades been interpreted with great caution, and final evaluations as to carcinogenicity have been deferred. The reason for this carefulness may be the lack of knowledge about a plausible mechanism. The purpose of this paper is to discuss the process of weighing epidemiological data, experimental data, and other background information into a synthesis such that the evaluation can be based on all data combined. A Bayesian approach to this weighing is discussed along with some alternatives. The Bayesian approach provides a structure for the pooling of evidence and points out where subjective judgments come into play.

INTRODUCTION

Uncertainty in risk assessment of environmental and occupational hazards may occur at different steps such as in the identification of a hazard, in specifying the dose-response relation between exposure and disease risk, and in assessing levels of exposure. The subject of this paper is the first of those, uncertainty in hazard identification. The methods and principles used to deal with uncertainty in hazard identification appear less sophisticated than those employed with respect to specification of dose-response relations or exposure assessment. When dealing with uncertainties in the latter two, one typically employs statistical and other quantitative methods; while uncertainties in hazard identification are most often dealt with in a more judgmental and informal way. As a consequence there may be more room for subjectivity when addressing uncertainties in hazard identification. The purpose of this paper is to discuss the reasons for and consequences of the lack of systematic and quantitative methods for dealing with uncertainties in hazard identification and also to discuss whether there are principles available that might be used to improve the situation. In doing so the case of extremely low frequency (EMF) radiation will be used as an example, and the potential of a Bayesian approach will be discussed.

[a]Address for correspondence: Anders Ahlbom, IMM, Karolinska Institute Box 210, S 171 77 Stockholm, Sweden. +46 8 728 74 70 (voice); +46 8 31 39 61 (fax).
anders.ahlbom@imm.ki.se (e-mail).

THE CASE OF EMF

The hypothesis that exposure to EMF might increase cancer risk was formulated in 1979 when Wertheimer and Leeper published their study on childhood cancer mortality and EMF radiation.[1] This publication was followed three years later by a paper looking at cancer mortality by job title, reporting that work in an "electrical occupation" was linked to an elevated risk of leukemia and brain cancer death.[2] These two studies have been followed by quite a number of studies that to a certain degree provide support to the original findings, in particular with regard to childhood leukemia and chronic and perhaps other leukemias as well as brain cancer in adults with occupational exposure. There is still, however, little support from experimental research for the hypothesis.

Since the strongest evidence appears to be for childhood leukemia, a rough summary of this literature is provided in TABLES 1 and 2. TABLE 1 displays those studies that have assessed EMF exposure on the basis of power lines near the home.[3] As can be seen from the table, the majority of the studies have RR values above unity, and the pooled RR across the studies is estimated at 1.6 (95% c.l., 1.3–2.1). TABLE 2 provides data on the small subset of studies that employed 24-hour EMF measurements in the homes of the study subjects. The results of these studies are relatively similar, and the pooled RR is 1.6 (1.1–2.4). The most recent review of the literature on EMF and cancer was published by a working group assembled by the United States National Institute of Environmental Health Sciences (NIEHS, 1998). The working group concluded that there is limited evidence for EMF exposure being a cause of childhood leukemia and adult chronic lymphatic leukemia. The overall conclusion by the working group was that electric and magnetic field exposure is a possible car-

TABLE 1. Summary of studies on childhood leukemia and residential magnetic field exposure estimated from power lines near the homes

Study	Exposure	RR	95% c.l.
Wertheimer	HCC/LCC	3.0	1.8–4.9
Fulton	VH/VL	1.0	0.6–1.8
Tomenius	220 kV visible	1.1	0.3–4.1
Savitz	VH/B	2.8	0.9–8.0
Coleman	50 m. subst.	1.5	0.7–3.4
Myers	0.1 µT calc.	0.8	0.1–9.6
London	VH/VL,UG	2.2	1.1–4.3
Feychting	0.2 µT calc.	2.7	1.0–6.3
Olsen	0.25 µT calc	1.5	0.3–6.7
Verkasalo	0.2 µT calc.	1.6	0.3–4.5
Tynes	0.2 µT calc.	0.5	0.1–2.2
Linet	VH/VL+UG	0.9	0.5–1.6
TOTAL		1.6	1.3–2.1

TABLE 2. Summary of studies on childhood leukemia and residential magnetic field exposure estimated from 24-hour magnetic field readings in homes

Study	RR (95% c.l.)
London	1.5 (0.7–3.3)
Michaelis	2.3 (0.8–0.7)
Linet	1.5 (0.9–2.6)
TOTAL	1.6 (1.1–2.4)

cinogen. This corresponds to classification in Group 2B according to the scheme applied by the International Agency for Research on Cancer (IARC).

All the epidemiological studies supporting a relation between EMF and cancer that have been published so far have been interpreted with great caution. Even those that have been acknowledged as being well designed and well conducted have been received with considerable carefulness. It was argued that the observed association with EMF might have come about through confounding, exposure misclassification, or selection bias, or through chance. Before a firm conclusion can be drawn, it has been argued, one therefore must await the next study to see whether or not it provides confirmation. This is in principle how the very first studies on this topic were received, and it is also how the latest studies have been received.

As an example of conservative interpretations, consider the latest study from the US.[5] Some of the findings in that study are summarized in TABLE 3. As can be seen, the study is entirely negative for wire codes and leukemia risk. However, that is not at all the case for 24-hour measurements, and particularly not so for the higher exposure level. Despite this, the paper is accompanied by an editorial that has the following conclusion:[6] "In this issue of the Journal, Linet *et al.* report the results of a major study showing that the risk of ALL does not increase with increasing electromagnetic field levels in the children's homes." That is, despite the risk elevations in the commented study and despite the previous literature, the editorial takes this opportunity to dismiss the hypothesis once and for all. The editorial even says: "It is time to stop wasting our research resources."

As another example of conservative interpretation, we refer to a later publication from the same US study that addresses the use of electrical appliances in relation to leukemia risk.[7,8] Results for some of the appliances are presented in TABLE 4. As can be seen, they are all linked to increased relative risks. The pattern, however, is not fully consistent: for other electrical appliances there is no risk elevation, and there is

TABLE 3. Summary of results on residential magnetic fields and childhood leukemia[a]

	Exposed cases	RR matched	RR unmatched
wire code VHCC vs. UG+VLC	24	0.9 (0.5–1.6)	n.a.
24-h measurement > 0.2 µT	83/58	1.2 (0.9–1.8)	1.5 (0.9–2.6)
24-h measurement > 0.3 µT	45/39	1.7 (1.0–2.9)	1.8

[a]From Linet *et al.* Ref.5.

TABLE 4. Summary of results on appliance use and childhood leukemia[a]

Exposure (ever used)	RR (95% c.l.)
electric blanket	2.75 (1.52–4.98)
hair dryer	1.55 (1.18–2.05)
video arcades	1.66 (1.18–2.33)
video games (TV)	1.91 (1.36–2.68)

[a]From Hatch et al. Ref.7.

some concern about the lack of dose response in some instances. Nevertheless, for the most important exposure source—electric blanket use—the relative risk is high, and there is a clear indication of dose response. The authors' conclusion, however, is careful: "Although not impossible, we think that a causal relation between magnetic fields from the appliances and acute lymphoblastic leukemia is unlikely.

WEIGHING SCIENTIFIC DATA AND BAYES' THEOREM

Thus, the epidemiological studies on EMF and cancer have been interpreted with considerable caution both by the investigators themselves and by reviewers. A plausible explanation for this carefulness is the lack of a known mechanism or a good candidate for a mechanism. When the literature on a topic is evaluated, the epidemiological data, the experimental data, and other relevant information have to be pooled together to form the basis for an overall conclusion. For pooling across studies within a discipline there exist systematic and quantitative methods, such as meta-analytic techniques, that can be employed. For pooling across disciplines no such method is readily available. Instead, this pooling is done in an informal and judgmental way that includes a considerable amount of subjectivity. The evaluators put subjective weights to the epidemiological evidence and to the experimental evidence and perform an informal weighing. It is conceivable that this is sometimes done without recognizing how conclusions are arrived at and that subjective judgments are involved.

Greenland reviews some Bayesian arguments in a recent publication that might help create a structure for this pooling.[9] A Bayesian approach, of course, may not lead to the avoidance of all subjective elements, but it may make them more visible. For example, some commonly used keywords may be given well-defined meanings with the help of Bayesian notations. If H is a hypothesis—e.g., that EMF causes cancer—and B a set of data—e.g., from an epidemiological study on EMF and cancer—the following notations can be defined:

B proves H:	$P(H|B) = 1$
B supports H:	$P(H|B) > P(H)$
B countersupports H:	$P(H|B) < P(H)$
B refutes H:	$P(H|B) = 0$

In common language this indicates, for example, that the study results, B, support the hypothesis, H, if the probability of the hypothesis given the study results is greater than that without the study results. It is easy to show that this is equivalent to the study supporting the hypothesis when the probability of the study results given the hypothesis is greater than the probability of the study results without conditioning the hypothesis. That is,

$$P(H|B) > P(H) \text{ is identical to } P(B|H) > P(B).$$

The essence of Bayes' theorem is an expression that explains how a prior probability is transformed into a posterior probability by consideration of new data:

$$P(H|B) = P(H) \times [P(B|H)/P(B)].$$

In this expression, as before, $P(H)$ is the prior probability that the hypothesis is true. The ratio in brackets is a way of formulating the strength of the study result—that is, how strongly the results support the hypothesis. The left-hand side is the probability of the hypothesis being true given the study results. That is, the original credibility of the hypothesis—say that EMF causes cancer—is transformed into a new such credibility by multiplication with a factor expressing the strength of the study result.

Two obstacles present themselves if one attempts to apply this relation numerically to a given situation. First, the prior probability of the hypothesis, $P(H)$, is a subjective probability that is not directly estimable from data. Second, determining the unconditional probability of the study results requires extensive computations in which one has to cover all possible states of nature that are alternatives to H. Therefore the main use of the expression may not be as the basis for the calculations of posterior probabilities.

The main use may instead be to provide a conceptual structure for how one's beliefs in a hypothesis should be altered by the advent of new data. First, the role of the prior belief is made clear. It is also made clear that the posterior belief will be related to the prior belief and that these are subjective and vary across evaluators. Second, according to the theorem the relative change in belief in the hypothesis due to new data should be the same for all evaluators and should be independent of the amount of credibility that the evaluator has to the hypothesis in the first place. That is, the relative change in the assessment of a hypothesis should be independent of the original assessment. This only holds, of course, on the assumption that the accuracy of the new data is judged similarly.

A question worth entertaining is whether new data also are evaluated according to the following principle:

$$P(H|B) = w \times P(H) + (1 - w) \times [P(B|H)/P(B)],$$

where w is a subjective weight indicating the importance that is put to the prior hypothesis, and $1 - w$ indicates the weight given to new data. It could be that evaluators differ in this respect, with some giving most of the weight to the prior beliefs and little to new data and others giving most of the weight to new data and little to the prior belief. This could apply to the pooling of epidemiological data with experimental data and other biological background information. It is not inconceivable that epidemiologists give more weight to epidemiology and biologists more weight to biology. However, this way of pooling new and old data or of pooling across disciplines is not consistent with Bayes' theorem. Indeed, it is a purely subjective approach to scientific evaluation.

DISCUSSION

When a new epidemiological study is published, it can be pooled with already existing epidemiological studies by means of metaanalytic techniques. However, there are no similar techniques in common use for pooling that also includes experimental and other background data. Instead, pooling across disciplines is done in an informal and less structured way. This may include subjective weighing of evidence from different scientific areas.

The Bayesian approach may offer a way of structuring this weighing procedure so that it becomes clear how the credibility that has been assigned to a hypothesis is being updated when new data become available. Even though the Bayesian theory may not easily lend itself to a quantitative approach to pooling across disciplines, it may still be useful because it clearly shows what is involved and what role subjective weights play.

Based on the Bayesian arguments a firmer conclusion regarding the hypothesis that EMF exposure is carcinogenic would be possible if new epidemiologic data turned out to provide better consistency, particularly with respect to dose-response patterns, end points for which effects are observed, or better consistency across various exposure measures. With such results $P(B|H)/P(B)$ would increase—that is, the amount of support from epidemiology would be greater.

Similarly, for experimental research to provide support for a firmer conclusion some data supporting a plausible mechanism would have to emerge. This would lead to an increase in the prior belief in the hypothesis—that is, to an increase in $P(H)$.

REFERENCES

1. WERTHEIMER, N. & E. LEEPER. 1979. Electrical wiring configurations and childhood cancer. Am. J. Epidemiol. **109:** 723–284.
2. MILHAM, S. 1982. Mortality from leukemia in workers exposed to electrical and magnetic fields (letter). N. Engl. J. Med. **307:** 249.
3. AHLBOM A & FEYCHTING M. 1998. Evidence of carcinogenic risk in children following residential exposure to extremely low frequency electromagnetic fields: focus on childhood leukaemia. Eur. J. Oncol. **3:** 111–114.
4. NIEHS. 1998. Assessment of health effects from exposure to power-line frequency electric and magnetic fields. National Institute of Environmental Health Sciences. Research Triangle Park, NC.
5. LINET, M.S., E.E. HATCH, R.A. KLEINERMAN, L.L. ROBISON, W.T. KAUNE, D.R. FRIEDMAN, R.K. SEVERSON, C.M. HAINES, C.T. HARTSOCK, S. NIWA, S. WACHOLDER & R. TARONE. 1997. N. Engl. J. Med. **337:** 1–7.
6. CAMPION, E. 1997. Power lines, cancer, and fear. Editorial. N. Engl. J. Med. **337:** 44–46.
7. HATCH, E., M.S. LINET, R.A. KLEINERMAN, R.E. TARONE, R.K. SEVERSON, C.T. HARTSOCK, C. HAINES, W.T. KAUNE, D. FRIEDMAN, L.L. ROBISON & S. WACHOLDER. 1998. Association between childhood acute lymphoblastic leukemia and use of electrical appliances during pregnancy and childhood. Epidemiology **9:** 234–245.

8. FEYCHTING, M., A. AHLBOM & D. SAVITZ. 1998. EMF and childhood leukemia. Editorial. Epidemiology **9:** 225–226.
9. GREENLAND, S. 1998. Probability logic and probabilistic induction. Epidemiology **9:** 322–332.

Mega-experiments to Identify and Assess Diffuse Carcinogenic Risks

MORANDO SOFFRITTI,[a] FIORELLA BELPOGGI, FRANCO MINARDI, LUCIANO BUA, AND CESARE MALTONI

European Ramazzini Foundation for Oncology and Environmental Sciences, Bologna, Italy

ABSTRACT: Diffuse carcinogenic risks, that is, those of low potency involving large areas of population and sometimes all mankind, pose a serious public health problem. Controlling these risks might help to reduce the incidence of, and mortality from, cancer. Because of their low expected carcinogenic potential, these risks are difficult to expose or assess. Epidemiologic investigation is of limited use in this field and yields its data too late to be useful. Experimental studies offer the only possible approach for assessing such risks. To increase experimental sensitivity and consistency of results, mega-experiments must be designed. That is, experiments that use a large number of animals with a well-known basic tumorigram, that extend the exposure and the biophase for as long as possible, that carefully observe the effects, and that are performed with suitable standardized methods. In the last 15 years the Ramazzini Foundation, in its Cancer Research Center at Bentivoglio, has conducted or planned five mega-experiments. Initial results indicate the great potential of these methods for identifying and assessing diffuse risks.

EXOGENOUS CARCINOGENIC AGENTS POSE A MAJOR HEALTH PROBLEM WITH A NEED FOR PRIMARY PREVENTION

It is a fact that the majority of tumors are caused by exogenous carcinogenic agents of natural or industrial origin that are present in the general and/or working environment, and/or that are linked to human life-styles. It is also a fact that industrial (man-made) carcinogens have increased during the last few decades as a result of the expansion of industry and life-styles linked to industrial development. Furthermore, environmental carcinogens, since they are exogenous and largely man-made, could in principle be removed. Thus, controlling these carcinogens (primary prevention) offers a means to contain them and, hence, lower the incidence of, and mortality from cancer. It must be stressed, however, that this preventive strategy is at present pursued far less than is needed.

[a]Address for correspondence: Cancer Research Center, European Ramazzini Foundation for Oncology and Environmental Sciences, Bentivoglio Castle, 40010 Bentivoglio (BO), Italy. 0039-051-06640143 (voice); 0039-051-06640223 (fax).
 e-mail: crcfr@tin.it

IDENTIFICATION AND ASSESSMENT OF EXOGENOUS RISKS AS A NECESSARY PREREQUISITE TO PRIMARY PREVENTION

Primary prevention calls for the identification of carcinogenic risks as a necessary prerequisite. The identification of exogenous carcinogenic agents and the assessment of the risks they represent is, therefore, a crucial area of research aimed at controlling cancer. Studies and research in this area have evolved historically, and now they must be prepared to face new challenges.

The First Three Eras

First Era. Carcinogenic agents were discovered by skilful observation of a self-emerging increase in certain tumors among population groups heavily exposed to strong carcinogens. Classic examples are: carcinoma of the scrotum in chimney-sweeps exposed to coal combustion products,[1] carcinoma of the lung in uranium miners exposed to radon,[2,3] carcinoma of the skin in sailors overexposed to sunlight,[4] carcinoma of the bladder in dyestuff industry workers exposed to aromatic amines,[5] and carcinoma of the skin among radiologists.[6,7] Some of these observations were subsequently confirmed by laboratory experiments in important, though limited, animal studies. For example, local treatment with soot extracts was found to cause skin carcinomas in mice[8] and administration of the aromatic amine, β-naphthylamine, was shown to induce bladder carcinomas in dogs.[9]

Second Era. The carcinogenic agents were identified by means of planned epidemiologic investigations (usually commenced as a result of medical observation of an unusual frequency of specific tumors) and also by studies on experimental animals. The epidemiologic investigations studied essentially high risk situations and did not attempt quantitative risk assessment as their primary goal. Experimental studies were continued, more with a view to confirming the positive epidemiology results, than to discover new factors or agents of risk. Only a few experimental studies provided quantitative data that could be used in public health regulations. During this era experiments were carried out on small numbers of animals, the biophase period was arbitrary, and the conduct of experiments was not codified or controlled. Paradigms for studies in this period are furnished by: (1) the epidemiologic investigations on leukemia among radiologists,[10,11] carcinoma of the nasal and paranasal cavities in workers exposed to nickel,[12] carcinoma of the bladder in workers exposed to aromatic amines,[13-15], and carcinoma of the lung in workers exposed to chromium[16]; and (2) experimental studies that demonstrated the carcinogenicity of benzidine,[17] nickel,[18,19] and chromium[20] in animals.

In both the first and second eras, the studies allowed only for the detection of major carcinogenic effects. In several cases, because of the nature of the carcinogens studied (such as nondiffusible chemical compounds that tended to concentrate in certain anatomical regions), these studies generated results suggesting that, for the various carcinogenic agents, there were specific target organs that varied from agent to agent.

Third Era. This era is characterized by important new facts and ideas. Epidemiology research became more adequate and was statistically based. It was geared to identifying the tumorigenic effects of exogenous carcinogens, not for a single specific tissue or organ, but for various anatomical sites of the human body. It also aimed at quantifying the risk in terms of the dose-response relationship. Classic examples are found in the epidemiologic investigations of exposure to asbestos from insulators in New York State,[21] and in the survivors of atom bombs in Nagasaki and Hiroshima.[22]

During the same period several studies demonstrated the potential of experimental bioassays as a tool for: (1) predicting the carcinogenicity of exogenous agents, particularly those of industrial origin; (2) providing information on the potential carcinogenic effects at various anatomical sites; and (3) providing quantitative risk assessments as a basis for regulatory action. The carcinogenicity of vinyl chloride provides a classic example. In this case experimental research led not only to prediction of the carcinogenicity of the compound and identification of its various target tissues and organs, but also provided quantitative data on carcinogenicity. This helped in making regulatory decisions on the permitted exposure levels.[23,24] These prerequisites form a basis for the two major projects employing carcinogenicity bioassays that started about 30 years ago and are still in progress: the project of the National Toxicology Program (NTP)[25,26]; and that of the European Ramazzini Foundation for Oncology and Environmental Sciences, at its Cancer Research Center (CRC) in the Castle of Bentivoglio/BT (Bologna).[27,28]

Epidemiologic and experimental studies conducted in this period have also indicated that, in humans and in animals, different carcinogenic agents may exert synergistic effects, such as is the case with the association of tobacco smoke and asbestos in humans,[29] and with various chemical agents in rodents.[30]

The Present Fourth Era and its New Challenges

The *fourth era* is just commencing. It is the result of new scientific knowledge and of newly emerging problems. Previous eras broadly evaluated the carcinogenicity of single agents, often known to be toxic and frequently shown to be strong carcinogens, by means of exposure to high doses. Apart from some pioneer research of the third era, studies generally measured carcinogenic effects on the basis of an increase in specific tumors. Both the scenario and the objective have now changed.

Basic and applied carcinogenic research has shown that: (1) Most carcinogenic agents are multipotential, that is, they may induce tumors of different types, in different tissues and organs. The types of induced tumors and their relative ratio may vary according to the type of exposure and host biological factors. (2) The most immediate and important (public health) parameter to employ in assessing carcinogenic effect is, therefore, represented by the total number of observed malignant tumors, whatever their type. (3) Carcinogenic agents with different natures, when delivered individually or in mixtures to the same organism in various sequences, may exert cumulative and multiplicative effects (syncarcinogenesis). (4) Because of the type of agent or use of a low dose, it is difficult to detect weak carcinogenic risks, due either to exposure to a single agent or to multiple agents or mixtures. This may only be possible by increasing the size of the human and animal populations studied and the duration of observation (epidemiologic follow up and experimental biophase, respectively). At the same time, new public health and social targets have become well-defined.

It is clear that, nowadays, risks must always be evaluated, not in terms of a single causal agent or a single tumor, but in terms of a multiplicity of agents that, singly or together, may determine multiple tumors (total risk burden). It is increasingly considered necessary: (1) to define the levels of risk in terms of total burden following marked exposure to strong carcinogenic agent(s), involving limited groups of individuals; (2) to define the effects at different exposure doses to single or multiple agents or mixtures of agents suspected to be carcinogenic, thereby arriving at a quantitative risk assessment; and (3) to deeply reconsider the potential carcinogenic risk of some forms of historical exposure hitherto considered innocuous in the absence of any specific contrary evidence. In our opinion, the new and most important problems of environmental and industrial carcinogenesis are expansion, identification, assessment, and control of diffuse carcinogenic risks.

DEFINITION AND DIMENSION OF THE PROBLEM AND METHODOLOGICAL APPROACHES FOR RISK IDENTIFICATION AND ASSESSMENT OF DIFFUSE CARCINOGENIC RISKS

Diffuse carcinogenic risk is defined as the exposure to single or multiple agents or mixtures that are expected to have limited carcinogenic potential because of the agent type (weak carcinogen) and/or dose/concentration (low), but that involve large groups of the population—in some cases, all of mankind. Probably, this type of exposure in quantitative terms contributes more to the worldwide increase in incidence of tumors than do strong carcinogenic risks involving limited categories of the population.

Diffuse carcinogenic risks are difficult to identify and assess, let alone control. At present this problem is underestimated, or even ignored. To identify and assess diffuse carcinogenic risks, medical science falls back on epidemiology and experimental tools. Faced with this new challenge, epidemiologic research must be made as *powerful* as possible by adjusting its programs, dimensions, and methodologies. However, one must take into account that, when dealing with weak carcinogenic potential and multiple confounding factors, epidemiology has only a limited capacity for identifying and quantifying diffuse risks as defined here. Moreover, epidemiology provides delayed results, which by the time they are available, preventive strategy is long overdue.

To expose low carcinogenic risks, the experiments envisaged must possess the following characteristics: (1) as far as possible they must reproduce the various conditions of human exposure; (2) they must include large groups of animals in order to express variations in the effects more sharply; (3) they must be protracted for the lifespan of the animals, to allow for maximum emergence of all latent neoplastic potentialities; and (4) they must likewise evaluate all the neoplastic and non-neoplastic pathologies, since the latter may be complementary or may interfere with the incidence of the former. Furthermore, these experiments must be conducted on animals with a spontaneous neoplastic pathology that is as similar as possible to the human equivalent (and, therefore, not be characterized by an *unreasonable* incidence of particular types of tumor). They must also be performed under highly standardized conditions. One important, perhaps decisive, aspect is the availability of historical data on spontaneous pathology in the animal systems employed, collected under the same standardized conditions as for the proposed experimental studies, in order to distinguish induced pathology from that expected. Experiments of this kind, in particular concerning the size of experimental groups, are called *mega-experiments*.

Positive results from these studies serve to identify the risk and to measure the level of that risk. Negative results do not necessarily mean no risk, but they do serve to determine the existence of a *safeguard* limit.

In the face of a proposal to activate mega-experiments of this type for evaluating diffuse risks (a task of great social importance), objections of an economic nature have been raised by various parties including, strangely enough, scientists working in the biomedical field. To these objections one may answer that the cost is considerable if compared with the economic resources allocated to biomedical studies in general, and to the research on cancer prevention in particular (which are unfortunately minimal and in no way compare with the budget for technological research). The cost, by contrast, becomes insignificant when compared with: (1) the consequences of pathology (even in economic terms) that may derive from ongoing particular risk situations; (2) the cost of health programmes of limited efficacy, which in several cases are promoted for clinical control; and (3) more specifically, the enormous business turnover and income, in the case of many industrial technologies and products.

The age of mega-experiments has already started, with the experimental projects of the Cancer Research Center of the Ramazzini Foundation (CRC/RF).

GENERAL DESCRIPTION, PLANS, AND SOME EARLY RESULTS FROM MEGA-EXPERIMENTS AT THE RAMAZZINI FOUNDATION CANCER RESEARCH CENTRE TO IDENTIFY DIFFUSE CARCINOGENIC RISKS

A wide-ranging program of experimental mega-projects (in some instances including several mega-experiments) to evaluate the effects of diffuse carcinogenic risks was started in 1985 by the CRC/RF. To date five projects have been undertaken, or are planned, that aim to study: (1) the carcinogenicity of vitamins A, C, and E; (2) the carcinogenicity of compounds that potentially migrate into mineral water from PVC bottles; (3) the carcinogenic effects of various doses of ionizing γ-radiation, with particular regard to low doses; (4) the carcinogenicity of extremely low frequency electromagnetic fields, sinusoidal-50 Hz magnetic fields (S-50 Hz MF); and (5) the carcinogenic effects of radiofrequency and microwave electromagnetic fields, 1.8 GHz-GSM microwave electromagnetic emissions (1.8 GHz-Mw). Because of the nature of the agents and/or because of the low doses tested, all such exposures may be expected to represent low risks and yet a large part of the population are nowadays exposed to these agents.

Basic Methodology of the CRC/RF Mega-Experiments

The routes of treatment reproduce the human exposure scenario. The doses tested include those to which humans may be exposed. All of these mega-experiments are being performed on Sprague-Dawley rats from the same colony used for more than 20 years. Data are available on about 15,000 historical controls kept under control for their life-span. The data include individual pedigree and behavioral, clinical, and pathologic observations. The mega-experiments are extended over the lifespan of the

TABLE 1 (Part I). Plan of first experimental project to evaluate the carcinogenic effects of various levels of vitamin A (retinol palmitate and acetate) administered in the diet, to male (M) and female (F) Sprague-Dawley rats

Vitamin	Experiment		Vitamin levels in the feed			Duration of diet regimen	Age at start	Animals			
	N	Identification	A (iu)[a]	C (mg)[a]	E (mg)[a]			Groups	M	F	M + F
A	1	BT 8002	150,000	30	75	LS[b]	12 day embryos[c]	I	110	110	220
			75,000	30	75	LS		II	110	110	220
			16,900	30	75	LS		III	110	110	220
			3,900	30	75	LS		IV	110	110	220
			3,900	5	35	LS		V	110	110	220
	2	BT 8004	150,000	30	75	13 weeks[d]	12 day embryos[c]	I	100	100	200
			75,000	30	75	13 weeks[d]		II	100	100	200
			16,900	30	75	LS		III	110	110	220
			3,900	30	75	13 weeks[d]		IV	100	100	200
			3,900	5	35	13 weeks[d]		V	100	100	200
	3	BT 8001	150,000	30	75	LS	6 weeks	I	210	210	420
			75,000	30	75	LS		II	210	210	420
			16,900	30	75	LS		III	210	210	420
			3,900	30	75	LS		IV	210	210	420
			3,900	5	35	LS		V	210	210	420
	4	BT 8003	150,000	30	75	LS	52 weeks	I	100	100	200
			75,000	30	75	LS		II	100	100	200
			16,900	30	75	LS		III	100	100	200
			3,900	30	75	LS		IV	100	100	200
			3,900	5	35	LS		V	100	100	200

[a] Per Kg of feed.
[b] LS, lifespan, from the commencement of the experiment until spontaneous death.
[c] Administered to pregnant mothers.
[d] The regimen is then followed by diet with historical vitamin levels, until spontaneous death.

TABLE 1 (Part II). Plan of first experimental project to evaluate the carcinogenic effects of various levels of vitamin C administered in the diet, to male (M) and female (F) Sprague-Dawley rats

Vitamin	Experiment		Vitamin levels in the feed			Duration of diet regimen	Age at start	Animals			
	N	Identification	A (iu)[a]	C (mg)[a]	E (mg)[a]			Groups	M	F	M + F
C	5	BT 8102	16,900	2,000	75	LS[b]	12 day embryos[c]	I	110	110	220
			16,900	30	75	LS		II	110	110	220
			16,900	5	75	LS		III	110	110	220
			3,900	5	35	LS		IV	110	110	220
	6	BT 8104	16,900	2,000	75	13 weeks[d]	12 day embryos[c]	I	100	100	200
			16,900	30	75	LS		II	110	110	220
			16,900	5	75	13 weeks[d]		III	100	100	200
			3,900	5	35	13 weeks[d]		IV	100	100	200
	7	BT 8101	16,900	2,000	75	LS	6 weeks	I	110	110	220
			16,900	30	75	LS		II	210	210	420
			16,900	5	75	LS		III	110	110	220
			3,900	5	35	LS		IV	210	210	420
	8	BT 8103	16,900	2,000	75	LS	52 weeks	I	100	100	200
			16,900	30	75	LS		II	100	100	200
			16,900	5	75	LS		III	100	100	200
			3,900	5	35	LS		IV	100	100	200

[a]Per Kg of feed.
[b]LS, lifespan, from the commencement of the experiment until spontaneous death.
[c]Administered to pregnant mothers.
[d]The regimen is then followed by diet with historical vitamin levels, until spontaneous death.

TABLE 1 (Part III). Plan of first experimental project to evaluate the carcinogenic effects of various levels of vitamin E administered in the diet, to male (M) and female (F) Sprague-Dawley rats

Vitamin	Experiment		Vitamin levels in the feed			Duration of diet regimen	Age at start	Animals			
	N	Identification	A (iu)[a]	C (mg)[a]	E (mg)[a]			Groups	M	F	M + F
E	9	BT 8202	16,900	30	2,000	LS[b]	12 day embryos[c]	I	110	110	220
			16,900	30	500	LS		II	110	110	220
			16,900	30	75	LS		III	110	110	220
			3,900	5	35	LS		IV	110	110	220
	10	BT 8204	16,900	30	2,000	13 weeks[d]	12 day embryos[c]	I	100	100	200
			16,900	30	500	13 weeks[d]		II	100	100	200
			16,900	30	75	LS		III	110	110	220
			3,900	5	35	13 weeks[d]		IV	100	100	200
	11	BT 8201	16,900	30	2,000	LS	6 weeks	I	110	110	220
			16,900	30	500	LS		II	110	110	220
			16,900	30	75	LS		III	210	210	420
			3,900	5	35	LS		IV	210	210	420
	12	BT 8203	16,900	30	2,000	LS	52 weeks	I	100	100	200
			16,900	30	500	LS		II	100	100	200
			16,900	30	75	LS		III	100	100	200
			3,900	5	35	LS		IV	100	100	200

[a]Per Kg of feed.
[b]LS, lifespan, from the commencement of the experiment until spontaneous death.
[c]Administered to pregnant mothers.
[d]The regimen is then followed by diet with historical vitamin levels, until spontaneous death.

animals. The treatment is started very early in life, thus allowing for observation of the treated animal for as long as possible. In some experiments the animals are exposed from embryos (by treating pregnant breeders). In one project (the γ-radiation project) the effect of the exposure of male breeders before mating has also been studied. The mega-experiments are being conducted by following Good Laboratory Practices (GLP) with highly standardized intra- and inter-experimental procedures. The animals are submitted to periodic controls on behavior, clinical status, and grossly detectable pathologic changes throughout the biophase, and then, at spontaneous death, to complete necropsy followed by systematic histopathology.

The Projects

First Experimental Project
Evaluating the Carcinogenic Effects of Vitamins A, C, and E

The aim of this project is to test the carcinogenic effects of three vitamins, A, C, and E, that are essential to the human organism. They are introduced into the body with the diet to a variable extent and they enjoy wide scale pharmacologic use and marketing (nowadays this includes their use for tumor intervention and prevention purposes). However, they have never been subjected to adequate, targeted carcinogenicity studies, either in general terms or in relation to dose. The vitamins studied at different dose-levels were supplied with the feed. The project plan is presented in TABLE 1. The biophase of this project has been completed and the pathology material is now under scrutiny. Preliminary data indicate that, when administered for the lifespan starting at six weeks of age, vitamin A causes an increase in the incidence of mammary cancer in females (see TABLE 2).

TABLE 2. Evaluation of the carcinogenic effects of various levels of vitamin A from first experimental project. Incidence of malignant mammary tumors in female Sprague-Dawley rats, six weeks old at the start of the experiment

Group	Vitamin A levels (iu/Kg in the feed)[a]	Animals N	Malignant mammary tumors			
			Animals with tumors		Tumors	
			N	%	N^b	per 100 animals
I	150,000	200	30	15.0	37^c	18.5
II	75,000	200	26	13.0	$32^{c,d}$	16.0
III	16,900	200	27	13.5	32^c	16.0
IV	3,900	200	11	5.5	$15^{c,d}$	7.5

[a]For the life span.
[b]One animal can bear more than one carcinoma.
[c]Adenocarcinomas.
[d]One with sarcomatous component.

Second Experimental Project
Evaluating the Carcinogenic Effects of Compounds that Migrate into Mineral Waters from PVC Bottles

This project was conducted to evaluate the carcinogenic effects of mixtures of chemical agents (in particular, vinyl chloride) that potentially migrate at low doses into drinking (mineral) water from the walls of PVC bottles.[31] At present bottles for beverages and other containers for food, formed from various plastic materials, are widely used. Apart from our studies on PVC bottles, other plastics have never been subjected to adequate long-term carcinogenicity studies.

The treatment consisted in supplying the experimental animals with drinking water with or without CO_2 addition, contained (stocked) in PVC bottles or in glass bottles for at least 30–60 days before use. The potential migration of chemicals from PVC was increased by treating the water contained in plastic bottles with granules of polymer (Benvic, 3–4 mm in diameter), in sufficient quantity to obtain a threefold increase in the contact surface with PVC. The granules were added at least 24 hours before the water was drunk, and filtered out before daily filling of the animal drinking bottles. The plan of the project is presented in TABLE 3. The experiment has ended and the most important results have been published.[31] The results did not show the onset of any unexpected specific tumors, nor variation in the relative incidence of different tumor types, within groups. No increase in the total number of malignant tumors was found in the animals drinking water from PVC bottles (see TABLE 4). On comparing the two groups drinking both types of water, with or without CO_2, contained either in glass or in PVC bottles, or likewise the two groups drinking the same water contained in both glass and PVC bottles, one finds practically no difference in the onset of total malignant tumors (see TABLE 5). These results do not exclude the fact that drinking water contained in PVC bottles may contain carcinogenic micropollutants but, because of the high detection potential of the experiment and because of the consistent stability of the data, they constitute a good safeguard level for public health.

Third Experimental Project
Evaluating the Carcinogenic Effects of Various Doses of γ-Radiation

This project was conducted to evaluate the carcinogenic effects of γ-radiation, in relation to dose (low doses in particular), schedule of treatment, and age of animals at the time of exposure. The project tested for any effect, on the tumorigram of descendents, of exposing male breeders before conception and females when pregnant, and the effect of direct exposure on six-week-old animals. One part of the project set out to assess the carcinogenic risks of food sterilized with high doses of γ-radiation. In the various project experiments the animals were randomized within the various groups by breeders, thus also affording information on the role of familial predisposition in γ-radiation carcinogenesis. The entire experimental population was composed of litters born within the same week. The plan of the experiment is presented in TABLE 6. The biophase of the experiment has ended and the pathology data is now under scrutiny.

Preliminary data from Experiment 3 show that γ-radiation delivered one-off to six eight-week-old female Sprague-Dawley rats at doses of 300, 100, and 10 rads are carcinogenic for the mammary gland. In fact, γ-radiation treatment causes: (1) a

TABLE 3. Plan of the second experimental project to evaluate the carcinogenic effects of compounds that migrate into drinking water from PVC bottles on male (M) and female (F) Sprague-Dawley rats

Experiment		Treatment (drinking water)			Groups	Animals		
							N	
N	Identification	Type	Duration	Start		M	F	M + F
1	BT 9001	Mineral water without CO_2 addition, contained in glass bottles	LS[a]	Since breeder matching	I	250	250	500
		Mineral water without CO_2 addition, contained in PVC bottles	LS	Since breeder matching	II	250	250	500
		Mineral water with CO_2 addition, contained in glass bottles	LS	Since breeder matching	III	250	250	500
		Mineral water with CO_2 addition, contained in PVC bottles	LS	Since breeder matching	IV	250	250	500

[a]LS, lifespan from the commencement of the experiment until spontaneous death.

TABLE 4. Evaluation of the carcinogenic effects of compounds migrating into drinking water from PVC bottles from the second experimental project. Total incidence of malignant tumors in male (M) and female (F) Sprague-Dawley rats

Group	Treatment (drinking water)	Animals		Malignant tumors			
		Sex	N	Animals bearing tumors		Tumors	
				N	%	N	per 100 animals
I	Mineral water without CO_2 addition, contained in glass bottles	M	250	100	40.0	118	47.2
		F	250	89	35.6	110	44.0
		M + F	500	189	37.8	228	45.6
II	Mineral water without CO_2 addition, contained in PVC bottles	M	250	92	36.8	103	41.2
		F	250	67	26.8	89	35.6
		M + F	500	159	31.8	192	38.4
III	Mineral water with CO_2 addition, contained in glass bottles	M	250	91	36.4	108	43.2
		F	250	72	28.8	86	34.4
		M + F	500	163	32.6	194	38.8
IV	Mineral water with CO_2 addition, contained in PVC bottles	M	250	88	35.2	106	42.4
		F	250	79	31.6	96	38.4
		M + F	500	167	33.4	202	40.4

TABLE 5. Evaluation of the carcinogenic effects of compounds migrating into drinking water from PVC bottles from the second experimental project. Total incidence of malignant tumors aggregated by type of water and by type of bottle

Group	Treatment (drinking water)	Animals		Malignant tumors		Tumors	
		Sex	N	Animals bearing tumors			
				N	%	N	per 100 animals
I	Mineral water with and without CO_2 addition, contained in glass bottles	M	500	191	38.2	226	42.5
		F	500	161	32.2	196	39.2
		M + F	1000	352	35.2	422	42.2
II	Mineral water with and without CO_2 addition, contained in PVC bottles	M	500	180	36.0	209	41.8
		F	500	146	29.2	185	37.0
		M + F	1000	326	32.6	394	39.4
III	Mineral water without CO_2 addition, contained in glass and PVC bottles	M	500	192	38.4	221	44.2
		F	500	156	31.2	199	39.8
		M + F	1000	348	34.8	420	42.0
IV	Mineral water with CO_2 addition, contained in glass and PVC bottles	M	500	179	35.8	214	42.8
		F	500	151	30.2	182	36.4
		M + F	1000	330	33.0	396	39.6
V	Both types of water in both types of containers	M	1000	371	37.1	435	43.5
		F	1000	307	30.7	381	38.1
		M + F	2000	678	33.9	816	40.8

TABLE 6. Plan of the third experimental project to evaluate carcinogenic effects from various doses of ionizing radiations

Experiment		Treatment (γ-rays)				Animals		
N	Identification	Type	Dose (rads)	Schedule	Groups	M	F	M + F
1	BT 3R	Irradiation of male breeders before matching	300	One off	I	154	167	321
			100	One off	II	401	398	799
			10	One off	III	743	694	1,437
			0		IV[a]	514	537	1,051
2	BT 2R	Irradiation of pregnant females at 12th day of pregnancy	100	One off	I	286	289	575
			50	One off	II	363	365	728
			10	One off	III	737	759	1,496
			0		IV[a]	514	537	1,051
3	BT 1R	Direct irradiation of 6–8 weeks old male and female rats	300	One off	I	211	205	416
			300	Fractionated[b]	II	83	107	190
			100	One off	III	318	301	619
			100	Fractionated[c]	IV	126	133	259
			10	One off	V	524	522	1,046
			10	Fractionated[d]	VI	220	215	435
			0		VII[a]	514	537	1,051
4	BT 4R	Irradiated feed since 12th day of embryonal life[f]	4,000,000	LS[e]	I	272	258	530
			1,000,000	LS[e]	II	292	317	609
			0		III[a]	514	537	1,051

[a]Control group common for four experiments.
[b]10 doses of 30 rads at four week intervals.
[c]10 doses of 10 rads at four week intervals.
[d]10 doses of 1 rad at four week intervals.
[e]LS, lifespan from the commencement of the experiment until spontaneous death.
[f]Administered to pregnant breeders.

TABLE 7. Evaluation of carcinogenic effects of various doses of ionizing radiations from the third experimental project. Incidence of fibroadenomas following one-off exposure of female Sprague-Dawley rats to γ-rays from Co^{60}

Group /dose (rad)	N of litters	N of animals	Fibroadenomas (FA)/fibroadenomas with glandular hyperplasia (FA+)																		
			FA							FA+							Total FA, FA+					
			Bearing litters		Bearing animals		Tumors			Bearing litters		Bearing animals		Tumors			Bearing litters		Bearing animals		Tumors	
			N	%	N	%	N	per 100 animals		N	%	N	%	N	per 100 animals		N	%	N	%	N	per 100 animals
I (300)	40	205	39	97.5	145	70.3	326	159.0		34	85.0	80	39.0	130	63.4		40	100.0	165	84.5	456	222.4
II (100)	58	301	54	93.1	162	53.8	266	88.4		48	82.7	107	35.5	165	54.8		58	100.0	217	72.1	441	146.5
III (10)	99	522	85	85.9	222	42.5	367	70.3		57	57.6	105	20.1	127	24.3		92	92.9	269	51.5	494	94.6
IV (0)	100	537	88	88.0	227	42.3	307	57.2		69	69.0	147	27.4	206	32.4		92	92.0	304	56.6	513	95.5

TABLE 8. Evaluation of carcinogenic effects of various doses of ionizing radiations from the third experimental project. Incidence of dysplasias in mammary gland/dysplasias in fibroadenomas following one-off exposure of female Sprague-Dawley rats to γ-rays from Co^{60}

Group N of /dose litters (rad)	N of animals	Dysplasias in mammary glands (DMG)/dysplasias in fibroadenomas (DFA)																	
		DMG						DFA						Total DMG, DFA				
		Bearing litters		Bearing animals		Dysplasias		Bearing litters		Bearing animals		Dysplasias		Bearing litters		Bearing animals		Dysplasias	
		N	%	N	%	N	per 100 animals	N	%	N	%	N	per 100 animals	N	%	N	%	N	per 100 animals
I (300) 40	205	3	7.5	4	1.9	4	1.9	13	32.5	19	9.3	20	9.7	14	35.0	23	11.2	24	11.7
II (100) 58	301	13	22.4	13	4.3	13	4.3	32	55.2	36	12.0	47	15.6	37	63.8	43	14.3	60	19.9
III (10) 99	522	34	34.3	48	9.2	69	13.2	47	47.5	68	13.0	80	15.3	59	59.6	96	8.4	149	28.5
IV (0) 100	537	5	5.0	5	0.9	5	0.9	25	25.0	30	5.6	35	6.5	29	29.0	35	6.5	40	7.4

TABLE 9. Evaluation of carcinogenic effects of various doses of ionizing radiations from the third experimental project. Incidence of mammary adenocarcinomas following one-off exposure of female Sprague-Dawley rats to γ-rays from Co^{60}

Group /dose (rad)	N of litters	N of animals	Adenocarcinomas (ADCA)/anaplastic adenocarcinomas (AADCA)															
			ADCA						AADCA						Total ADCA, AADCA					
			Bearing litters		Bearing animals		Tumors		Bearing litters		Bearing animals		Tumors		Bearing litters		Bearing animals		Tumors	
			N	%	N	%	N	per 100 animals	N	%	N	%	N	per 100 animals	N	%	N	%	N	per 100 animals
I (300)	40	205	36	90.0	80	39.0	108	52.7	4	10.0	4	1.9	5	2.4	37	92.5	82	40.0	113	55.1
II (100)	58	301	46	79.3	77	25.6	107	35.5	1	1.7	1	0.3	1	0.3	47	81.0	78	25.9	108	35.9
III (10)	99	522	50	50.5	73	13.9	96	18.4	1	1.0	2	0.4	3	0.6	50	50.5	74	14.2	99	19.0
IV (0)	100	537	42	42.0	68	12.6	86	16.0	0	—	0	—	0	—	42	42.0	68	12.6	86	16.0

TABLE 10. Evaluation of carcinogenic effects of various doses of ionizing radiations from the third experimental project. Number of aggregated mammary adenocarcinomas and their precursors (dysplasias) per 100 animals resulting from one-off exposure to γ-rays from Co^{60}

Group/ dose (rad)	Mammary adenocarcinomas plus their precursors N per 100 animals
I (300)	66.8
II (100)	55.8
III (10)	47.5
IV (0)	23.4

dose-related increase in mammary fibroadenomas at 300 and 100 rads (see TABLE 7); (2) a non dose-related increase in mammary gland dysplasia at 300, 100, and 10 rads (see TABLE 8), probably because a higher percent of such lesions evolve to carcinomas in the groups exposed to the higher dose levels; (3) a dose-related increase in mammary carcinomas at 300, 100, and 10 rads, as a percentage of bearing litters and of bearing animals, and number of adenocarcinomas per 100 animals (see TABLE 9). When the number per 100 animals of mammary adenocarcinomas and their precursors (dysplasias) are aggregated, a clear cut dose-response relationship can be observed. The carcinogenic risk of the lowest tested dose (10 rads) is shown in TABLE 10.

Fourth Experimental Project
Evaluating the Carcinogenicity of Extremely
Low Frequency Electromagnetic Fields

This project aims to study the carcinogenic potential of extremely low frequency, sinusoidal, 50 Hz magnetic fields (S-50 Hz MF) at different doses, as well as their carcinogenic potential in association with known carcinogenic exposure. In all the experiments exposure to S-50 Hz MF will start from the 12th day of pregnancy of the breeder and continue throughout the lifespan of the offspring. In the project experiments, the animals are to be randomly placed into various groups by breeders, thus helping to assess the role of family factor(s) in the response. The plan of the project is shown in TABLE 11. This project is on the verge of commencing.

Fifth Experimental Project
Evaluating the Carcinogenicity of
Radiofrequency/Microwave Electromagnetic Fields

The fifth experimental project is intended to test the carcinogenicity of 1.8 GHz-GSM microwave electromagnetic emissions (1.8 GHz-Mw) at different doses. Ex-

TABLE 11. Plan of the fourth experimental project to evaluate carcinogenic effects of extremely low-frequency electromagnetic fields on male (M) and female (F) Sprague-Dawley rats

Experiment		Treatment			Duration	Groups	Animals			End points to be evaluated
N	Identification	Exposure to S-50 Hz MF (μTesla)[a]	Other exposures				M	F	M+F	
			Type	Dose						
1	BT 1CMS	1000 C	—	—	LS	I	250	250	500	carcinogenic effects
		1000 O/O	—	—	LS	II	250	250	500	carcinogenic effects
		100 C	—	—	LS	III	500	500	1000	carcinogenic effects
		20 C	—	—	LS	IV	500	500	1000	carcinogenic effects
		2 C	—	—	LS	V	500	500	1000	carcinogenic effects
		0	—	—	LS	VI	500	500	1000	(control)
		1000 C	• Low frequency (200 KHz), C[b,c]	10 μTesla	LS	VII	150	150	300	synergic carcinogenic effects
			• 1.8 GHz-Mw[c]	400 mwatt/ kg b.w.						
		1000 C	• Low frequency (200 KHz), C[b]	10 μTesla	LS	VIII	250	250	500	synergic carcinogenic effects
		1000 C	• γ-rays[d]	10 rads	LS	IX	100	100	200	synergic carcinogenic effects
		20 C	• γ-rays[d]	10 rads	LS	X	100	100	200	synergic carcinogenic effects
2	BT 2CMS	1000 C	• Aflatoxin B1[e]	70 μg/rat	IS[f]	I	100	100	200	increase in the incidence of hepatic preneoplastic foci induced by Aflatoxin B1
		0	• Aflatoxin B1[e]	70 μg/rat	IS	II	100	100	200	
		0	—	—	IS	III	100	100	200	

[a]The exposure is to be performed 20 hours daily, continuously (C) or intermittently, 30 minutes on and 30 minutes off (O/O), 7 days weekly, starting during embryo life by irradiating the pregnant breeders from the 12th day of pregnancy and continuing on the offspring for their lifespan (LS).
[b]Continuous (C) and concomitant exposure along with S-50 Hz MF exposure.
[c]Radiofrequency/microwave electromagnetic fields: 1.8 GHz-GSM microwave electromagnetic emissions (1.8 GHz-Mw).
[d]Administered one-off at the age of six weeks, as an initiating treatment.
[e]Administered by gavage nine times in two weeks, at age 6–7 weeks, as an initiating treatment.
[f]IS, interim sacrifices.

TABLE 12. Plan of the fifth experimental project to evaluate carcinogenic effects of radiofrequency/microwave electromagnetic fields, 1.8 GHz-GSM microwave electromagnetic emissions, on male (M) and female (F) Sprague-Dawley rats

Experiment		Treatment			Animals		
N	Identification	Exposure to 1.8 GHz-Mw (mwatt/kg b.w.)^a			N		
					M	F	M + F
1	BT 1 Mw	2000	LS	I	250	250	500
		400	LS	II	500	500	1000
		80	LS	III	500	500	1000
		4	LS	IV	500	500	1000
		0	LS	V	500	500	1000

^{a}The exposure is to be performed 20 hours daily, seven days weekly, starting during embryo life by irradiating the pregnant breeders from the 12th day of pregnancy and continuing for the lifespan (LS) of the offspring.

posure to 1.8 GHz-Mw is to be performed starting from the 12th day of pregnancy of the breeder and continued through the lifespan of the offspring. In the experiments the animals are randomly placed into various groups by breeders so as to throw light on the role of family factor(s) in the responses. The plan of the project is shown in TABLE 12. This project is about to commence.

CONCLUSIONS

Mega-experiments, as defined in this report, are the most adequate instruments at present available for identifying and assessing diffuse potentially carcinogenic exposure. In our experience they are feasible, they can detect low and extremely low risk situations, and they produce consistent results that may resolve uncertainties in risk assessment.

The problem with diffuse carcinogens is enormous and it is of increasing concern. It forms one of our main public health issues. This calls for an increase in the use of mega-experiments to investigate industrial and environmental carcinogenesis. The Ramazzini Foundation leads the way in this research field and will give it priority in years to come.

REFERENCES

1. POTT, P. 1775. Chirurgical observations relative to the cataract, the polypus of the nose, the cancer of the scrotum, the different kinds of ruptures and the mortification of the toes and feet. Hawes, Clarke & Collins, London.
2. HARTING, F.H. & W. HESSE. 1879. Lung cancer, the disease of miners in the Schneeberg mines. Vierteljahreschrift für gerichtliche medizin **30**: 296–309.
3. PELLER, S. 1939. Lung cancer among mine workers in Joachimsthal. Hum. Biol. **11**: 130–143.

4. UNNA, P.G. 1894. Carcinom der seemanshaut. In Histopathologie der hautkrankheiten. Hirschwald, Berlin.
5. REHN, L. 1895. Blasengeschwülste bei Fuchsin-Arbeitern. Arch. Clin. Chir. **50:** 588–600.
6. FRIEBEN, A. 1902. Demonstration eines cancroids des rechten handrückens, das sich nach hangdauernder einwirkung von röntgenstrahlen entwickelt hatte. Fortschr Röntgenstr **6:** 106.
7. WOLBACK, S.R. 1909. The pathological histology of chronic X-ray dermatitis and early X-ray carcinoma. J. Med. Res. **21:** 415–449.
8. PASSEY, R.D. 1922. Experimental soot cancer. Br. Med. J. **ii:** 539.
9. HUEPER, W.C., F.H. WILEY & H.D. WOLFE. 1938. Experimental production of bladder tumors in dogs by administration of beta-naphthylamine. J. Ind. Hyg. Tox. **20:** 46–84.
10. MARCH, H.C. 1944. Leukemia in radiologists. Radiology **4:** 275–278.
11. MARCH, H.C. 1950. Leukemia in radiologists in a 20 year period. Am. J. Med. Sci. **220:** 282–286.
12. BARNETT, G.P. 1948. Annual report of the chief inspector of factories for the year 1948. 93. H.M.S.O. London.
13. CASE, R.A.M., M.E. HOSKER, D.B. MCDONALD & J.T. PEARSON. 1954. Tumours of the urinary bladder workmen engaged in the manufacture and use of certain dyestuff intermediates in the British chemical industry. Part I. The role of aniline, benzidine, alpha-naphthylamine, and beta-naphthylamine. Br. J. Ind. Med. **11:** 75–104.
14. CASE, R.A.M. & J.T. PEARSON. 1954. Tumours of the urinary bladder in workmen engaged in the manufacture and use of certain dyestuff intermediates in the British chemical industry. Part II. Further consideration of the role of aniline and of the manufacture of auramine and magenta (fuchsine) as possible causative agents. Br. J. Ind. Med. **11:** 213–216.
15. CASE, R.A.M. & M.E. HOSKER. 1954. Tumour of the urinary bladder as an occupational disease in the rubber industry in England and Wales. Br. J. Prev. Soc. Med. **8:** 39–50.
16. MANCUSO, T.F. & W.C. HUEPER. 1951. Occupational cancer and other health hazards in a chromate plant: a medical appraisal. I. Lung cancers in chromate workers. Ind. Med. Surg. **20:** 358–363.
17. SPITZ, S., W.H. MAGUIGAN & K. DOBRINER. 1950. The carcinogenic action of benzidine. Cancer **3:** 789–804.
18. HUEPER, W.C. 1952. Experimental studies in metal cancerogenesis. I. Nickel cancers in rats. Texas Rep. Biol. Med. **10:** 167–186.
19. SUNDERMAN, F.W., A.J. DONNELLY, B. WEST & J.F. KINCAID. 1959. Nickel poisoning. IX. Carcinogenesis in rats exposed to nickel carbonyl. Arch. Ind. Health **20:** 36–41.
20. HUEPER, W.C. 1958. Experimental studies in metal cancerogenesis. X. Cancerogenic effects of chromite ore roast deposited in muscle tissue and pleural cavity of rats. Arch. Ind. Health **18:** 284–291.
21. SELIKOFF, I.J., E.C. HAMMOND & H. SEIDMAN. 1979. Mortality experience of insulation workers in the United States and Canada, 1943-1976. *In* Health Hazards of Asbestos Workers. I.J. Selikoff & E.C. Hammond, Eds. Ann. N.Y. Acad. Sci. **330:** 91–116.
22. KATO, H. & W.J. SCHULL. 1982. Studies of the mortality of A-bomb survivors. 7. Mortality, 1950–1978: Part I. Cancer mortality. Radiat. Res. **90:** 395–432.
23. MALTONI, C., G. LEFEMINE, A. CILIBERTI, G. COTTI & D. CARRETTI. 1981. Carcinogenicity bioassays of vinyl chloride monomer: a model of risk assessment on experimental basis. Environ. Health Perspect. **41:** 3–29.

24. MALTONI, C., G. LEFEMINE, A. CILIBERTI, G. COTTI & D. CARRETTI. 1984. Experimental research on vinyl chloride carcinogenesis. In Archives of Research on Industrial Carcinogenesis, Vol. II. C. Maltoni & M.A. Mehlman, Eds.: Princeton Scientific Publishers, Princeton.
25. HUFF, J.E., J. CIRVELLO, J. HASEMAN & J. BUCHER. 1991. Chemicals associated with site-specific neoplasia in 1394 long-term carcinogenesis experiments in laboratory rodents. Environ. Health Perspect. **93:** 247–270.
26. FUNG, V.A., J. C. BARRETT & J. HUFF. 1995. The carcinogenesis bioassays in perspective: application in identifying human cancer hazards. Environ. Health Perspect. **103:** 680–683.
27. MALTONI, C., M. SOFFRITTI, C. PINTO, P. CARMENTANO, A. PALAZZINI & F. MINARDI. 1991. Models of development, environment and cancer. In Update in oncology. F. Pannuti & G. Robustelli della Cuna, Eds.: 107–158. Edizioni Medico-Scientifiche, Pavia.
28. MALTONI, C., M. SOFFRITTI, F. BELPOGGI, F. MINARDI & A. PALAZZINI. 1999. La ricerca primaria in oncologia con particolare riguardo agli studi sperimentali. Gli Ospedali della Vita **25:** 19–37.
29. SELIKOFF, I.J., E.C. HAMMOND & J. CHURG. 1968. Asbestos exposure, smoking and neoplasia. J.A.M.A. **204**(2): 106–112.
30. BERGER, M.R., D. SCHMÄHL & H. ZERBAN. 1987. Combination experiments with very low doses of three genotoxic N-nitrosamines with similar organotropic carcinogenicity in rats. Carcinogenesis **8:** 1635–1643.
31. MALTONI, C., G. LEFEMINE, F. BELPOGGI, M. SOFFRITTI, A. LENZI, A. CILIBERTI & F. MINARDI. 1997. Risultati di saggi sperimentali di cancerogenicità di acque minerali contenute in bottiglie di PVC, su ratti Sprague-Dawley. Eur. J. Oncol. **2:** 531–551.

Long-Term Chemical Carcinogenesis Bioassays Predict Human Cancer Hazards

Issues, Controversies, and Uncertainties

JAMES HUFF[a]

[a]*National Institute of Environmental Health Sciences, Research Triangle Park, North Carolina 27709, USA*

> *We're going to outwork, outwalk, outtalk, outfast, outlast them. The best is yet to come! I don't need any alarm clock to wake me up in the morning—I'm driven by purpose.*
>
> Jackson, The New Yorker, *3 February, 1992*

ABSTRACT: Long-term carcinogenesis bioassays are the most valued and predictive means for identifying potential carcinogenic hazards of various agents to humans. Agents may be chemicals, chemical mixtures, multiple chemicals, combinations of chemicals, residues and contaminants, commercial products and formulations, and various exposure circumstances. Life-styles, dietary factors, and occupational exposure circumstances are very difficult, but not totally impossible, to evaluate experimentally. Historically, the first chemical bioassay took place in the early part of this century: Yamagiwa and Ichikawa[1] in 1915, showed that coal tar applied experimentally to rabbit ears caused skin carcinomas. Since then, nearly 1500–2000 bioassays of one sort or another have been carried out. Importantly, however, some of these bioassays must be considered inadequate for judging the absence of carcinogenicity, since there were various limitations on the way they were performed: too few animals, too short a duration, too low exposure concentrations, too limited pathology, as examples. Thus, each bioassay must be critically evaluated, especially those reported to be *negative*, because "false negatives" are certainly more hazardous to human health than are "false positives". Likewise, one must be careful not to discount bioassay results simply because a target organ in rodents may not have a direct counterpart in humans (e.g., Zymbal glands[2]), or because an organ site in rodents may not be a major site of cancers in humans (e.g., mouse liver). The design and conduct of a bioassay is not simple, however, and one must be fully aware of possible pitfalls as well as viable and often necessary alternatives. Similarly, evaluating results and interpreting findings must be approached with the utmost objectivity and consistency. These and other select issues, controversies, and uncertainties possibly encountered in long-term bioassays are covered in this paper. One fact remains abundantly clear: for every known human carcinogen that has been tested adequately in laboratory animals, the findings of carcinogenicity are concordant.

[a]Address for correspondence: 919-541-3780 (voice); 919-558-7055 (fax).
e-mail: huff1@niehs.nih.gov

INTRODUCTION

> Epidemiological observation is certainly not the method of choice for detecting new chemical hazards, which should be avoided by laboratory investigation of new agents before they are introduced. Epidemiology cannot tell us that any particular material is safe in the absolute sense and it is much more likely than laboratory science to overlook small effects of the many thousands of chemicals that are used in modern society. (R. Doll, Ref. 3.)

Certain human diseases have been traced to exposures to environmental and occupational chemicals, mixtures of chemicals, physical agents, life styles, socioeconomic conditions, dietary factors, and/or workplace conditions. Concerning carcinogens, in many instances the first evidence of potential adverse effects, including cancer, came from experimental studies on animals; and only subsequently were these adverse effects discovered in humans.[4] Associations of human cancers, a diverse group of 200 or more diseases, with chemicals and occupations have been made since the middle 1700s.[5–8] Subsequently, an enormous amount of information has become available and a veritable avalanche of important findings have been published. However, not all published bioassay results are equally reliable for protecting public health. Each must be scrutinized for adequacy of design, experimental conduct, pathology, reporting, and interpretation.[9–10]

A plethora of chemical carcinogenesis information has accumulated since the seminal bioassay performed on trichloroethylene by the National Cancer Institute[11] in the United States, as well as previous and subsequent work carried out in Italy,[12–17] France,[18–22] Japan,[23–28] and other countries.[29] Conversely, during the last 10 to 15 years, the number of bioassays commenced, completed, and reported has drastically declined, resulting in a growing number of chemicals with little or no toxicity or carcinogenicity data.

I present here a personal perspective of several purported issues, controversies, and uncertainties most often opined concerning the long-term bioassay.

BACKGROUND ON ISSUES

> As crude a weapon as the cave man's club, the chemical barrage has been hurled against the fabric of life. (R. Carson, Ref. 30.)

The chemical burden of modern society continues to increase dramatically. A few facts are provided in TABLE 1 to emphasize the numbers and quantities of chemicals being used and produced in the United States, and the most common exposure situations encountered by individuals and populations. Instead of than allowing these unwanted and often unnecessary exposures to endure unchecked, more efforts need to be directed toward reduction of these myriad exposures and exposure situations.

The number of chemicals being tested in various parts of the world for possible carcinogenicity in laboratory rodents seems to have declined considerably during the last decade or more.[29,31] For instance, whereas bioassays are currently being conducted or have recently been completed on 160 agents, in 18 institutions, in nine countries (personal communication, Julian Wilbourn, December, 1998), the number of ongoing or recently started bioassays is much lower than the number started in the 1960s, 1970s, and 1980s.[29] The real number of bioassays may be somewhat higher

TABLE 1. Background to the problem of chemicals and cancer

1. 13,000,000 synthesized or characterized chemical entities: 65,000–85,000 in common and/or commercial use in the United States.
2. Millions of combinations, mixtures, consumer products, and formulations.
3. 2,000 agents (±?) have been tested for carcinogenicity.
4. 177,800,000,000 Kg or 391,200,000,000 lb of synthetic organic chemicals produced annually in the U.S.
5. Top 50 U.S. chemical production, 650,000,000 lb.
   (64% inorganics; 36% organics).
6. Uncharacterized, unidentified, and unpredictable exposures:
   (1) occupational workplace circumstances,
   (2) pollution of air, water, and soil,
   (3) waste sites and facilities.
7. Local unique exposures and hot spots:
   (1) arsenic smelter, refineries;
   (2) chemical plants;
   (3) accidents/spills, TCDD, methyl isocyanate, pesticides, solvents, and gases.
8. Individual or personalized multiplicative exposures: workplace, drugs and over-the-counter products, herbs and vitamins, tobacco smoking, alcohol, life style, social, pesticides, chlorinated and fluorinated drinking water, smog, diet, acid rain, home environment (insulation, formaldehyde, solvents, etc.), cosmetics, fuel exhausts, nature, hobbies, pollution burdens, occupation, and others.
9. Toxic chemical releases. In 1992, U.S. manufacturers released 3.18 billion pounds of toxic chemicals into the environment.

because not all those doing bioassays communicate this information to the IARC, and many bioassays—especially those performed on commercial or proprietary products, pesticides, and drugs—are never, or only rarely, published. Unfortunately, the excellent and valuable IARC Directories of ongoing bioassays <http://193.51.164.11/htdocs/Directory/index.html> and of ongoing epidemiological studies have both been discontinued.

Furthermore, many of the long-term studies being conducted and reported lack certain characteristics that hinder their power of detecting a carcinogenic effect in laboratory animals,[31-34] and, hence, reduce their ability to predict likely carcinogenic hazards to humans. Some of these limitations are: (1) using only one sex of a single strain and species, or only a single species of laboratory rodents; (2) exposing rodents, especially mice, for short durations of only 18 months, or sometimes less; (3) not extending the length of long-term experiments beyond two years (for many chemicals and weaker carcinogens, responses are manifest and observed only after age 30 months or more); (4) an increasing trend to use lower exposure concentrations, based ostensibly on more and more subtle and often irrelevant neurologic observations, or histologic lesions observed in shorter-term studies; (5) not using appropriate age- and survival-adjusted statistics; (6) limited histopathology; (7) inappropriate use of historical tumor control data; (8) inadequate attention to dietary factors;[35–37] and (9) others.[38–41]

One tragic public health omission in current bioassays is not attempting to study and evaluate realistic combinations of chemicals that better mimic actual human exposure conditions. Undoubtedly this is a desperate need and one that is extremely difficult to undertake. Nonetheless, the necessary scientific, public health, and practical efforts must be made.[42]

Certain biologic issues have become more prominent for purportedly discounting studies that show positive chemical-induced carcinogenic effects.[10,43–45] Conspicuous among these are: (1) attempting to disregard certain rodent-specific organs showing carcinogenic effects (e.g., forestomach and Zymbal glands);[2] (2) using hypotheses as proven mechanisms to neglect carcinogenic responses in rodents (e.g., α_2u-globulin and kidney tumors in male rats);[43,46–48] (3) utilizing observed chemical toxic lesions to discount induced tumor responses (e.g., forestomach inflammation, ulcers, and hyperplasia as rationale for tumor induction rather than the chemical agent itself);[43,44] (4) suggesting that chemically induced benign tumors are immaterial to human cancer hazard alerts;[49] (5) implying that rodent liver tumors (and especially mouse liver tumors) can be ignored in cancer risk assessments;[50–52] (6) promoting the notion that rodent cancer effects are due mainly to high exposure phenomena.[53–55]

PURPORTED UNCERTAINTIES IN LONG-TERM BIOASSAYS

> I have no data yet. It is a capital mistake to theorize before one has data. Insensibly one begins to twist facts to suit theories, instead of theories to suit facts. (Sherlock Holmes [Arthur Conan Doyle, 1891].)

While there are avowed uncertainties in the use and interpretation of long-term carcinogenesis bioassays,[10,38,40,42,56] one should not take a single characteristic, or even collective instances, to mean automatically that particular bioassay results are meaningless or inappropriate for predicting potential human risks associated with exposure to chemical carcinogens. The tendency to do this seems to be increasing in those with vested interests, or those having relatively little knowledge or experience in the area of chemical carcinogenesis.[45] Of course, this does not mean significant identified and accepted uncertainties should be ignored when making predictions of carcinogenic risks to humans. Several selected uncertainties are given in the following discourse, with personal experience rebuttals.

Animal Carcinogenicity Findings Accord with Human Cancer Risks

> Prevention is obviously the most practical method of dealing with problems of health. Not having a disease at all is far better than the most effective treatment. (Blumberg, Ref. 57.)

Prospective bioassay results compared with retrospective epidemiological findings show convincingly that bioassays predict with reasonably certainty that cancers will occur in humans exposed to the offending carcinogenic agent.[4,45,56,58] Any doubts of this should have been dismissed long ago. In the early days of bioassays there appeared to be little more than scientific inquisitiveness about results obtained from animal studies. In more modern times, bioassay findings became a veritable truth, and caused considerable discontent among groups with vested interests in any chemical that was judged to be carcinogenic in laboratory animals. Today, both industry and, apparently, regulatory agencies have taken a more entrenched view that animal data are not to be "trusted" as predictors of similar fates in humans. Steady and persistent lobbying by industrial interests during the past 10 to 15 and even 20 years has tended to "spook" and, hence, convince regulators and others that rodents, not being humans, cannot be used as surrogates with past impunity. This repetitious strategy has worked quite successfully, especially when couched in "scientific" and "mechanistic" gobbledegook and misinformation.[42,43,48,56,59–62]

We should learn better from the past, given that many chemicals now considered carcinogenic to humans by epidemiologic methods were first shown to cause cancers in laboratory animals.[4,22] Many of the Group 1 IARC human carcinogens (carcinogenic to humans) that were previously shown to be carcinogenic in experimental animals, and only later to cause cancer in humans, are listed in TABLE 2. Not uncommonly, epidemiology data were often not even contemplated until unequivocal carcinogenesis was established in animals. Unfortunately, we continue to repeat this adamantine attitude today, by ignoring animal data until cancer deaths occur in humans. Recent examples include 1,3-butadiene, trichloroethylene, gasoline, silica, fiberglass (glass wool), and environmental tobacco smoke.

Considering bioassays of relatively recent vintage on chemicals causing cancers in laboratory animals, the following are of utmost concern, relating to exposures and potential human cancers:

TABLE 2. Chemicals first shown to cause cancer in laboratory animals and only subsequently in humans

1.	aflatoxins	14.	diethylstilbestrol
2.	4-aminobiphenyl	15.	melphalan
3.	asbestos	16.	methoxypsoralen + UVA
4.	azathioprine	17.	mustard gas
5.	betel quid with tobacco	18.	myleran
6.	1,3-butadiene	19.	nonsteroidal estrogens
7.	chlorambucil	20.	silica, crystalline
8.	chlornaphazine	21.	solar radiation
9.	chloromethyl methyl ether (tech. grade)	22.	steroidal estrogens
10.	ciclosporin	23.	2,3,7,8-TCDD
11.	coal tar pitches	24.	thiotepa
12.	coal tars	25.	trichloroethylene
13.	cyclophosphamide	26.	vinyl chloride

- 2,2-bis(bromomethyl)-1,3-propanediol (a fire retardant).[63,64]
- cobalt sulfate (naturally occurring, used in electroplating; as a coloring agent for ceramics; drying agent in inks, paints, varnishes; animal feed as a mineral supplement).[65,66]
- chlorination and chlorination byproducts (water chlorination).[67–76]
- chloroprene (manufacture of neoprene—polychloroprene).[77–81]
- 2,3-dibromo-1-propanol (a flame retardant and chemical intermediate).[82,83]
- ethylbenzene (manufacture of styrene).[84–86]
- isoprene (naturally occurring, in making rubber).[87–91]
- methyl *tert*-butyl ether (MTBE; oxygenate added to gasoline).[92–95]
- methylenegenol (naturally occurring, flavoring agent in foods, and fragrance.[96]
- phenolphthalein (naturally occurring, laxative).[97–101]
- tetrafluoroethylene (production of polytetrafluoroethylene, Teflon®, and other polymers).[102,103]
- tetranitromethane (formed during manufacture of TNT; used as a rocket fuel).[104–107]

Even when selecting and testing chemicals with a relatively strong likelihood of predicting cancer in laboratory animals, we were correct only two-thirds of the time.[108,109] Importantly, and often ignored by those who tabulate data by simple pluses and minuses, these carcinogens are not equally carcinogenic; some cause cancers in multiple sites in both sexes of two rodent species, whereas most others tend to be much less potent, inducing cancers in fewer organ-sex-species combinations. Thus, when using qualitative information one must be careful in grouping chemicals according to posed cancer risks. Conversely, only 1 in 5 chemicals chosen randomly on the basis of human exposure and production volume proved to be carcinogenic in animals. Using this information and findings from others we opined that less than 5–10% of all chemicals tested would present a carcinogenic hazard to humans.[110,111]

Clearly we still do not know enough about predicting chemical carcinogenesis and will continue to be surprised.[108,109,112] Wasting lives to chemical carcinogens is not a good strategy; thus, we must strive to reduce exposures to chemicals and agents shown to cause cancers in humans and in experimental animals.[113] History has shown us the way, but we appear not to be convinced or perhaps uncommitted; this attitude must change to best protect human health.

Liver Tumors in Rodents and Relevance to Humans

> It is important to recognize that the target site for human carcinogens is not always the same as in rodents. (Williams, Ref. 114.)

The argument that rodent liver carcinogenesis, especially as shown by live mouse tumors, does not indicate carcinogenicity in humans represents perhaps the earliest and most consistent criticism to be leveled against the relevance of bioassays for use in protecting public health. This tactic gained momentum (and actually spawned considerable and worthy research) when so-called nongenotoxic carcinogenic agents were shown to induce *only* liver tumors in rodents and particularly in mice. One of the first cries of discontent espoused the notion that if liver tumors in rodents were relevant to humans, why then is there no epidemic of liver cancers in the population. This, of course, is obvious: tumor site concordance is not necessary, or obligatory, in identifying chemical cancer hazards for humans.[115] One example is benzene and tumors of the Zymbal gland (an organ of vestigial presence in humans), the first cancer discovered in animals exposed to the human carcinogen benzene.[2,116–118] Now we have shown that benzene, in addition to being clastogenic, is mutagenic as well.[119]

Trichloroethylene.

A early example is trichloroethylene (TCE), a high–production volume short-chain chlorinated aliphatic solvent ($CCl_2=CHCl$), used at one time as an anesthetic, to decaffeinate coffee, and as a dry-cleaning agent, and still used as a general solvent and as a degreasing solvent.[120] The testing history of this chemical is reviewed here to remind us that all too often a preconceived certainty may turn out not to be so certain.

In 1976 the National Cancer Institute published a technical report on the carcinogenicity of TCE[11] with these conclusions:

> The results of this carcinogenesis test of trichloroethylene clearly indicate that trichloroethylene induced a hepatocellular carcinoma response in mice. While the absence of a similar effect in rats appears most likely attributable to a difference in sensitivity between the Osborne-Mendel rat and the B6C3F1 mouse, the early mortality of rats due to toxicity must also be considered.

Also noted in that first bioassay report by the NCI was the admission of alleged differences in sensitivity between the strains of rats and mice used in that bioassay for developing chemically induced liver tumors. An equally interesting and not uncommon feature of earlier bioassays was the use of positive controls, quite unique today:

> Carbon tetrachloride (CCl_4) was used as a positive control for the series of chlorinated chemicals which included trichloroethylene. While virtually all male and female mice developed hepatocellular carcinomas following carbon tetrachloride treatment, the response in the Osborne-Mendel rats was considerably less. Only about 5% developed hepatocellular carcinomas.

Although these findings of liver tumors were quite clear, they were challenged because a small amount of stabilizing agent was in the commercial product, epichlorohydrin. Interestingly, epichlorohydrin had not been shown to induce liver tumors, but caused application-site tumors of the forestomach after oral administration and of the nasal cavity after inhalation. Nonetheless, a subsequent bioassay on TCE without epichlorohydrin was performed.[121] with these confirmatory results:

> Under the conditions of these studies, epichlorohydrin-free trichloroethylene caused renal tubular-cell neoplasms in male F344/N rats, produced toxic nephrosis in both sexes, and shortened the survival time of males. This experiment in male F344/N rats was considered to be inadequate to evaluate the presence or absence of a carcinogenic response to trichloroethylene [note: toxicity and shortened survival]. For female F344/N rats receiving trichloroethylene, containing no epichlorohydrin, there was no evi-

TABLE 3. Chemicals carcinogenic to humans causing liver tumors in rodents

A. Chemicals causally associated with cancer in humans
IARC Group 1: carcinogenic to humans[a]

1.	aflatoxins	8.	estrogens (ethinyl estradiol)
2.	4-aminobiphenyl	9.	2-naphthylamine
3.	benzene	10.	oral contraceptives, combined
4.	benzidine	11.	tamoxifen
5.	1,3-butadiene[b]	12.	trichloroethylene[b]
6.	cyclophosphamide	13.	tetrachlorodibenzo-p-dioxin
7.	diethylstilbestrol	14.	vinyl chloride

B. Chemicals strongly suspected to be associated with cancer in humans
IARC Group 2A: probably carcinogenic to humans[b]

1.	azacitidine	11.	N-methyl-N´-nitro-N-nitroso-guanidine (MNNG)
2.	androgenic (anabolic) steroids, e.g., oxymetholone	12.	N-nitrosodiethylamine
3.	benz(a)anthracene	13.	N-nitrosodimethylamine
4.	benzidine-based dyes	14.	polybrominated biphenyls[b]
5.	captafol	15.	polychlorinated biphenyls
6.	chloramphenicol	16.	styrene-7,8-oxide
7.	chloroprene[b]	17.	tetrachloroethylene
8.	ethylene bromide, dibromoethane	18.	1,2,3-trichloropropane
9.	IQ (2-amino-3-methylimidazo-[4,5-f]quinoline)	19.	tris[2,3-dibromopropyl]PO$_4$
10.	4,4´-methylenebis(2-chloroaniline) (MOCA)	20.	vinyl bromide
		21.	vinyl fluoride

[a]There are 75 Group 1 human carcinogens identified by IARC; subtracting the 13 industrial processes known to cause cancer in humans that typically cannot be tested in animals, and subtracting human infectious agents, solar radiation, and radon leaves 50 agents that have been or can be tested in laboratory animals. Of these 50, 14 (28%) human carcinogens caused liver tumors in laboratory rodents.

[b]These entries have been upgraded or added by the author.

[c]There are 59 Group 2A probable human carcinogens identified by IARC; subtracting the four industrial processes, three mixtures, four infectious agents, and ultraviolet radiation A, B, C that typically cannot be tested in animals leaves 45 agents that have been or can be tested in laboratory animals. Of these 45, 21 (47%) caused liver tumors in laboratory rodents.

TABLE 4. Selected key findings and conclusions from long-term chemical carcinogenicity studies

1. All known human carcinogens that have been tested adequately in laboratory animals are likewise carcinogenic to experimental animals.[19,42,45,58,137,139,140,142]
2. Carcinogenesis findings from studies in laboratory animals are scientifically reasonable for identifying potential carcinogenic hazards to humans.[42,45,56,58,140,141]
3. Most chemicals are not considered potentially carcinogenic to humans.[9,58,108,111,137]
4. Approximately 5–10% of all chemicals might be predicted to be potentially carcinogenic to humans.[110,111]
5. Chemicals can be grouped by qualitative strength-of-evidence based on empirical indicators of potency: numbers of tumor sites; consistency of dose-response relationships; correlations between sexes, strains, or species; multiplicity of tumors; site responses; others.
6. Malignant and benign tumors (same site or cell type) can be combined to evaluate and interpret carcinogenicity.[49]
7. Benign tumors are relevant for judging carcinogenicity; few chemicals induce only benign tumors.[49]
8. Site-specific tumor analysis is useful to determine chemically induced carcinogenesis.[155]
9. Comparing total malignant tumor incidences between control and exposed animals might be useful to identify select carcinogens for further study.[84,138]
10. Liver neoplasia is valid for identifying potential cancer hazard to humans.[50,52]
11. Rodent-specific organs are useful for identifying potential cancer risks to humans: Zymbal glands, forestomach, Harderian gland, preputial gland.[2]
12. Chemically induced cellular toxicity and chemical carcinogenesis are not reliably correlated.[43,44]
13. Cellular proliferation per se does not cause cancer.[43,44,62,156,157]
14. Chemically induced cell replication per se cannot be used to predict carcinogenesis.[158–160]
15. Most chemical carcinogens do not cause cancer only at the highest doses or exposure levels used.[10,45,53,55,56]
16. Purported mechanisms of carcinogenesis are not yet well enough understood for generic utilization.[45,62,161]
17. Mechanisms of carcinogenesis are not sufficiently well developed to discount carcinogenic effects observed in rodents from predicting potential cancer hazards to humans.[2,46,47,48,52,134]
18. A single, complete mechanism of chemical carcinogenesis has yet to be fully defined.

TABLE 4/continued.

19.	Evidence for associating chemically induced stones in the urinary bladder as causative for tumors is weak, and typically empirical.[43,59,162,163]
20.	Route of exposure has little or no effect on the innate carcinogenic potential of chemicals.[164]
21.	Corn oil or olive oil used in oral studies has little or no influence on chemical carcinogenesis.[39]
22.	Rodent interspecies concordance in carcinogenic response is good. Correlations between sexes of the same strain and species are even better.[142,165]
23.	Known human carcinogens induce carcinogenesis in animals, with at least one concordant tumor site.[19,58,135]
24.	Concordance between *in vitro* genetic toxicity and *in vivo* carcinogenesis is relatively low.
25.	Caging and cage location exhibit no impact on chemical carcinogenesis.
26.	Chemical structure alone typically does not allow cancer prediction.[108,109,112]
27.	False-positive rates are relatively low; little is known about false-negative rates.[166]
28.	Nearly 30% of chemicals shown to cause cancer in humans were first observed in laboratory animals.[4,22,56]
29.	Regulatory decisions made using animal data are prudent public health practices.
30.	Epidemiological investigations should be considered on those chemicals considered carcinogenic in multiple species and causing cancers at multiple sites.[9,31,42,142]
31.	Cancer prevention is strengthened by avoiding or eliminating exposure to agents causing cancers in laboratory animals and/or in humans.[113,114,138]

dence of carcinogenicity. Trichloroethylene (without epichlorohydrin) was carcinogenic for B6C3F1 mice, causing increased incidences of hepatocellular carcinomas in males and females and of hepatocellular adenomas in females.

To get at the issues of strain difference in rats and whether or not TCE caused tumors of the kidney, another multistrain bioassay was accomplished,[122] with these somewhat disappointing but still useful results:

Under the conditions of these two-year gavage studies of trichloroethylene in male and female ACI, August, Marshall, and Osborne-Mendel rats, trichloroethylene administration caused renal tubular cell cytomegaly and toxic nephropathy in both sexes of the four strains. However, these are considered to be inadequate studies of carcinogenic activity because of chemically induced toxicity, reduced survival, and deficiencies in the conduct of the studies. Despite these limitations, tubular cell neoplasms of the kidney were observed in rats exposed to trichloroethylene and interstitial cell neoplasms of the testis were observed in Marshall rats exposed to trichloroethylene.

Thus, these studies confirm the kidney and the liver as TCE-induced tumor target sites for rodents, with a new target site of TCE being the testis. Others have likewise reported carcinogenicity of TCE in rodents,[123–128] including the lung and lymphoma. Additionally, we now know that both major metabolites of TCE—dichloroacetic acid and trichloroacetic acid—are each carcinogenic to rodents.[129,130]

Recent epidemiologic evidence,[131,132] coupled with earlier cancer findings in humans,[133] leads to the logical conclusion that TCE is carcinogenic to humans. Organ-associated cancers identified in humans exposed to TCE were all shown first in animals: liver and biliary tract, non-Hodgkin's lymphoma, and kidney. Thus, here we have a chemical that was first shown to cause cancer of the liver in mice in the early to middle 1970s, which results were critically challenged as being irrelevant to humans; subsequently other organs in rodents were shown to develop cancer when exposed to TCE; and finally, TCE is now considered to be carcinogenic to humans, causing tumors of the liver, biliary tract, and kidney, and non-Hodgkin's lymphoma.[131-134]

Other examples of agents that were shown to cause cancer of the liver in rodents and are now also evaluated as human carcinogens include those shown in TABLE 3, taken from the International Agency for Research on Cancer listings of Group 1 (carcinogenic to humans) and Group 2A (probably carcinogenic to humans). Thus, before discounting liver cancer (or any cancer) findings in bioassays as being irrelevant to humans, one must do considerably more research to prove this contention.

TABLE 5. Basic NTP design protocol for long-term chemical carcinogenesis studies in laboratory animals

1.	Purpose	Identify chronic toxicity (nonneoplastic) and carcinogenic (neoplastic) effects of chemicals.
2.	Animals	a. Fischer 344 hybrid rats. b. B6C3F1 inbred mice (C3H × C57Bl/6). These are the overwhelming choices of the NTP for toxicity and carcinogenicity experiments, although on occasion other species and strains are used where appropriate.
3.	Groups and group sizes	a. Both males and females of each species and strain. b. 50 to 60 or more animals/sex-species group. c. Concurrent controls and 2 to 4 experimental groups.
4.	Exposure levels	Chosen to show some minimal yet obvious chemical-associated effects of a degree not to compromise well-being or growth and survival.
5.	Exposure duration	24 months (approximately 2/3 life span of these strains).
6.	Routes of exposure	Priority typically given to mimic human exposures. Historically, via feed (43%), oral intubation (26%), inhalation (10%), skin (9%), drinking water (7%), i.p. inj. (2%).
7.	Pathology	All animals, controls and exposed; complete gross and histologic examination. Special target organs may be step-sectioned.

The point of this historical TCE reminiscence is to stress that results in animals should always be taken seriously, and rather than attempt to argue away the relevancy of the findings for humans, perhaps a better approach would be to reduce exposures. That is, we should strive to eliminate or reduce exposures not only to known human and animal carcinogens, but to all chemicals regardless of any evidence of toxicity or carcinogenicity.

Some see fit to place other chemicals into this same accusatory paradigm of carcinogenicity to rodents not being relevant to humans, leading some to adopt a wait-and-see attitude, relying on purported or hypothetical mechanisms of action posed as different between rodents and humans, and ending in simply delay, delay, delay for protecting public health. Chemicals that have in the past been deemed, or even currently are deemed, rodent-only hazards include: 1,3-butadiene, dichloromethane (methylene chloride), formaldehyde, gasoline, and others shown in TABLE 2. For the chemicals listed, the evidence of carcinogenicity was seen first in laboratory animals and only subsequently in humans.

Meanwhile, the right thing to do is reduce exposures to any carcinogenic or toxic agents. TCE and the chemicals listed in TABLES 2 and 3 should certainly give us pause as we attempt to discount cancer findings in animals.

Key Findings from Long-Term Chemical Carcinogenesis Bioassays

During two decades of planning, doing, interpreting, and evaluating long-term bioassays, my colleagues and I have come to accept and endorse a number of conclusions. Some have been easy to sanction, using the database of facts on close to 500 sets of bioassays; whereas other deductions reflect our collective experience over the years. Many of these are given in TABLE 4. The 31 listed key findings pertain in most instances to the value and validity of bioassays for identifying carcinogenic risks to humans. For more information on a particular finding, see the cited references.

A Typical NTP Protocol and Suggested Alternatives for Bioassay Designs

The National Cancer Institute initiated their carcinogenesis bioassay testing program in the 1960s; the program became part of the NTP in the late 1970s. During these 25 years or so the bioassay core design has changed little. That is, it entails using both sexes of two species of rodents exposed to chemicals for 104 weeks.[32–34] The B6C3F1 hybrid mouse has been used routinely for these studies, with several exceptions for dermal studies. The initial choice of rats was Osborne-Mendel, but shortly thereafter this was replaced by the currently and long-time used Fischer 344 inbred rat. Some details of the standard design for testing chemicals for potential carcinogenicity are given in TABLE 5. Using core standards of species and strains and two-year exposure regimens tends to limit flexibility and innovation, but it does provide better consistency and comparability.

Suggested modifications or alternatives to this typical design are listed in TABLE 6. Foremost among these is to extend the duration of a bioassay to 30 or more months. Some (C. Maltoni, personal communication, February, 1999) expose animals for 24 months and then let the animals live their natural life span. Others con-

TABLE 6. Alternative protocol design considerations for long-term chemical carcinogenesis studies

1. *Animals*. Chemical and target site specific. For example, for a potential leukemogen or testicular carcinogen *do not use* Fischer 344 rats, as this strain has very high control background incidences. Also, for a possible mammary carcinogen *do not use* Sprague-Dawley rats, which have a high background incidence. For skin carcinogens *do not use* insensitive B6C3F1 mice, or rats in general. For potential lung chemical carcinogens *do not use* hamsters. Thus, one needs to know the control tumors incidences of animals before selection.

2. *Sex-Species*. Instead of using both sexes, consider a single sex of two species. For example, male Fischer rats and female B6C3F1 mice. For short-chain aliphatic halogenated solvents use two strains of mice (rats appear to be resistant or generally not responsive to these solvents).

3. *Groups and Group Sizes*. At least 100 per group, with up to 1000 per group for a predictably weak environmental carcinogen (e.g., electromagnetic fields), or a chemical with extensive human population exposures (e.g., fluoride or aspartame).

4. *Exposures*. Highest concentration, or dose, at the MTE (minimal toxic exposure level observed from shorter-term toxicology studies); lower exposure levels could be selected at *metabolic saturation point* or at *pharmacokinetic inflection*. Lowest levels may be a few or several multiples of human exposures or environmental levels. Consider intermittent regimens of exposures rather than continuous (feed or drinking water) or six hours per day for five days per week (inhalation). Consistent with more realistic exposure patterns, except drugs.

5. *Routes*. Mimic main route of human exposure, where possible. However, because inherent carcinogenic potential is typically irrelevant to route of exposure, perhaps the easiest and cheapest route should be used; that is, food. Use multiple routes when appropriate: for example, chemical(s) could be given by inhalation and in drinking water and by skin painting and by gavage to better simulate actual human exposures (e.g., pesticides, solvents, water supply contaminant such as trihalomethanes, and added chemicals such as fluoride).

6. *Duration*. Flexible: (a) at least two years for unknowns; (b) longer periods for metals (e.g., cadmium carcinogenesis was not apparent before 30 months) and most other chemicals; (c) supplemental routine shorter exposure groups (e.g., 13 or 25 or 52 weeks of exposure and then stop exposures for remaining duration) to determine tumor progression/regression; (d) preconception, gestation, lactation, and F1 generations exposures for 30–36 months if large human populations are exposed (e.g., fluoride, food additives, EMF, drugs, ozone) intermittent and random exposures for solvents.

7. *Chemicals*. Multiple exposures and mixtures more close to human exposure patterns. For example, oxazapam by gavage, fluoride by drinking water, pesticides by feed, and solvents by skin. Combinations need to be evaluated versus single chemicals with high purity.

8. *Pathology*. More selective; in general, standard histopathology is costly, excessive, and unproductive. More effort needs to be directed at lesions observed grossly. Species-specific high-background tumor organs should be avoided—testicular interstitial cell tumors in Fischer rats, for example. More effort should be given to multiple sections for predicted or grossly observed target organs—for example, solvents and kidney; hormones and glands; aniline dyes and spleen; halogenated hydrocarbons and liver; site of application such as nose and lung via inhalation, stomach, and forestomach by gavage, oral via drinking water.

tinue exposure until 10–20% of animals remain. This extension of duration allows more opportunities for discovering late-stage or weak carcinogens.

Regardless of the design, we need to devote more effort and resources to testing multiple chemicals. Testing single chemicals came largely from occupational exposure circumstances, but even there workers received multiple chemical exposures (resulting in typical confounding factors in most epidemiological studies). Drugs, of course, were another reason for single-chemical testing, but here again most people taking drugs even for chronic conditions never relay on a single agent. So we must now forge ahead in our attempt to mimic real-life exposure situations. Regulators as well need to rethink policies and strategies of setting exposure limits on single chemicals, because safe levels of chemicals (sometimes marginally safe levels) may not be safe when all the so-called safe levels are aggregated for the many chemicals to which we are routinely and consistently exposed.

PERSONAL REMARKS

The betterment of public health can be accomplished only by commitment—commitment to the ideas and practices of neighborly goodness, integrity, and fairness. The numbness that has set in the conflict between industrial and environmental issues must stop. The idea that chemicals are only good for us is untenable. As an example, those who proselytize that pesticides are safe and have made our lives undeniably better do not know the facts or history. In truth, the nation's farms lose more to pestilence today, as a percentage of crops, than was lost in the early 1940s before the current rage and scourge of pesticide growth. Newer ideas of farming have reduced our reliance on chemicals somewhat, but pollution of soil, air, and waterways remains rampant.

New information that signals yet another chemical harm engenders yet another argument that the harm is not real. Some argue on behalf of a chemical because it is produced, sold, and used at a rate of 25,000,000,000 pounds per year even though it has been clearly shown to induce multiple cancers in animals. The arguments become more far fetched each time; for MTBE (methyl *tert*-butyl ether, an oxygenate used in gasoline) the rationale used to ignore the animal findings and center on the what appear to be fabricated opinions. Thus, in the three MTBE studies reported, the results were unequivocal: carcinogenic in both sexes in each of the species and strains of rodents exposed. Yet, panel after panel of individual scientists argue that the results are irrelevant to humans because of (1) who performed one of the studies (not relevant), (2) a purported lack of tumor site concordance between the studies (not true and also not a relevant criterion), and (3) the suggestion that one of the tumor sites developed via a mechanism not present in humans (not true). Answers: (1) industry reported two of the studies, and both were clearly positive for carcinogenicity; the second was done by a respected scientist in chemical carcinogenesis; (2) at least two tumor sites were common among the studies (testicular tumors and kidney tumors); and (3) $\alpha_2 u$-globulin is a hypothesis mechanism for male rat kidney tumors.

The issue of discounting tumors in rodents that have no apparent counterpart in humans is equally unwise. One need only examine tumor patterns of known human carcinogens that have been tested adequately in animals to realize that: (1) tumor concordance is not a common or necessary attribution across species, although there is in all cases a single site concordance between animals and humans;[58,135] and (2) obviously one reason is that animals receive complete necropsies and histopathology examination of about 30 to 40 tissues and organs while humans are rarely autopsied, and cause of cancer death is usually apparent (and thus other tumor sites remain undiscovered).

CONCLUSIONS AND SUMMARY

> While high uncertainty may obscure both the probability of a risk and the magnitude of harm, uncertainty does not eliminate risk. Unrecognized risks are still risks; uncertain risks are still risks; and denied risks are still risks. (Cairns, Ref. 149.)

Chemicals—both natural and synthetic—cause cancer. Because not all or even a majority of chemicals cause cancer, we must be able to identify with reasonable certainty those proportionately few that do. Carcinogenesis bioassays using laboratory animals have a solid history of identifying those agents most likely to be carcinogenic to humans: natural and synthetic chemicals, mixtures of chemicals, drugs, and commercial products.[9,31,34,58,108,111,135–141] Tellingly, nearly 30 agents causing cancer in humans were first found to induce cancer in animals (see TABLE 2 and Refs. 4, 22, 42, 45, 56, and 142). Unfortunately, however, bioassays have not been, nor can they be, used to evaluate or discover industrial processes or occupational exposure circumstances that cause or might cause cancer in humans.[19,42,139–141] Equally difficult to test for carcinogenesis are environmental mixtures, dietary factors, foods, and actual human exposures to myriad and multiple chemicals, coupled with varied life styles and socioeconomic situations.[42,56,113,143,144] Thus, we are obligated most often to test single or simple combinations of chemicals for possible carcinogenesis, which make it all the more important to select the most appropriate and public health-warranted chemicals to test.

Despite these obstacles, all chemicals known to cause cancer in humans that can be tested in animals are likewise carcinogenic in animals.[19,42,45,56,58,137,140,142] Does this imply that any chemical that causes cancer in animals will be carcinogenic in humans? No. Carcinogens are not equal; each must be evaluated using all relevant information and especially the strength of the carcinogenesis evidence. In fact, using a multifactorial matrix approach including mechanistic information, exposures, and degrees and potency of responses, we have predicted that only 5–10% of all chemicals would eventually be reasonably anticipated to cause cancer in humans.[109] The absolute number of carcinogens would, indeed, be large; yet, importantly, most agents tested in animals do not cause cancer under conditions of long-term bioassays.[10,42,45,56,110,136,140,142] Conversely, several experimental anticarcinogens have been identified in routine bioassays (e.g., see Refs. 146–150), that could be pursued for purposes of preventing cancer. Likewise, in foods there may be mutagens and carcinogens as well as antimutagens and anticarcinogens—especially in fruits and vegetables—that in composite tend to be preventative (e.g., see Refs. 151–153). Moreover, to test only one ingredient of a food (e.g., D-limonene in oranges), without testing or considering all factors in that food, can lead to incomplete or misleading conclusions. Thus, under most circumstances, composite foods, rather than selected constituents, should be tested for possible carcinogenic effects.

Prudent public health policy obligates us to continue with the rational strategy of reducing or eliminating exposures to chemical carcinogens, to chemicals in general, and to unhealthy workplace conditions.[113,114] Additionally, we need to persevere in our efforts to reduce or eliminate unnecessary industrial emissions (more than 2.2 billion pounds are released per year in the U.S.) and chemical contaminations of our air, animal and plant life, land and food crops, water and fish, and diets.[138] Consequently, cancer incidence and mortalities related to and influenced by chemicals, as well as other chemically associated diseases, could be restricted, reduced, or eradicated. This goal we must continue to approach. Because few if any of the causes of the major cancers in humans have been identified, we must rely on what we know about chemicals and carcinogenesis, and thereby have little doubt that exposure to animal and human carcinogens plays some role—whether minimal or significant—in cancer causation.

After all, does not public health and human decency commit us to keep individual and corporate wastes confined, or at least to use and dispose of these dangerous materials properly and safely without undue harm to others? Performing these recovery or recycling processes more faithfully would substantially reduce the amounts of hazardous chemicals being released to our environments. Likewise, continued distribution of carcinogens in consumer products needs to be curtailed. The resultant subsequent reduction in exogenous cancer risk factors would lead to lessened morbidity and mortality from cancer. Reduction of exposures to both toxic and carcinogenic (and all) chemicals is simply the right thing to do.

ACKNOWLEDGMENTS

I appreciate the comments and suggestions by Kamal Abdo, John Bucher, and Po Chan, National Institute of Environmental Health Sciences; and by Jerrold Ward, National Cancer Institute. I thank Jackie Stillwell for helping to reorganize the reference formatting from the author-year style to numerical citations.

REFERENCES

1. YAMAGIWA, K. & K. ICHIKAWA. 1918. Experimental study of the pathogenesis of carcinoma. Cancer Res. **3:** 1–29.
2. HUFF, J.E. 1992. Applicability to humans of rodent-specific sites of chemical carcinogenicity: tumors of the forestomach and of the harderian, preputial, and zymbal glands induced by benzene. J. Occup. Med. Toxicol. **1:** 109–141.
3. DOLL, R. 1987. The role of epidemiology in the detection and reduction of cancer risks. In Cancer Risks. Strategies for Elimination. P. Bannasch, Ed.: 14–23. Springer-Verlag.
4. HUFF, J.E. 1993. Chemicals and cancer in humans: first evidence in experimental animals. Environ. Health Perspect. **100:** 201–210.
5. SHIMKIN, M.B. 1977. Contrary to nature. DHEW Pub. No. (NIH) 79-720. National Institutes of Health, Bethesda.
6. SHIMKIN, M.B. 1980. Some classics of experimental oncology. 50 selections, 1775–1965. DHEW Pub. No. (NIH) 80-2150. National Institutes of Health, Bethesda.

7. TOMATIS, L. & J.E. HUFF. 1999. Evolution of research in cancer etiology. *In* The Molecular Basis of Human Cancer: Genomic Instability and Molecular Mutation in Neoplastic Transformation. W.B. Coleman & G.J. Tsongalis, Eds. Humana Press, Totowa. In press.
8. HUFF, J.E. 1999. Historical milestones of chemical carcinogenesis: a personal selection. Environ. Health Perspect. Submitted.
9. HUFF, J.E., J.K. HASEMAN & D.P. RALL. 1991. Scientific concepts, value, and significance of chemical carcinogenesis studies. Ann. Rev. Pharmacol. Toxicol. **31:** 621–652.
10. HUFF, J.E. 1993. Issues and controversies surrounding qualitative strategies for identifying and forecasting cancer causing agents in the human environment. Pharmacol. Toxicol. **72**(Suppl. 1): 12–27.
11. NCI. 1976. Carcinogenesis bioassay of trichloroethylene (CAS No. 79-01-6). TR-2. National Cancer Institute, Bethesda.
12. MALTONI, C., A. DEL GAUDIO & D. CARRETTI. 1966. Cutaneous tumors of various types induced in the rat with local applications of 9,10-dimethyl-1,2-benzanthracene. Cancro **19**(4): 383–392. (Article in Italian.)
13. MALTONI, C., S. PERETTI & G. GHETTI. 1968. Synergic oncogenic effect of 2-N-fluorenylacetamide and carbon tetrachloride on rat liver. Cancro **21**(1): 63–72. (Article in Italian.)
14. MALTONI, C., G. LEFEMINE, P. CHIECO & D. CARRETTI. 1974. Vinyl chloride carcinogenesis: current results and perspectives. Med. Lav. **65**(11–12): 421–444.
15. MALTONI, C. 1976. Occupational carcinogenesis. Predictive value of carcinogenesis bioassays. Ann. N.Y. Acad. Sci. **271:** 431–443.
16. VIOLA, P.L. 1970. Pathology of vinyl chloride. Med. Lav. **61**(3): 147–180.
17. VIOLA, P.L., A. BIGOTTI & A. CAPUTO. 1971. Oncogenic response of rat skin, lungs, and bones to vinyl chloride. Cancer Res. **31**(5): 516–522.
18. TOMATIS, L., C. PARTENSKY & R. MONTESANO. 1973. The predictive value of mouse liver tumour induction in carcinogenicity testing—a literature survey. Int. J. Cancer **12**(1): 1–20.
19. TOMATIS, L., A. AITIO, J. WILBOURN & L. SHUKER. 1989. Human carcinogens identified so far. Jpn. J. Cancer Res. **80:** 795–807.
20. TOMATIS, L. 1976. The IARC program on the evaluation of the carcinogenic risk of chemicals to man. Ann. N.Y. Acad. Sci. **271:** 396–409.
21. TOMATIS, L. 1977. Validity and limitations of long-term experimentation in cancer research. IARC Sci. Publ. **16:** 299–307.
22. Tomatis, L. 1979. The predictive value of rodent carcinogenicity tests in the evaluation of human risks. Ann. Rev. Pharmacol. Toxicol. **19:** 511–530.
23. ITO, N. 1973. Experimental studies on tumors of the urinary system of rats induced by chemical carcinogens. Acta Pathol. Jpn. **23**(1): 87–109.
24. ITO, N. & E. Farber. 1966. Effects of trypan blue on hepatocarcinogenesis in rats given ethionine or N-2-fluorenylacetamide. J. Natl. Cancer Inst. **37**(6): 775–785.
25. ITO, N., I. JOHNO, M. MARUGAMI, Y. KONISHI & Y. HIASA. 1966. Histopathological and autoradiographic studies on kidney tumors induced by N-nitrosodimethylamine in rats. Gann **57**(6): 595–604.
26. ITO, N., Y. HIASA, Y. KONISHI & M. MARUGAMI. 1969. The development of carcinoma in liver of rats treated with m-toluylenediamine and the synergistic and antagonistic effects with other chemicals. Cancer Res. **29**(5): 1137–1145.
27. ITO, N., H. NAGASAKI, M. ARAI, S. MAKIURA, S. SUGIHARA & K. HIRAO. 1973. Histopathologic studies on liver tumorigenesis induced in mice by technical polychlorinated biphenyls and its promoting effect on liver tumors induced by benzene hexachloride. J. Natl. Cancer Inst. **51**(5): 1637–1646.
28. ITO, N., T. SHIRAI & R. HASEGAWA. 1992. Medium-term bioassays for carcinogens. *In* Mechanisms of Carcinogenesis in Risk Identification. H. Vainio, P. Magee, D. McGregor & A. McMichael, Eds. IARC Sci. Pub. **116:** 353–388. International Agency for Research on Cancer, Lyon.
29. IARC. 1996. Directory of agents being tested for carcinogenicity. No **17:** 1–247. International Agency for Research on Cancer, Lyon.

30. CARSON, R. 1962. Silent Spring. Houghton Mifflin, New York.
31. HUFF, J.E., E.E. MCCONNELL, J.K. HASEMAN, G.A. BOORMAN, S.L. EUSTIS, B.A. SCHWETZ, G.N. RAO, C.W. JAMESON, L.G. HART & D.P. RALL. 1988. Carcinogenesis studies: results from 398 experiments on 104 chemicals from the U.S. National Toxicology Program. Ann. N.Y. Acad. Sci. **534:** 1–30.
32. HUFF, J.E. & J.A. MOORE. 1984. Carcinogenesis studies design and experimental data interpretation/evaluation at the National Toxicology Program. Prog. Clin. Biol. Res. **141:** 43–64.
33. CHHABRA, R.S., J.E. HUFF, B.S. SCHWETZ & J. SELKIRK. 1990. An overview of pre-chronic and chronic toxicity/carcinogenicity experimental study designs and criteria used by the National Toxicology Program. Environ. Health Perspect. **86:** 313–321.
34. HUFF, J.E. 1992. Design strategies, results and evaluations of long-term chemical carcinogenesis studies. Scand. J. Work Environ. Health. **18**(Suppl.1): 31–37.
35. RAO, G.N., J. EDMONDSON & M.R. ELWELL. 1993. Influence of dietary protein concentration on severity of nephropathy in Fischer-344 (F-344/N) rats. Toxicol. Pathol. **21**(4): 353–356.
36. RAO, G.N. 1996. Influence of diet on tumors of hormonal tissues. Prog. Clin. Biol. Res. **394:** 41–56.
37. RAO, G.N. 1996. New diet (NTP-2000) for rats in the National Toxicology Program toxicity and carcinogenicity studies. Fundam. Appl. Toxicol. **32**(1): 102–108.
38. HASEMAN, J.K., J.E. HUFF & J.A. MOORE. 1983. Shortcomings of rodent carcinogenicity studies. Fundam. Appl. Toxicol. **3**(3): 3a–7a.
39. HASEMAN, J.K., J.E. HUFF, G.N. RAO, J.E. ARNOLD, G.A. BOORMAN & E.E. MCCONNELL. 1985. Neoplasms observed in untreated and corn oil gavage control groups of F344/N rats and (C57BL/6N X C3H/HeN)F1 (B6C3F1) mice. J. Natl. Cancer Inst. **75**(5): 975–984.
40. HASEMAN, J.K., J.E. HUFF, G.N. RAO & S.L. EUSTIS. 1989. Sources of variability in rodent carcinogenicity studies. Fundam. Appl. Toxicol. **12**(4): 793–804.
41. RAO, G.N. & J.E. HUFF. 1990. Refinement of long-term toxicity and carcinogenesis studies. Fundam. Appl. Toxicol. **15**(1): 33–43.
42. HUFF, J.E. 1999. Cancer hazards and risk assessments in chemical carcinogenesis. *In* Patty's Industrial Hygiene and Toxicology, 5th edit. Chapter 6. John Wiley & Sons, Inc. New York. In press.
43. HUFF, J.E. 1992. Chemical toxicity & chemical carcinogenesis. Is there a causal connection? A comparative morphological evaluation of 1500 experiments. *In* Mechanisms of Carcinogenesis in Risk Identification. H. Vainio, P. Magee, D. McGregor & A. McMichael, Eds. IARC Sci. Pub. **116:** 437–475. International Agency for Research on Cancer, Lyon.
44. HUFF, J.E. 1993. Absence of morphologic correlation between chemical toxicity and chemical carcinogenesis. Environ. Health Perspect. **101**(Suppl. 5): 45–53.
45. HUFF, J.E. 1999. Value, validity, and historical development of carcinogenesis studies for predicting and confirming carcinogenic risks to humans. *In* Testing, Predicting, and Interpreting Chemical Carcinogenicity, Chapter 2. K.T. Kitchin, Ed.: 21–123. Marcel Dekker, New York.
46. HUFF, J.E. 1996. α_2u-Globulin nephropathy, posed mechanisms, and white ravens. Environ. Health Perspect. **104**(12): 1264–1267.
47. MELNICK, R.L., M.C. KOHN & J. HUFF. 1997. Weight of evidence versus weight of speculation to evaluate the alpha2u-globulin hypothesis. Environ. Health Perspect. **105**(9): 904–906.
48. MELNICK, R.L. & M.C. KOHN. 1999. Possible mechanisms of induction of renal tubular cell neoplasms in rats associated with α_2u-globulin: role of protein accumulation versus ligand delivery to the kidney. IARC Scientific Publications. In press.
49. HUFF, J.E., S.L. EUSTIS & J.K. HASEMAN. 1989. Occurrence and relevance of chemically induced benign neoplasms in long-term carcinogenicity studies. Cancer Metastasis Rev. **8**(1): 1–22. (Published erratum appears in Cancer Metastasis Rev. **8**(3): 281.)

50. MARONPOT, R.R., J.K. HASEMAN, G.A. BOORMAN, S.E. EUSTIS, G.N. RAO, J.E. HUFF. 1987. Liver lesions in B6C3F1 mice: the National Toxicology Program, experience and position. Arch. Toxicol. Suppl. **10:** 10–26.
51. CARMICHAEL, N.G., H. ENZMANN, I. PATE & F. WAECHTER. 1997. The significance of mouse liver tumor formation for carcinogenic risk assessment: results and conclusions from a survey of ten years of testing by the agrochemical industry. Environ. Health Perspect. **105:** 1196–1203.
52. HUFF, J.E. 1999. Chemically induced liver tumors in rodents and relevance to human carcinogenesis. Submitted.
53. HASEMAN, J.K. & A. LOCKHART. 1994. The relationship between use of the maximum tolerated dose and study sensitivity for detecting rodent carcinogenicity. Fundam. Appl. Toxicol. **22**(3): 382–391.
54. BUCHER, J.R., C.J. PORTIER, J.I. GOODMAN, E.M. FAUSTMAN & G.W. LUCIER. 1996. Workshop overview. National Toxicology Program Studies: principles of dose selection and applications to mechanistic based risk assessment. Fundam. Appl. Toxicol. **31**(1): 1–8.
55. BUCHER, J.R. 1999. Doses in rodent cancer studies: sorting fact from fiction. Drug Metab. Rev. In press.
56. HUFF, J.E. 1999. Cancer hazards for humans predicted from long-term carcinogenesis bioassays. Drug Metab. Rev. In press.
57. BLUMBERG, B.S. 1993. Accomplishments in Cancer Research for 1992. Preface. Lippincott.
58. HUFF, J.E. 1994. Chemicals causally associated with cancers in humans and in laboratory animals: A perfect concordance. *In* Carcinogenesis, Chapter 2. M.P. Waalkes & J.M. Ward, Eds.: 25–37. Raven Press, New York.
59. HUFF, J.E. 1999. Control tumor incidence data from NTP and NCI for kidney, urinary bladder, and thyroid glands. *In* IARC Meeting on Rodent Specific Tumors, Lyon. 3–7 November, 1997. In press.
60. IARC. 1999. IARC meeting on rodent specific tumors. IARC Sci. Pub., Lyon. 3–7 November, 1997. In press.
61. HOEL, D.G., J.K. HASEMAN, M.D. HOGAN, J.E. HUFF & E. MCCONNELL. 1988. The impact of toxicity on carcinogenicity studies: implications for risk assessment. Carcinogenesis **9:** 2045–2052.
62. HUFF, J.E. 1995. Mechanisms, chemical carcinogenesis, and risk assessment: cell proliferation and cancer. Am. J. Ind. Med. **27**(2): 293–300.
63. NTP. 1996. Toxicology and carcinogenesis studies of 2,2-bis(bromomethyl)-1,3-propanediol (FR-1138®) (CAS No. 3296-90-0) in F344 Rats and B6C3F1 mice (feed studies). TR-452. National Toxicology Program, Research Triangle Park.
64. DUNNICK, J.K., J.E. HEATH, D.R. FARNELL, J.D. PREJEAN, J.K. HASEMAN & M.R. ELWELL. 1997. Carcinogenic activity of the flame retardant, 2,2-bis(bromomethyl)-1,3-propanediol in rodents, and comparison with the carcinogenicity of other NTP brominated chemicals. Toxicol. Pathol. **25**(6): 541–548.
65. NTP. 1998. Toxicology and carcinogenesis studies of cobalt sulfate heptahydrate (CAS No. 10026-24-1) in F344/N rats and B6C3F1 mice (inhalation studies). TR-471. National Toxicology Program, Research Triangle Park.
66. BUCHER, J.R., J.R. HAILEY, J.D. ROYCROFT, J.K. HASEMAN, R.C. SILLS, S.L. GRUMBEIN, P.W. MELLICK & B.J. CHOU. 1999. Inhalation toxicity and carcinogenicity studies of cobalt sulfate. Toxicol. Sci. Submitted.
67. NTP. 1992. Toxicology and carcinogenesis studies of chlorinated water (CAS Nos. 7782-50-5 and 7681-52-9) and chloraminated water (CAS No. 10599-90-3) (deionized and charcoal-filtered) in F344/N rats and B6C3F1 mice (drinking water studies). TR-392. National Toxicology Program, Research Triangle Park.
68. MORRIS, R.D., A.M. AUDET, I.F. ANGELILLO, T.C. CHALMERS & F. MOSTELLER. 1992. Chlorination, chlorination by-products, and cancer: a meta-analysis. Am. J. Public Health **82**(7): 955–963. (Published erratum appears in Am. J. Public Health **83**(9): 1257, 1993.)

69. DUNNICK, J.K. & R.L. MELNICK. 1993. Assessment of the carcinogenic potential of chlorinated water: experimental studies of chlorine, chloramine, and trihalomethanes. J. Natl. Cancer Inst. **85**(10): 817–822.
70. MELNICK, R.L., J.K. DUNNICK, D.P. SANDLER, M.R. ELWELL & J.C. BARRETT. 1994. Trihalomethanes and other environmental factors that contribute to colorectal cancer. Environ. Health Perspect. **102**(6–7): 586–588.
71. MORRIS, R.D. 1995. Drinking water and cancer. Environ. Health Perspect. **103**(Suppl. 8): 225–231.
72. MELNICK, R.L., G.A. BOORMAN & V. DELLARCO. 1997. Water chlorination, 3-chloro-4-(dichloro-methyl)-5-hydroxy-2(5H)-furanone (MX), and potential cancer risk. J. Natl. Cancer Inst. **89**(12): 832–833.
73. SOFFRITTI, M., F. BELPOGGI, A. LENZI & C. MALTONI. 1997. Results of long-term carcinogenicity studies of chlorine in rats. Ann. N.Y. Acad. Sci. **837**: 189–208.
74. CANTOR, K.P. 1997. Drinking water and cancer. Cancer Causes Control **8**(3): 292–308.
75. KOIVUSALO, M., T. HAKULINEN, T. VARTIAINEN, E. PUKKALA, J.J. JAAKKOLA & J. TUOMISTO. 1998. Drinking water mutagenicity and urinary tract cancers: a population-based case-control study in Finland. Am. J. Epidemiol. **148**(7): 704–712.
76. YANG, C.Y., H.F. CHIU, M.F. CHENG & S.S. TSAI. 1998. Chlorination of drinking water and cancer mortality in Taiwan. Environ. Res. **78**(1): 1–6.
77. TICE, R.R., R. BOUCHER, C.A. LUKE, D.E. PAQUETTE, R.L. MELNICK & M.D. SHELBY. 1988. Chloroprene and isoprene: cytogenetic studies in mice. Mutagenesis **3**(2): 141–146.
78. MELNICK, R.L., M.R. ELWELL, J.H. ROYCROFT, B.J. CHOU, H.A. RAGAN & R.A. MILLER. 1996. Toxicity of inhaled chloroprene (2-chloro-1,3-butadiene) in F344 rats and B6C3F(1) mice. Toxicology **108**(1–2): 79–91.
79. NTP. 1998. Toxicology and carcinogenesis studies of chloroprene (CAS No. 126-99-8) in F344/N rats and B6C3F1 mice (inhalation studies). TR-467. National Toxicology Program, Research Triangle Park.
80. BULBULYAN, M.A., O.V. CHANGUINA, D.G. ZARIDZE, S.V. ASTASHEVSKY, D. COLIN & P. BOFFETTA. 1998. Cancer mortality among Moscow shoe workers exposed to chloroprene. Cancer Causes Control **9**(4): 381–387.
81. MELNICK, R.L., R.C. SILLS, C.J. PORTIER, J.H. ROYCROFT, B.J. CHOU, S.L. GRUMBEIN & R.A. MILLER. 1999. Multiple organ carcinogenicity of inhaled chloroprene (2-chloro-1,3-butadiene) in F344/N rats and B6C3F1 mice and comparison of dose-response with 1,3-butadiene in mice. Carcinogenesis. In press.
82. NTP. 1993. Toxicology and carcinogenesis studies of 2,3-dibromo-1-propanol (CAS No. 96-13-9) in F344/N rats and B6C3F1 mice (dermal studies). TR-400. National Toxicology Program, Research Triangle Park.
83. EUSTIS, S.L., J.K. HASEMAN, W.F. MACKENZIE & K.M. ABDO. 1995. Toxicity and carcinogenicity of 2,3-dibromo-1-propanol in F344/N rats and B6C3F1 mice. Fundam. Appl. Toxicol. **26**: 41–50.
84. MALTONI, C., A. CILIBERTI, C. PINTO, M. SOFFRITTI, F. BELPOGGI & L. MENARINI. 1997. Results of long-term experimental carcinogenicity studies of the effects of gasoline, correlated fuels, and major gasoline aromatics on rats. Ann. N.Y. Acad. Sci. **837**: 15–52.
85. CHAN, P.C., J.K. HASEMAN, J. MAHLER & C. ARANYI. 1998. Tumor induction in F344/N rats and B6C3F1 mice following inhalation exposure to ethylbenzene. Toxicol. Lett. **9**(1): 23–32.
86. NTP. 1999. Toxicology and carcinogenesis studies of ethylbenzene (CAS No. 100-41-4) in F344/N rats and B6C3F1 mice (inhalation studies). TR-466. National Toxicology Program, Research Triangle Park. In press.
87. MELNICK, R.L., R.C. SILLS, J.H. ROYCROFT, B.J. CHOU, H.A. RAGAN & R.A. MILLER. 1994. Isoprene, an endogenous hydrocarbon and industrial chemical, induces multiple organ neoplasia in rodents after 26 weeks of inhalation exposure. Cancer Res. **54**(20): 5333–5339.

88. MELNICK, R.L., R.C. SILLS, J.H. ROYCROFT, B.J. CHOU, H.A. RAGAN & R.A. MILLER. 1996. Inhalation toxicity and carcinogenicity of isoprene in rats and mice: comparisons with 1,3-butadiene. Toxicology **113**(1–3): 247–252.
89. PLACKE, M.E., L. GRIFFIS, M. BIRD, J. BUS, R.L. PERSING & L.A. COX, JR. 1996. Chronic inhalation oncogenicity study of isoprene in B6C3F1 mice. Toxicology **113**(1–3): 253–262.
90. HONG, H.L., T.R. DEVEREUX, R.L. MELNICK, S.R. ELDRIDGE, A. GREENWELL, J. HASEMAN, G.A. BOORMAN & R.C. SILLS. 1997. Both K-ras and H-ras protooncogene mutations are associated with Harderian gland tumorigenesis in B6C3F1 mice exposed to isoprene for 26 weeks. Carcinogenesis **18**(4): 783–789.
91. NTP. 1999. Toxicology and carcinogenesis studies of isoprene (CAS No. 78-79-5) in F344/N rats (inhalation studies). TR-486. National Toxicology Program, Research Triangle Park. In press.
92. BELPOGGI, F., M. SOFFRITTI & C. MALTONI. 1995. Methyl-tertiary-butyl ether (MTBE)—a gasoline additive—causes testicular and lymphohaematopoietic cancers in rats. Toxicol. Ind. Health **11**(2): 119–149.
93. BELPOGGI, F., M. SOFFRITTI, F. FILIPPINI & C. MALTONI. 1997. Results of long-term experimental studies on the carcinogenicity of methyl *tert*-butyl ether. Ann. N.Y. Acad. Sci. **837:** 77–95.
94. BELPOGGI, F., M. SOFFRITTI & C. MALTONI. 1998. Pathological characterization of testicular tumours and lymphomas-leukemias and of their precursors observed in Sprague-Dawley rats exposed to methyl-teritary-butyl-ether [MTBE]. Eur. J. Oncol. **3:** 201–206.
95. BIRD, M.G., H.D. BURLEIGH-FLAYER, J.S. CHUN, J.F. DOUGLAS, J.J. KNEISS & L.S. ANDREWS. 1997. Oncogenicity studies of inhaled methyl tertiary-butyl ether (MTBE) in CD-1 mice and F-344 rats. J. Appl. Toxicol. **17**(Suppl. 1): S45–S55.
96. NTP. 1999. Toxicology and carcinogenesis studies of methyleugenol (CAS NO. 93-15-2) in F344/N rats and B6C3F1 mice (gavage studies). TR-491. National Toxicology Program, Research Triangle Park. In press.
97. NTP. 1996. Toxicology and carcinogenesis studies of phenolphthalein (CAS No. 77-09-8) in F344/N rats and B6C3F1 mice (feed studies). TR-465. National Toxicology Program, Research Triangle Park.
98. DUNNICK, J.K. & J.R. HAILEY. 1996. Phenolphthalein exposure causes multiple carcinogenic effects in experimental model systems. Cancer Res. **56**(21): 4922–4926.
99. DUNNICK, J.K., J.F. HARDISTY, R.A. HERBERT, J.C. SEELY, E.M. FUREDI-MACHACEK, J.F. FOLEY, G.D. LACKS, S. STASIEWICZ & J.E. FRENCH. 1997. Phenolphthalein induces thymic lymphomas accompanied by loss of the p53 wild type allele in heterozygous p53-deficient (+/−) mice. Toxicol. Pathol. **25**(6): 533–540.
100. LONGNECKER, M.P., D.P. SANDLER, R.W. HAILE & R.S. SANDLER. 1997. Phenolphthalein-containing laxative use in relation to adenomatous colorectal polyps in three studies. Environ. Health Perspect. **105**(11): 1210–1212.
101. TSUTSUI, T., Y. TAMURA, E. YAGI, K. HASEGAWA, Y. TANAKA, A. UEHAMA, T. SOMEYA, F. HAMAGUCHI, H. YAMAMOTO & J.C. BARRETT. 1997. Cell-transforming activity and genotoxicity of phenolphthalein in cultured Syrian hamster embryo cells. Int. J. Cancer **73**(5): 697–701.
102. NTP. 1997. Toxicology and carcinogenesis studies of tetrafluoroethylene (CAS No. 116-14-3) in F344 rats and B6C3F1 mice (inhalation studies). TR-450. National Toxicology Program, Research Triangle Park.
103. HONG, H.L., T.R. DEVEREUX, J.H. ROYCROFT, G.A. BOORMAN & R.C. SILLS. 1998. Frequency of ras mutations in liver neoplasms from B6C3F1 mice exposed to tetrafluoroethylene for two years. Toxicol. Pathol. **26**(5): 646–650.
104. STOWERS, S.J., P.L. GLOVER, S.H. REYNOLDS, L.R. BOONE, R.R. MARONPOT & M.W. ANDERSON. 1987. Activation of the K-ras protooncogene in lung tumors from rats and mice chronically exposed to tetranitromethane. Cancer Res. **47**(12): 3212–3219.
105. NTP. 1990. Toxicology and carcinogenesis studies of tetranitromethane (CAS No. 509-14-8) in F344/N rats and B6C3F1 mice (inhalation studies). TR-386. National Toxicology Program, Research Triangle Park.

106. BUCHER, J.R., J.E. HUFF, M.P. JOKINEN, J.K. HASEMAN, M. STEDHAM & J.M. CHOLAKIS. 1991]. Inhalation of tetranitromethane causes nasal passage irritation and pulmonary carcinogenesis in rodents. Cancer Lett. **57**(2): 95–101.
107. YOU, M., Y. WANG, A. LINEEN, G.D. STONER, L.A. YOU, R.R. MARONPOT & M.W. ANDERSON. 1991. Activation of protooncogenes in mouse lung tumors. Exp. Lung Res. **17**(2): 389–400.
108. FUNG, V.A., J.E. HUFF, E. WEISBURGER & D.G. HOEL. 1993. Predictive strategies for selecting 379 NCI/NTP chemicals evaluated for carcinogenic potential: scientific and public health impact. Fund. Appl. Toxicol. **20:** 413–36.
109. HUFF, J., E. WEISBURGER & V.A. FUNG. 1996. Multicomponent criteria for predicting carcinogenicity: dataset of 30 NTP chemicals. Environ. Health Perspect. **104** (Suppl. 5): 1105–1112.
110. HUFF, J.E., E.E. MCCONNELL & J.K. HASEMAN. 1985. On the proportion of positive results in carcinogenicity studies in animals. Environ. Mutagen. **7**(4): 427–428.
111. FUNG, V.A., J.C. BARRETT & J.E. HUFF. 1995. The carcinogenesis bioassay in perspective: application in identifying human cancer hazards. Environ. Health Perspect. **103:** 680–683.
112. BRISTOL, D.W., J.T. WACHSMAN & A. GREENWELL. 1996. The NIEHS predictive-toxicology evaluation project: chemcarcinogenicity bioassays. Environ. Health Perspect. **104S**(5): 1001–1010.
113. TOMATIS, L., J.E. HUFF, I. HERTZ-PICCIOTTO, D. SANDLER, J. BUCHER, P. BOFFETTA, O. AXELSON, A. BLAIR, J. TAYLOR, L. STAYNER & J.C. BARRETT. 1997. Avoided and avoidable risks in cancer. Carcinogenesis **18:** 97–105.
114. WILLIAMS, G.M. 1995. Tamoxifen experimental carcinogenicity studies: implications for human effects. Proc. Soc. Exp. Biol. Med. **208**(2): 141–143.
115. HUFF, J., J. CIRVELLO, J. HASEMAN & J. BUCHER. 1991. Chemicals associated with site-specific neoplasia in 1394 long-term carcinogenesis experiments in laboratory rodents. Environ. Health Perspect. **93:** 247–270. (Published erratum in Environ. Health Perspect. **95:** 213, 1991.)
116. MALTONI, C. & C. SCARNATO. 1979. First experimental demonstration of the carcinogenic effects of benzene; long-term bioassays on Sprague-Dawley rats by oral administration. Med. Lav. **70**(5): 352–357.
117. HUFF, J.E., J.K. HASEMAN, D.M. DEMARINI, S. EUSTIS, R.R. MARONPOT, A.C. PETERS, R.L. PERSING, C.E. CHRISP & A.C. JACOBS. 1989. Multiple-site carcinogenicity of benzene in Fischer 344 rats and B6C3F1 mice. Environ. Health Perspect. **82:** 125–163.
118. MALTONI, C., A. CILIBERTI, G. COTTI, B. CONTI & F. BELPOGGI. 1989. Benzene, an experimental multipotential carcinogen: results of the long-term bioassays performed at the Bologna Institute of Oncology. Environ. Health Perspect. **82:**109–124.
119. TSUTSUI, T., N. HAYASHI, H. MAIZUMI, J. HUFF & J.C. BARRETT. 1997. Benzene-, catechol-, hydroquinone-, and phenol-induced cell transformation, gene mutations, chromosome aberrations, aneuploidy, sister chromatid exchanges and unscheduled DNA synthesis in Syrian hamster embryo cells. Mutat. Res. **373**(1): 113–123.
120. WATERS, E.M., H.B. GERSTNER & J.E. HUFF. 1977. Trichloroethylene. I. An overview. J. Toxicol. Environ. Health **2**(3): 671–707.
121. NTP. 1990. Carcinogenesis studies of trichloroethylene (without epichlorohydrin) (CAS No. 79-01-6) in F344/N rats and B6C3F1 mice (gavage studies). TR-243. National Toxicology Program, Research Triangle Park.
122. NTP. 1988. Toxicology and carcinogenesis studies of trichloroethylene (CAS No. 79-01-6) in four strains of rats (ACI, August, Marshall, Osborne-Mendel) (gavage studies). TR-273. National Toxicology Program, Research Triangle Park.
123. FUKUDA, K., K. TAKEMOTO & H. TSURUTA. 1983. Inhalation carcinogenicity of trichloroethylene in mice and rats. Ind. Health **21**(4): 243–254.
124. HENSCHLER, D., E. EDER, T. NEUDECKER & M. METZLER. 1977. Carcinogenicity of trichloroethylene: fact or artifact? Arch. Toxicol. **37**(3): 233–236.
125. HENSCHLER, D., W. ROMEN, H.M. ELSASSER, D. REICHERT, E. EDER & Z. RADWAN. 1980. Carcinogenicity study of trichloroethylene by long term inhalation in three animal species. Arch. Toxicol. **43**(4): 237–248.

126. HENSCHLER, D., H. ELSASSER, W. ROMEN & E. EDER. 1984. Carcinogenicity study of trichloroethylene, with and without epoxide stabilizers, in mice. J. Cancer Res. Clin. Oncol. **107**(3): 149–156.
127. MALTONI, C., G. LEFEMINE & G. COTTI. 1986. Experimental research on trichloroethylene carcinogenesis. *In* Archives of Research on Industrial Carcinogenesis Series, Volume 5. C. Maltoni & M.A. Mehlman, Eds. Princeton Scientific Pub. Co. Princeton.
128. MALTONI, C., G. LEFEMINE, G. COTTI & G. PERINO. 1988. Long-term carcinogenicity bioassays on trichloroethylene administered by inhalation to Sprague-Dawley rats and Swiss and B6C3F1 mice. Ann. N.Y. Acad. Sci. **534**: 316–342.
129. PEREIRA, M.A. 1996. Carcinogenic activity of dichloroacetic acid and trichloroacetic acid in the liver of female B6C3F1 mice. Fundam. Appl. Toxicol. **31**(2): 192–199.
130. DEANGELO, A.B., F.B. DANIEL, B.M. MOST & G.R. OLSON. 1996. The carcinogenicity of dichloroacetic acid in the male Fischer 344 rat. Toxicology **114**(3): 207–221.
131. HENSCHLER, D., S. VAMVAKAS, M. LAMMERT, W. DEKANT, B. KRAUS, B. THOMAS & K. ULM. 1995. Increased incidence of renal cell tumors in a cohort of cardboard workers exposed to trichloroethene. Arch. Toxicol. **69**(5): 291–299.
132. VAMVAKAS, S., T. BRUNING, B. THOMASSON, M. LAMMERT, A. BAUMULLER, H.M. BOLT, W. DEKANT, G. BIRNER, D. HENSCHLER & K. ULM. 1998. Renal cell cancer correlated with occupational exposure to trichloroethene. J. Cancer Res. Clin. Oncol. **124**(7): 374–382.
133. IARC. 1995. Trichloroethylene. Dry cleaning, some chlorinated solvents and other industrial chemicals. *In* IARC Monographs on the Evaluation of Carcinogenic Risk to Humans **63**: 75–158. International Agency for Research on Cancer, Lyon.
134. HUFF, J.E. 1999. Trichloroethylene: clear evidence of carcinogenicity in animals and in humans. Submitted.
135. WILBOURN, J., L. HAROUN, E. HESELTINE, J. KALDOR, C. PARTENSKY & H. VAINIO. 1986. Response of experimental animals to human carcinogens: an analysis based upon the IARC Monographs programme. Carcinogenesis **7**(11): 1853–1863.
136. HUFF, J.E. & D.G. HOEL. 1992. Perspective and overview of the concepts and value of hazard identification as the initial phase of risk assessment for cancer and human health. Scand. J. Work Environ. Health. **18**(Suppl. 1): 83–89.
137. HUFF, J.E. & D.P. RALL. 1992. Relevance to humans of carcinogenesis results from laboratory animal toxicology studies. *In* Maxcy-Rosenau-Last's Public Health & Preventive Medicine, 13th edit. J.M. Last & R.B. Wallace, Eds.: 433–440 and 453–457. Appleton & Lange, Norwalk.
138. MALTONI, C. 1997. Biomedical research as a science for development: the case of gasoline. Ann. N.Y. Acad. Sci. **837**: 1–14.
139. IARC. 1999. IARC Monographs on the Evaluation of Carcinogenic Risks to Humans, Volumes 1–73. International Agency for Research on Cancer, Lyon.
140. HUFF, J.E. 1998. Carcinogenesis results in animals predict cancer risks to humans. *In* Maxcy-Rosenau-Last's Public Health & Preventive Medicine, 14th edit. R.B. Wallace, Ed.: Appleton-Lange, Norwalk.
141. HUFF, J.E. 1998. NTP Report on Carcinogens: history, concepts, procedures, progress. Eur. J. Oncol. **3**: 343–355.
142. HUFF, J.E., S. SOWARD. 1999. Carcinogenesis bioassays of 500 chemicals: results, evaluations, tumor site specificity, prevalence categories, and human risk potential. Submitted.
143. HUFF, J.E., J.A. BOYD & J.C. BARRETT, Eds. 1996. Cellular and molecular mechanisms of hormonal carcinogenesis: environmental influences. Prog. Clin. Biol. Res. **134**: 1–479.
144. HUFF, J.E. 1994. Carcinogenic hazards from eating fish and shellfish contaminated with disparate and complex chemical mixtures. *In* Toxicology of Chemical Mixtures: From Real Life Examples to Mechanisms of Toxicological Interactions, Chapter 9: 157–194. Academic Press, New York.
145. HUFF, J.E. & J.C. BARRETT. 1999. Breast cancer and associated environmental risk factors. Environ. Health Perspect. Submitted.

146. ABDO, K.M., S.L. EUSTIS, J.K. HASEMAN, J.E. HUFF, A. PETERS & R. PERSING. 1988. Toxicity and carcinogenicity of rotenone given in the feed to F344/N rats and B6C3F1 mice for up to two years. Drug Chem. Toxicol. **11:** 225–235.
147. DOUGLAS, J.F. & J.E. HUFF. 1984. No evidence of carcinogenicity of l-ascorbic acid in rodents. J. Toxicol. Environ. Health **14:** 605–609.
148. CHHABRA, R.S., J.E. HUFF, J.K. HASEMAN, A. HALL, G. BASKIN & M. COWAN. 1988. Inhibition of some spontaneous tumors by 4-hexylresorcinol in F344/N rats and B6C3F1 mice. Fundam. Appl. Toxicol. **11:** 685–690.
149. HASEMAN, J.K. & F.M. JOHNSON. 1996. Analysis of National Toxicology Program rodent bioassay data for anticarcinogenic effects. Mut. Res. **350:** 131–141.
150. CHAN, P.C., R.C. SILLS, A.G. BRAUN, J.K. HASEMAN & J.R. BUCHER. 1996. Toxicity and carcinogenicity of Δ^9-tetrahydrobcannabinol in Fischer rats and B6C3F1 mice. Fundam. Appl. Toxicol. **30:** 109–117.
151. WATTENBERG, L.W. 1992. Inhibition of carcinogenesis by minor dietary constituents. Cancer Res. **52**(Suppl. 7): 2085s–2091s.
152. WATTENBERG, L.W. 1996. Inhibition of tumorigenesis in animals. IARC Sci. Pub. **139:** 151–158.
153. WATTENBERG, L.W. 1997. An overview of chemoprevention: current status and future prospects. Proc. Soc. Exp. Biol. Med. **216**(2): 133–141.
154. CAIRNS, J. 1999. Absence of certainty is not synonymous with absence of risk. Environ. Health Perspect. **107:** A56–A57.
155. HASEMAN, J.K., E.C. THARRINGTON, J.E. HUFF & E.E. MCCONNELL. 1986. Comparison of site-specific and overall tumor incidence analyses for 81 recent National Toxicology Program carcinogenicity studies. Regul. Toxicol. Pharmacol. **6**(2): 155–170.
156. FARBER, E. 1995. Cell proliferation as a major risk factor for cancer: a concept of doubtful validity. Cancer Res. **55**(17): 3759–3762.
157. FARBER, E. 1996. Cell proliferation is not a major risk factor for cancer. Mod. Pathol. **9**(6): 606.
158. MELNICK, R.L. & J.E. HUFF. 1993. Liver carcinogenesis is not a predicted outcome of chemically induced hepatocyte proliferation. Toxicol. Ind. Health **9**(3): 415–438.
159. MELNICK, R.L., J. HUFF, J.C. BARRETT, R.R. MARONPOT, G. LUCIER & C.J. PORTIER. 1993. Cell proliferation and chemical carcinogenesis: a symposium overview. Mol. Carcinog. **7**(3): 135–138.
160. MELNICK, R.L., M.C. KOHN, J.K. DUNNICK & J.R. LEININGER. 1998. Regenerative hyperplasia is not required for liver tumor induction in female B6C3F1 mice exposed to trihalomethanes. Toxicol. Appl. Pharmacol. **148**(1): 137–147.
161. MELNICK, R.L., M.C. KOHN & C.J. PORTIER. 1996. Implications for risk assessment of suggested nongenotoxic mechanisms of chemical carcinogenesis. Environ. Health Perspect. **104**(Suppl. 1): 123–134.
162. BARRETT, J.C. & J.E. HUFF. 1991. Cellular and molecular mechanisms of chemically induced renal carcinogenesis. Ren. Fail. **13**(4): 211–225.
163. MELNICK, R.L., G.A. BOORMAN, J.K. HASEMAN, R.J. MONTALI & J.E. HUFF. 1984. Urolithiasis and bladder carcinogenicity of melamine in rodents. Toxicol. Appl. Pharmacol. **72**(2): 292–303.
164. PERERA, F., T. BRENNAN & J.R. FOUTS. 1989. Comment on the significance of positive carcinogenicity studies using gavage as the route of exposure. Environ. Health Perspect. **79:** 315–321.
165. HASEMAN, J.K. & J.E. HUFF. 1987. Species correlation in long-term carcinogenicity studies. Cancer Lett. **37**(2): 125–132. (Published erratum appears in Cancer Lett. **38**(3): 365, 1988.)
166. HASEMAN, J.K. 1999. Using the NTP database to assess the value of rodent carcinogenicity studies for determining human cancer risk. Drug Metab. Rev. In press.

Uncertainty in Biomonitoring and Kinetic Modeling

LUTZ EDLER[a,b]

Biostatistics Unit, German Cancer Research Center, Heidelberg, Germany

ABSTRACT: Uncertainty in exposure assessment and uncertainty in kinetic models of early effects after exposure to a toxin are addressed in this paper. Sources of uncertainty in the determination of exposure of workers in chemical industry exposed to dioxins are exhibited and a simple kinetic model for biomonitor measurements of the concentrations from occupational exposure is derived. Model uncertainty, and uncertainty in the model parameters of physiologically-based pharmacokinetic models (PBPK models) are addressed when these models are used to estimate the effective dose in risk assessment. Uncertainty in the model parameters originating from the use of different statistical analysis methods is exhibited for Hill type nonlinear kinetics of enzyme induction mediated by a toxin.

INTRODUCTION

Uncertainty is prevalent throughout the process of risk assessment at various levels. Uncertainty concerning the exposure assessment particularly influences dose estimates. Uncertainty in dose-response modeling, mostly caused by limited knowledge of how to model the relationship, exaggerates these effects. Both types of uncertainties are propagated to the risk estimation procedure and finally to risk management decisions.[1] Therefore, careful analysis is required so as to identify sources of uncertainty and remove them. An estimate of the impact of uncertainty on risk estimates and on management conclusions is required for the establishment of efficient public health protection strategies.

Human exposure data show a large measure of uncertainty when estimated indirectly from life style—sojourn measurements in general population studies, or estimated from job-exposure matrix information in occupational studies. To circumvent the problems associated with indirect exposure measurements, one attempts to determine exposure by biomonitor measurements of the toxin in humans. The measurement of the toxin concentration in blood has become the preferred method. However, this procedure is not without uncertainty, as is shown below. When biomonitor data are used for exposure assessment, uncertainty becomes an issue since the these data are incorporated in a dose-response model as independent variables that trigger a toxic response.

---

[a]Address for correspondence: Biostatistics Unit, Research Programme Genome Research and Bioinformatics, German Cancer Research Center, Im Neuenheimer Feld 280, D-69120 Heidelberg, Germany. +49 6221 42 2392 (voice); +49 6221 42 2397 (fax).
  e-mail:edler@dkfz-heidelberg.de
[b]This work was performed in connection with the authors participation in the CCHS/NATO Pilot Study: Advanced Cancer Risk Assessment.

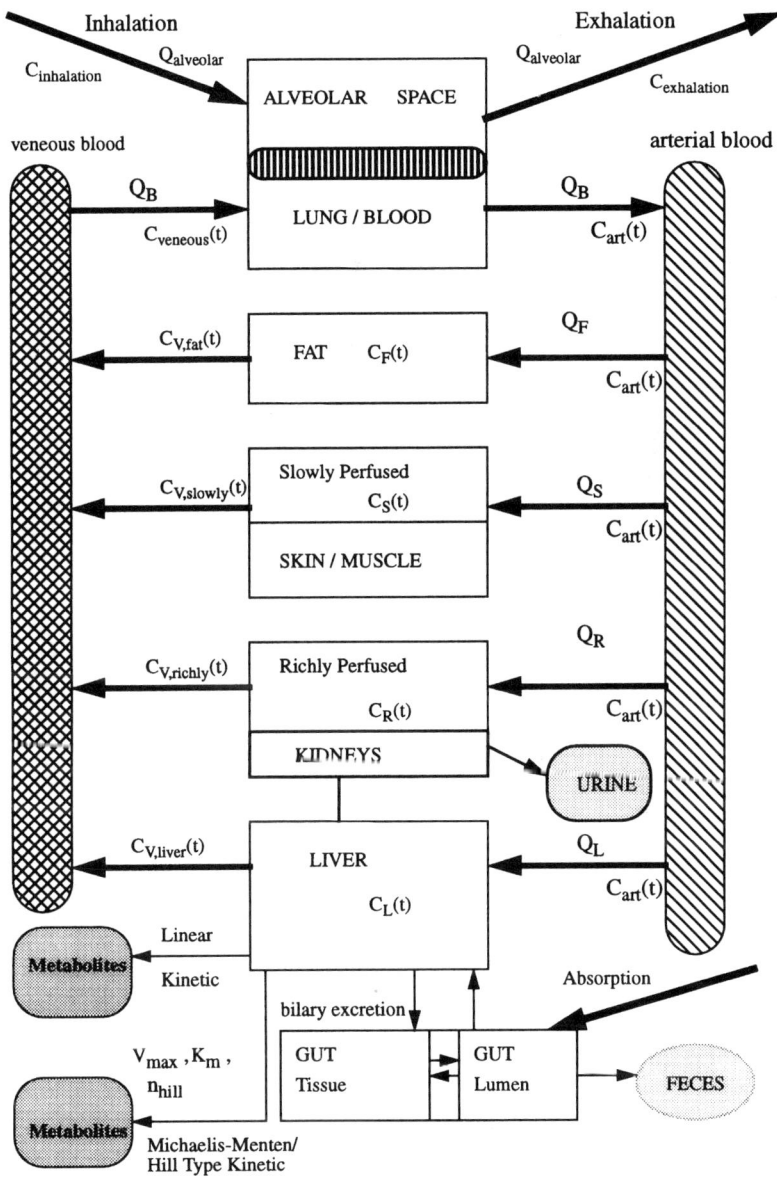

FIGURE 1. A typical PBPK (physiologically-based pharmacokinetic) model with the body compartments fat, liver, richly and slowly perfused organs, alveolar and ingestinal absorption routes, and metabolization and elimination paths. $C(t)$ denotes the concentration in the compartments; $C_V(t)$, the concentration in blood plasma within a compartment, equivalent to the concentration in venous blood leaving a compartment; $C_{art}(t)$, the concentration in arterial blood entering a compartment; and Q, flow rate.

When the toxin concentration is not a direct dose parameter, kinetic models are applied to describe the effective dose (DNA adducts, metabolites, induced enzymes, etc.). The degree of uncertainty in the kinetic models themselves, and in the effective dose estimates obtained by using them as endpoints, needs to be investigated for a valid exposure assessment and for an honest judgement of exposure parameters in the dose-response model.

PBPK models define drug kinetic processes in terms of the physiology, anatomy, and biochemistry of the organism. They comprise a series of compartments that represent body organs and tissues,[2,3] all body compartments linked together by a flow network. A mass conservation law is applicable to the quantity of a chemical introduced, eliminated, and remaining in the organism. The mathematical counterpart of mass conservation is a system of deterministic kinetic equations (mass-balance equations) that account for the quantity (concentration) of the chemical in each compartment as a function of time and dose. Practical application of a PBPK model requires specification of a large number of model parameters. Naturally, there is uncertainty about the correct physiological parameters. It is an important task to assess both the gain obtained through a biologically more accurate model and the cost associated with increased uncertainty. This raises the need to evaluate the additional variability introduced. The typical PBPK model consists of body compartments, the blood flow system, the alveolar and ingestinal absorption routes, and the metabolizing and elimination paths, as illustrated in FIGURE 1.

In the next section we give a schematic outline of the role of kinetics in the process of risk assessment. Uncertainty is then defined in the light of recent statistical work and its role in pharmacokinetic modeling. The main body of the paper is subdivided into three parts. The first offers a simple kinetic model for biomonitor data obtained in humans after occupational exposure to dioxins and this exhibits sources of uncertainty. The second addresses model uncertainty and uncertainty of PBPK model parameters when used to estimate the biologically effective target dose. The third discusses the Hill equation as a class of nonlinear kinetic models for receptor mediated processes, again exemplified by the dioxin problem. We show how uncertainty in model parameters originates from the use of different statistical analysis methods. A second example, from mechanistic carcinogenesis research in which the uncertainty is one order of magnitude lower, is included to indicate the influence of the design of an experiment.

METHODS AND SUBJECTS STUDIED

Kinetics Models in Risk Assessment

In the process of risk assessment, kinetic models play the role of mediators and interfaces.[4,5] FIGURE 2 shows this function schematically for an epidemiology approach to modeling disease incidence, and for an animal-to-human extrapolation scenario. In the latter, the animal model is used to determine a dose response model $\overline{P}(d)$ and a human model is derived by analogy to the animal model using human specific information as far as is available. Biologically, it is much more plausible that the dose $E(d)$ delivered to the target tissue, rather than the administered dose d, is responsible for effects. The metabolites, induced enzymes, or hormones may serve

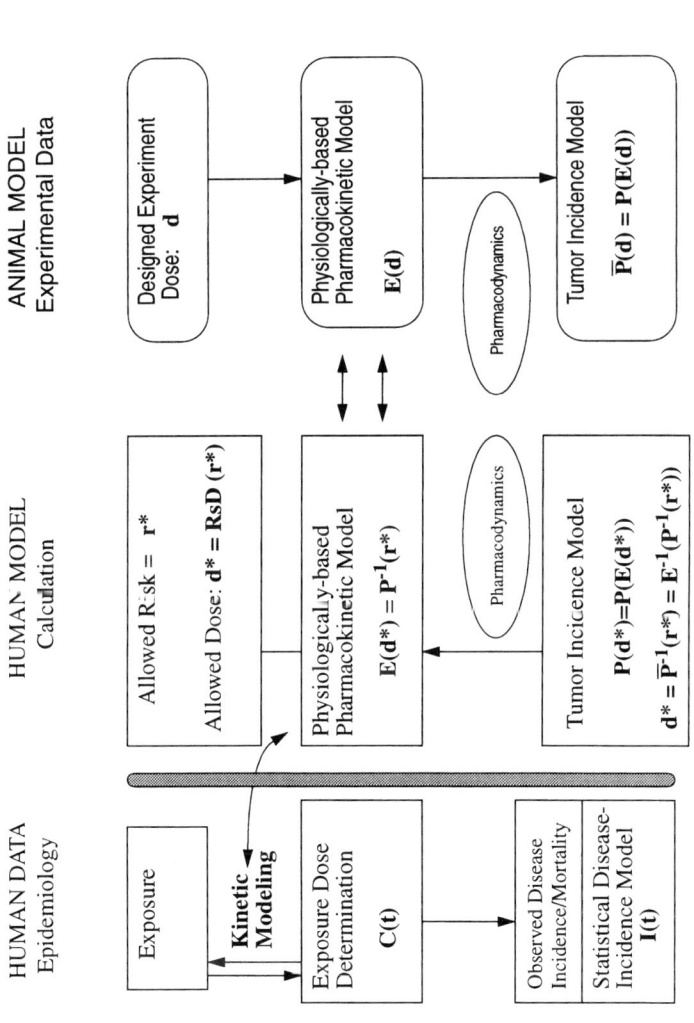

FIGURE 2. Physiologically-based pharmacokinetic models envisaged as an interface between the administered dose/exposure dose and the pharmacodynamic effect model. The scheme shows a toxicokinetic-to-toxicodynamic perspective on the epidemiological approach of modeling disease incidence, and on animal-to-human extrapolation. The animal model is used to determine a dose response model $P(d)$ and a human model is derived in analogy to the animal model. From an allowed level of risk r^*, the allowed maximum dose d^* is obtained by inverting the dose-response model established for the animal.

as target tissue doses. The PBPK model provides a means for obtaining better estimates of the ultimate effective dose E. The starting point of risk assessment is the definition of an allowed level of risk $r*$ defined by the regulators. Estimation of the corresponding allowed maximum dose $d* = R_s D(r*)$ is obtained by inverting the dose-response model, $d* = \overline{P}^{-1}(r*)$. Thus, PBPK models have become the interface between the administered dose/exposure dose and the pharmacodynamic effect model. For a long time the role of kinetic models in epidemiology studies was less developed than in animal studies. Recently, kinetic models have enjoyed more recognition for application in human models,[6,7] and they are now used both for modeling the exposure process and for deriving an effective dose in disease incidence models. If limited information is available for humans it can be supplemented by information available for animals.

An Elementary PBPK Model for Dioxin

We give an example of uncertainty analysis, using the PKPB model for dioxin (2,3,7,8 tetrachlorodibenzo-*p*-dioxin, TCDD) due to Leung *et al.*[8] (as described in Ref. 9). That PBPK model treats the liver compartment as two *subcompartments* representing binding sites for TCDD: a cytosolic Ah-receptor of high affinity and low capacity, and a hypothetical second microsomal binding protein of low affinity and high capacity. The reversible high-affinity binding is modeled by a Michaels-Menten type kinetic. The receptor-ligand complex translocates to the cell nucleus, mediates gene expression, and initiates transcription of regulatory and structural genes. Among the first genes expressed are those that code for CYP1A1 and CYP1A2. For an extension of this model see Kohn *et al.*[10] The distribution within the liver is assumed to be governed by a nonlinear capacity-limited binding of TCDD in venous blood flowing through the liver (free TCDD) and binding to the cytosolic and the microsomal subcompartments. The model is computationally represented as a linear system of first-order ordinary differential equations for the amount of TCDD in the five compartments: blood, liver, fat, viscera, and muscle/skin. However, the liver involves nonlinear Michaelis-Menten kinetics.[9]

Concepts of Uncertainty

The conceptual approach to uncertainty underlying this work is motivated by the work of Hodges[11] and it distinguishes among structural, statistical, and technical uncertainty. *Structural uncertainty* in risk assessment often arises from incomplete or insufficient biological and toxicological knowledge about the mechanisms involved. This leads to the uncertainty about the true, or the best, model. Edler and Portier[12] describe three PBPK-models for dioxin. More structure can be discovered by information extraction using modern data-analysis methods. Following this line, Chatfield[13] distinguishes among model misspecification, model classes, and sets of different models. Bayesian methods for propagation of model uncertainty were described by Draper.[14]

The second type of uncertainty in the classification of Hodges[11] is *error type uncertainty*. This is standard in statistical analysis when the estimation of parameters, confidence regions, or posterior distributions are the goal of statistical inference and when predictions need to be made on the basis of uncertainty in the data. This type of uncertainty is viewed as a variation, conditional on structure.

The third type under the Hodges classification addresses *technical uncertainty*, arising because of inaccuracies introduced by repeatedly manipulating (or processing) the raw data, numerical instability, and by analytical and numerical approximations when fitting models. In the context of PBPK models, technical uncertainty arises from the numerical solution of the differential equations $\dot{y} = f(t, y)$ involving the concentration value $y(t)$ at time t, given initial conditions $y(t_0) = y_0$. Optional solution methods are one-step procedures, such as Euler-Cauchy, Heun, and Runge-Kutta; or multistep procedures, such as Adams-Bashforth and Adams-Moulton.[9] The choice of the step size in solving the equations is of influence on the results. A small step size leads to a higher rounding error, and a larger step size to a higher local error in the solution of the differential equation. The choice of software also falls into this category of uncertainty. The range of models selected is strongly conditioned by the set of models for which the analyst has software available and by his/her desire or ability to spend time and money in developing or purchasing software.

Uncertainty Analysis of PBPK Models

Uncertainty analysis in PBPK models aims at evaluating the degree of uncertainty in tissue dose prediction induced by uncertainty in model parameters.[15] The goal is to characterize the extent of uncertainty propagation and to identify those parameters to which the endpoint is particularly sensitive. The kinetic endpoint C is a function of the model parameters p, the dose x, and the time t in a structural equation of the general form

$$C(t;x, p) - f(t;x, p). \tag{1}$$

The data are modeled by

$$c_{ij} = c(t_j;x_i, p) = f(t_j;x_j, p) + g(x_i, \beta)\varepsilon_{ij}, \tag{2}$$

where g is a weight applied to the error term ε. Two situations can be distinguished in modeling and uncertainty analysis: (1) all parameters p are determined in advance, the model is simulated and the resulting concentrations are compared with the observed data, and (2) only a subset of the parameters are determined in advance, the remaining parameters are estimated with the observed data. Most uncertainty analyses performed so far have dealt only with the first of these.

Analysis of model uncertainty is formalized by assuming a random distribution for the parameter with a density $h(p)$ and an expected value equal to the scalar value p. Uncertainty can be modeled additively by using a normal, a triangular, or even a uniform distribution, or multiplicatively by using a log-normal distribution. This stochastic uncertainty approach yields a random concentration C with a distribution determined by that of the parameter. Uncertainty in the tissue distribution C as a function, $c(p) = (p_1, \ldots, p_m)$, of the model parameters is defined by Krewski *et al.*[15] as

$$\begin{aligned} U(C|X_j) &= Var_{X_j}[E_{X_1, \ldots, X_{j-1}, X_{j+1}, \ldots, X_m}(C|X_j)] \\ &= Var_{X_1, \ldots, X_m}[C] - E_{X_j}[Var_{X_1, \ldots, X_{j-1}, X_{j+1}, \ldots, X_m}(C|X_j)], \end{aligned} \tag{3}$$

where X denotes the vector of random variables attributed to the model parameter vector p. Relative uncertainty is given as a coefficient of variation,

$$RU(C, X_j) = \frac{\sqrt{U(C|X_j)}}{E(C)} \cdot 100 \tag{4}$$

and overall uncertainty by $Var(C)$. The concept of uncertainty is related to sensitivity analysis, which investigates directly the result of changes of the model parameters on C. Sensitivity of C to changes of the parameter p_j is so generally defined by

$$S(C, p_j^*) = \left.\frac{\partial c(p)}{\partial p_j}\right|_{p=p^*}, \tag{5}$$

as function of $p = (p_1, ..., p_m)$. Relative sensitivity, $RS(C, P_j)$, is related to relative uncertainty, $RU(C, P_j)$, at $p_j = p_j^*$ by[15]

$$RS(C, p_j^*) = \frac{\left.\frac{\partial c(p_1, ..., p_m)}{\partial p_j}\right|_{p=p^*}}{\frac{c(p^*)}{p_j^*}} \cong \frac{RU(C, X_j)}{\sqrt{Var(X_j)}/p_j^*}. \tag{6}$$

In practice, uncertainty is determined numerically by means of Monte Carlo (MC) simulations, randomly varying the parameter p and determining the empirical distribution of C. MC sampling of model parameters is defined by the chosen distribution, its truncation and ranges of acceptable values, and correlations of the components of the parameter vector. Physiological parameters are often directly related to the body weight (BW) with the allometric power function $p = aBW^b$, where a power index b of about 0.75 is common. Dependent sampling can be achieved by a deterministic relationship with random multipliers. Thus, the cardiac output QB is, for example, given by $QB = F_{QB}BW^{0.74}$ as a function of BW with scaling coefficient F_{QB}.

An MC sample of the concentration C is analyzed by standard statistical methods. The variance-covariance matrix and coefficients of variation are used below to describe the uncertainty in C. Linear regression measures, such as the measure of determination of C by p_j (standardized regression, rank regression coefficients, and partial or partial rank correlation coefficients) are methods that have been employed.

Biomonitor TCDD Data in an Occupational Cohort

Polychlorinated dibenzodioxins (PCDDs) belong chemically to the class of halogenated aromatic hydrocarbons. The most toxic PCDD of a group of 22 TCDD isomers is 2,3,7,8-TCDD (abbreviated to TCDD here) or commonly *dioxin*. TCDD is believed to be responsible for a series of toxic effects in mammals.[16] This toxic environmental pollutant is widespread, resistant to degradation, and accumulates in the food chain. Incidents of poisoning have occurred in industrial and agricultural workers, military personnel, and the general population. Environmental sources occur in the production and use of herbicides containing 2,4,5-T-trichlorphenol (TCP), pentachlorphenol (PCP), hexachlorophene, and also the pulp and paper industry, incineration of municipal and industrial waste, transformer/capacitor fires involving chlorinated biphenyls and benzenes, burning wood in the presence of chlorine, disposal of chlorinated chemical waste, and spraying phenoxy herbicides. Human exposure is via food ingestion (about 98%), air breathing (about 2%) and skin absorption (unknown). In humans TCDD occurs in body fat, blood serum, and maternal milk.

TCDD has been found to increase the incidence of liver tumors in female rats.[17,18] Epidemiology studies have shown a dose-dependent increase in cancer mortality.[19–21] These studies relied heavily on occupational cohorts. Among them were workers in the German chemical industry who were subjected to accidental and chronic exposure to dioxins. Measurement of TCDD levels in humans enabled the determination of a dose-response relationship.[22,23] When dose parameters are determined from biomonitor data, uncertainty becomes an issue.

We have examined exposure data of a subcohort of the so-called Boehringer cohort[19,22] of individuals who were severely exposed to dioxins by virtue of handling TCDD contaminated chemicals between 1952 and 1984. A second medical in-

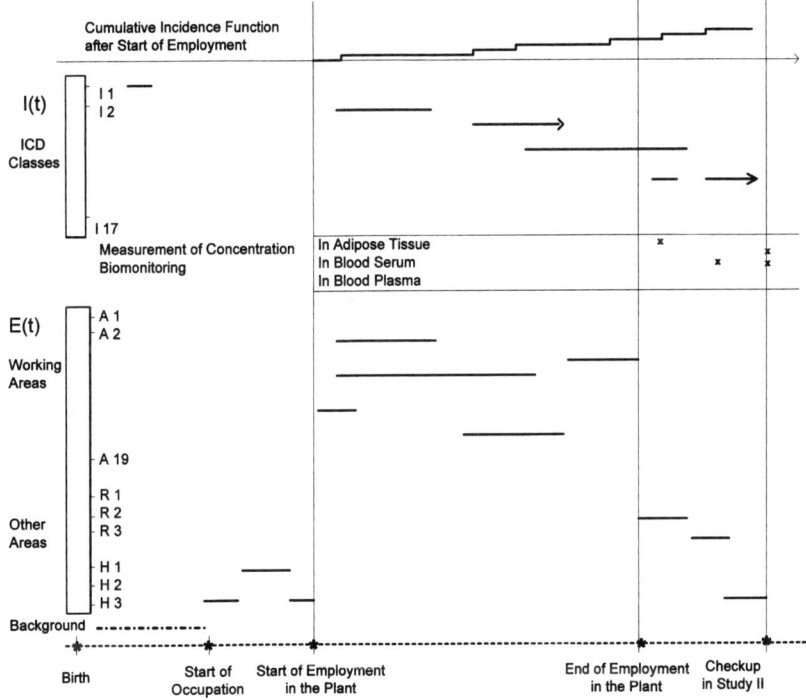

FIGURE 3. Schematic presentation of the exposure and disease events occurring to a person during his/her occupation and inclusion of the biomonitoring. Exposure is possible some time after birth and start of occupational life. A_i denotes a working area; R_i and H_i denote other sources of exposure. When changing the working area, exposure may change, and further changes may occur until the end of employment. I_i denotes the type of disease of an individual, categorized, for example, by the International Classification for Diseases (ICD). Biomonitor data is obtained after employment.

vestigation program was launched in 1992, by addressing a total of 375 former employees of the company who had worked at plants and facilities where exposure to dioxins was probable. In this comprehensive morbidity study a cohort of 192 people responded and they were examined between 1992 and 1994 for individual dioxin levels.[24,25] The aim of the study was to relate the occurrence of diseases, during and after the occupation, to previous exposure to dioxin in a dose related manner. This required the determination of the exposure dose function and the disease incidence function on an individual basis. FIGURE 3 shows schematically the events that may occur to an individual during his/her occupation. Some time after birth and start of occupational life, exposure may have commenced in one working area, after entry into the plant. When the working area is changed, exposure may change, and further changes may occur until the end of employment. Measurements of dioxin concentrations have been available only since the plant closed in 1984.

RESULTS

Uncertainty in the Measurement of Dioxin Concentrations

Uncertainty in the dioxin concentration among workers in a cohort was assessed from a total of 379 dioxin measurements that were available for the 192 workers: 37 from adipose tissue samples from an initial medical examination during 1985–1986, 44 samples from an investigation guided by an occupational insurance fund between 1989 and 1990, 164 samples elicited from a local governmental agency, and 134 samples obtained during an investigation by the US CDC.[25] The majority of the samples originated from the final examination period. Assuming a half-life of 7.1 years, all earlier measurements were extrapolated forward to the medical examination date, between 1992 and 1994, assuming an exponential decay according to a linear first order kinetic. Thus, ideally, all multiple concentration values for each individual should be identical. The divergence among these synchronized individual measurements is illustrated by plotting the multiple data against the corresponding mean concentration for each individual. The plot in FIGURE 4a shows the divergence of individual values and thus partially illustrates the uncertainty of the biomonitor data. Part of this divergence may be caused by differences between analytical methods in the determination of dioxin concentrations, the difference between adipose tissue concentrations, and blood serum concentrations. Inadequacy of the linear kinetics could have provided a further source of uncertainty. A subset of concentration values was obtained by splitting one sample into two subsamples. These two subsamples were analyzed in two different laboratories using basically the same technique. FIGURE 4b demonstrates that in a number of cases the paired dioxin concentration measurements were quite different. From these observations we may conclude that there is also uncertainty in biomonitor data due to the laboratory method used to determine the concentration in the sample.

Uncertainty in the Back-Calculation Results

To establish a dose-response relationship in a disease-incidence model, an appropriate dose metric was determined using the method of back-calculation. This procedure reconstructs the exposure process for an individual on the basis of current and, if available previous, dioxin measurements, and from information about lifetime working history, as illustrated in FIGURE 3. An elementary kinetic model of absorption, accumulation and elimination of the toxin is used. The working history is partitioned into a small number of time intervals I_j, with the exposure rate d_j given by the working area A_j corresponding to I_j. Piecewise linear first-order kinetics are applied to estimate the exposure rate d_i from each working area A_i. Additionally, a background exposure rate d_0 is introduced. Assuming linear first-order kinetics for TCDD elimination from the body at a rate k_e and a constant exposure through the respective working area at a rate d, the kinetic equation for the concentration in the body is given by

$$\frac{dC(t)}{dt} = d - k_e C(t). \quad (7)$$

The initial condition is given by $C(t_0) = c_0$, where exposure starts at time t_0 and the body concentration at that time is c_0. We postulate exposure for a total of m intervals, I_i, each lasting from time t_i to time t_{i+1} ($i = 0, 1, ..., m - 1$). Assuming background exposure for the interval $[t_0, t_1)$ from birth at $t_0 = 0$ and starting with $C(0) = c_0 = 0$, then the dioxin concentration in the body during the interval I_i is given by

$$C(t) = A_i - (A_i - c_i)\exp[-k_e(t - t_i)], \quad t_i \le t \le t_{i+1}, \quad (8)$$

where $C(t_i) = c_i$. Also

$$A_i = \frac{d_i}{k_e} \quad (9)$$

TABLE 1. Variation in basic physiological parameters for a human PBPK model among different research groups[a]

PBPK Parameters	TuMa[27]	KiRo[29]	RaAn[31]	PoKa[35]	BOIS[32]	FARR[33]	HET[34]
BW	70	70	83	70	70	70	70
Volume (% BW)							
V_{liver}	1.7	1.49	4.0	3.14	2	2.6	2.2
V_{fat}	10.1	13.4	9.4	23.1	20	23	16.2
$V_{richly\ perfused}$	—	2.6	5.0	3.71	5	5	2.6
$V_{slowly\ perfused}$	38.2	28.5	73	62.1	63	62	43.5
Flow (% QB)							
(QB)		(290)	(347.9)	(264.3)		(348)	(372)
Q_{liver}	39.2	37	24	37		24	26
Q_{fat}	5.4	9	5	9		5	5
$Q_{richly\ perfused}$	—	42	52	42		52	36.7
$Q_{slowly\ perfused}$	16.2	12	19	12		19	25

[a]Volumes V_i are given as a percentage of body weight (BW) and flow rates Q_i are given as a percentage of cardiac output (QB), QB values in parentheses.

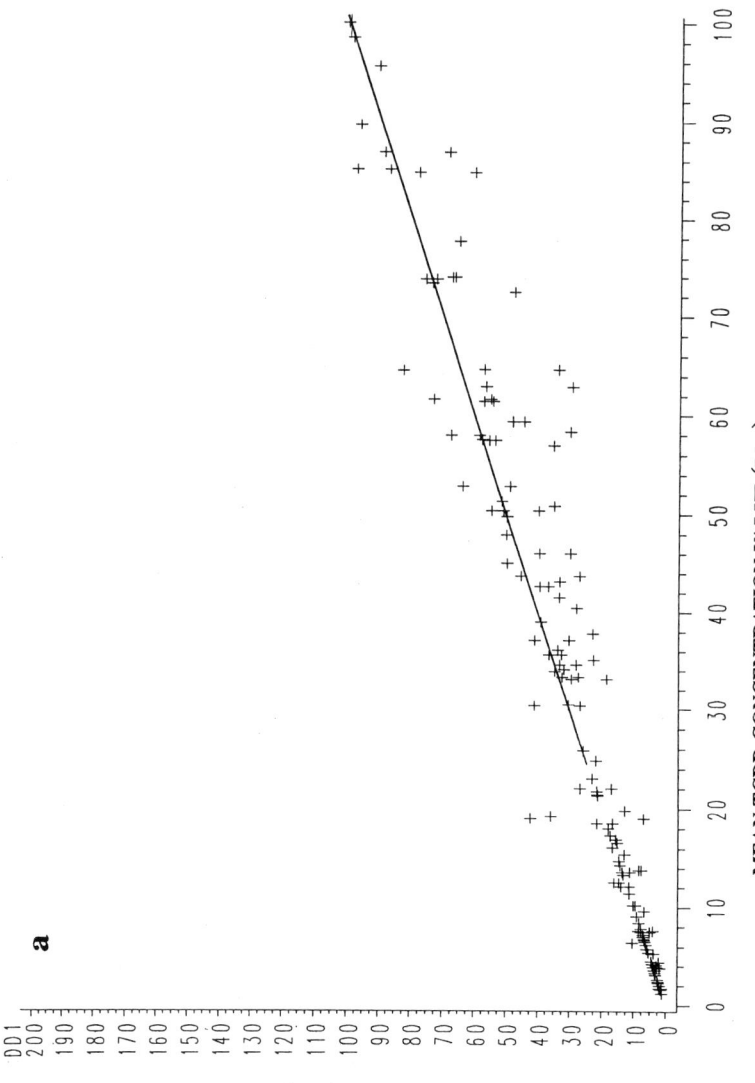

FIGURE 4. See legend on opposite page.

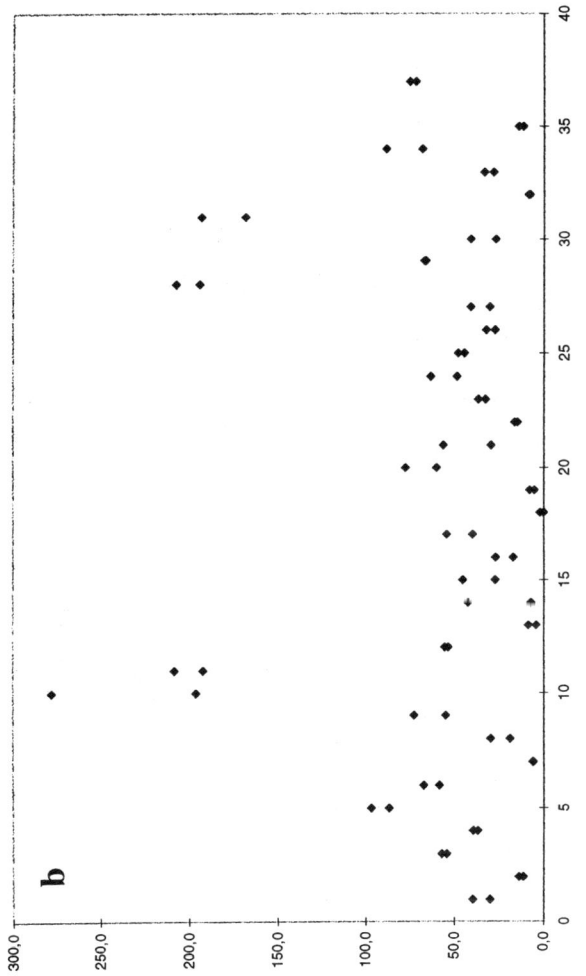

FIGURE 4. Uncertainty in the biomonitor data of dioxin concentration measurements in human blood serum from a sample of 192 workers. **Part a** shows individual repeated measurements synchronized by a first-order kinetics, forward calculation to the date of medical examination plotted against the corresponding individual mean value. The presentation is limited to subjects with mean TCDD values less than 100 ppt for convenience of presentation. **Part b** shows the divergence of split sample determinations in two laboratories. This presentation is limited to individuals with TCDD concentrations below 300 ppt. The plot shows pairs of measurements from the two laboratories. The *horizontal axis* gives the case number, the *vertical axis* the TCDD concentrations.

where d_i is the dose rate in the time interval $[t_i, t_{i+1})$. The general form for $C(t)$ is a function of all exposure rates d_i, the background exposure rate d_0, and the elimination rate k_e is

$$C(t) = C(t, d_1, d_2, ..., d_{19}, d_0, k_e). \tag{10}$$

The parameters in (10) are estimated by the least squares method from the available data on the working history and all concentration values from the biomonitor times $t_{m+i} \geq t_m$, $i = 1, 2, ...$ Measurements of dioxin concentrations in humans are in lipid adjusted ppt units. Therefore, $C(t)$ represents the TCDD concentration in body fat (BF), and exposure must be scaled for that. From estimates of $C(t)$ for all times, one can derive life-time exposure measures. Useful metrics are provided by the area under the dioxin concentration curve, peak values, and values reached after a minimum length of occupation. Because of the availability of multiple measurements from different biomonitor times $t_{m+i} \geq t_m$, $i = 1, 2, ...$, we are able to estimate background exposure rate and half-life for 2,3,7,8-TCDD, and most of its important congeners.

The estimate of $C(t)$ contains additional uncertainty from the assessment of working history according to the scheme shown in FIGURE 3, which was based on infor-

TABLE 2a. Results of a Monte Carlo simulation for a two year study with dose 0.1 μg/Kg BW using independent sampling, with truncated normal distribution, and narrow truncation (752 simulations)[a]

Endpoint[b]	Mean	S.D.	CV (%)	Pearson Product Correlation		
				CL	CF	AHH
CL	34,551	7,605	22	0.74	0.39	0.59
CF	7,470	1 232	16		0.37	0.28
AHH	22.9	1.5	6.6			0.29
MIC	167	13.5	8.1			

[a]Mean, standard deviation (S.D.), and coefficient of variation (CV) for Monte Carlo sample.
[b]Concentrations in liver (CL), in fat (CF), and in binding proteins (AHH and MIC).

TABLE 2b. Results of a Monte Carlo simulation for a two year study with dose 0.1 μg/Kg BW using independent sampling, with uniform distribution, and narrow truncation and only absorption, excretion, binding and enzymatic induction varied (253 simulations)

Endpoint	Mean	S.D.	CV (%)	Pearson Product Correlation		
				CF	AHH	MIC
CL	40,055	10,412	26	0.88	0.36	0.51
CF	8,116	1,640	20		0.37	0.28
AHH	24.9	2.2	8.8			0.57
MIC	177.8	17.4	9.8			

mation from questionnaires completed by the company and by workers. When, for a subsample of individuals, we compared the data on the working history from the second examination (1992–1994) with data obtained during the first examination (1984–1986) we found different statements on the type of the working area in about 30% of the cases, and different sojourn times in about 50% of the case. Some of these

TABLE 2c. Results of a Monte Carlo simulation for a one week study with dose 0.1 μg/Kg BW using independent sampling with four different distribution scenarios

Endpoint	Distribution	Truncation	Mean	S.D.	CV (%)
CL	normal	narrow ($N = 999$)	3,364	453	13.5
	uniform	narrow ($N = 1167$)	3,437	843	24.5
	normal	wide ($N = 999$)	3,692	1,213	32.9
	uniform	wide ($N = 622$)	3,408	2,580	75.7
CF	normal	narrow ($N = 999$)	612	78	12.7
	uniform	narrow ($N = 1167$)	611	124	20.3
	normal	wide ($N = 999$)	573	165	28.9
	uniform	wide ($N = 622$)	762	363	47.6
AHH	normal	narrow ($N = 999$)	11.6	1.3	11.2
	uniform	narrow ($N = 1167$)	11.6	1.6	13.8
	normal	wide ($N = 999$)	11.8	2.9	24.6
	uniform	wide ($N = 622$)	12.8	5.3	41.4
MIC	normal	narrow ($N = 999$)	94.5	9.0	9.5
	uniform	narrow ($N = 1167$)	94.6	11.4	12.1
	normal	wide ($N = 999$)	96.4	20.4	21.2
	uniform	wide ($N = 622$)	108	35	32.4

TABLE 2d. Results of a Monte Carlo simulation for a 30-week study with dose 0.1 μg/Kg BW using independent sampling with truncated normal distribution

Endpoint	Parameters Varied	Mean	S.D.	CV (%)
CL	all	42,233	9,626	22.8
	only partition coefficients	41,168	1,396	3.4
AHH	all	23.6	1.5	6.4
	only partition coefficients	23.7	0.01	0.04
MIC	all	171	13.7	8.0
	only partition coefficients	171	0.06	0.04

differences were substantial, others were insubstantial with respect to the degree and impact on exposure.

Uncertainty in PBPK Models for Dioxin

PBPK models have been applied to the analysis of animal data and extrapolation to humans, as is mentioned above. A source of uncertainty is the choice of the PBPK model itself. Model uncertainty for dioxin arising from three different models[8,26-29] is described Reference 12. For more recently proposed models see References 10 and 30. Here we will consider uncertainty in the model parameters p and its impact on the concentrations $C(t;x, p)$, where x denotes the dose. Imprecise knowledge of the physiological, physicochemical, and biochemical constants leads to imprecise estimates of C. TABLE 1 exhibits the uncertainties in these kinetic parameters for humans as they were used by different groups of modelers.[27,29,31-36]

Portier and Kaplan[35] analyzed uncertainty in the Ramsey-Andersen PBPK[31] of methylene chloride and its transmission to the pharmacodynamic endpoint of cancer incidence. Three models for benzene with similar structure were compared by Bois *et al.*[32] Seven PBPK models for chloroethylene were examined by Hattis *et al.*[36] Ranges of model parameters were determined using multiplicative factors. Hetrick *et al.*[34] examined PBPK models for styrene, methylchloroform, and methylene chloride in an hypercube sampling MC simulation of uncertainty for the biochemical and the metabolic parameters. Coefficients of variation were calculated for the endpoints by using a normal distribution model.

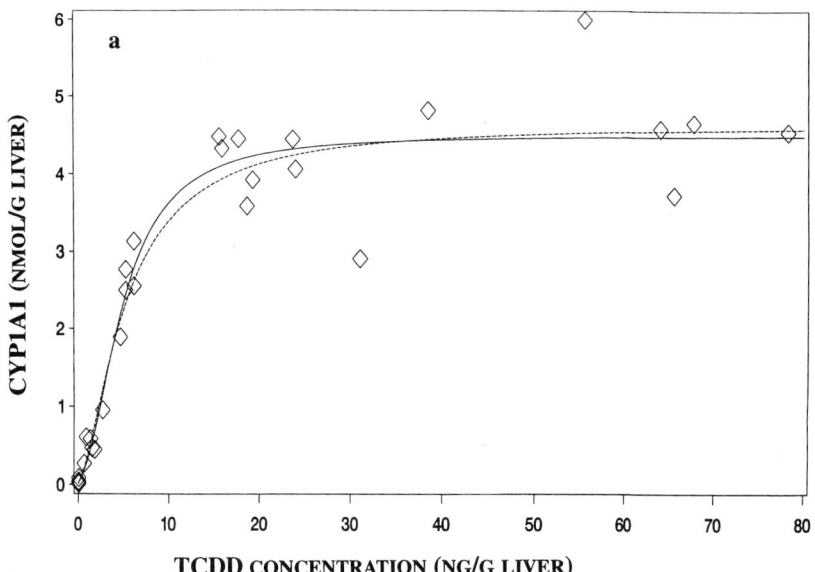

FIGURE 5. Legend see opposite page.

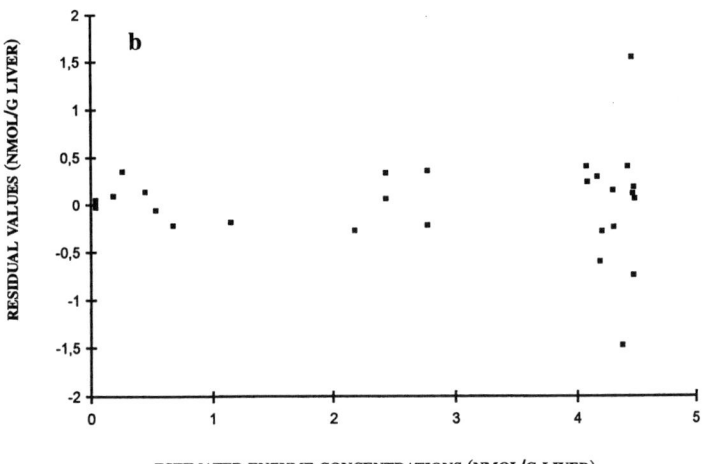

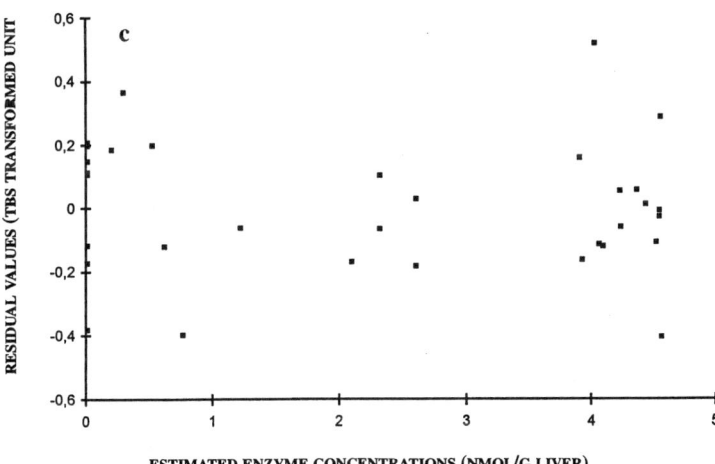

FIGURE 5. Analysis of the kinetic of the induction of CYP1A1 by TCDD in rat liver in the 31 week experiment of Tritscher et al.[38] after initiation with diethylnitrosamin. The CYP1A1 concentration (nmol/g liver) is plotted versus the TCDD concentration (ng/g liver) in (**a**) for the four dose groups and the controls. The *solid line* indicates the fit of the standard nonlinear regression, the *broken line* the fit of the weighted TBS model. Parts (**b**) and (**c**) exhibit the respective residual plots for nonlinear regression and weighted TBS regression.[16]

Elementary Uncertainty Analysis in a PBPK Model for Dioxin Using MC Simulation

A Monte Carlo simulation study of the PBPK model of Leung et al.,[8] described above was conducted for three dose conditions

(A) 0.1 µg per Kg BW per day, five days per week, and two days off, for seven days,

(B) 0.1 µg per Kg BW per day for two years,

(C) 1.4 µg per Kg BW per day in two weeks for 30 weeks.

The time after each bolus dose was partitioned into the following intervals, one hour the remaining 23 hours of the first day, and interval until the next bolus. In each subinterval the differential equations were solved by using Runge-Kutta methods. Blood concentration was evaluated with higher precision than that of the other compartments. Sets of parameters values were generated by using Monte Carlo methods, sampling each parameter univariately and independently, with a distribution specified by its mean, standard deviation, and range of allowed values (truncation) in the case of the normal distribution, and by the range in the case of the uniform distribution.[37] We report here the results from two truncations: a narrow range of approximately one standard deviation, and a wider range. The kinetic model parameters p were volumes, flow rates, partition coefficients, absorption coefficients, elimination and transition rates, binding constants, and induction constants.

The resulting uncertainty depends strongly on the simulation assumptions and on the exposure model used. This is illustrated in TABLE 2 by the results of four analyses. Initially, a two year study with a daily oral dose of 0.1 µg/kg BW given five days per week and with two days off was simulated. The full set of 28 parameters in the model of Leung et al.[8] was simulated by using independent sampling from a normal distribution with a narrow truncation (752 simulations). Means, standard deviations, and coefficients of variation for four endpoints are shown in TABLE 2a together with their correlation coefficients. Variability in terms of the coefficient of variation was lower for the enzymatically induced concentrations than it was for TCDD concentration in the fat and the liver. Correlations between the tissue concentrations in the compartments ranged between 0.54 and 0.88. A limited study (TABLE 2b) was performed with the same dose design but varying the absorption, excretion, binding, and enzymatic parameters according a uniform distribution (253 simulations). The greater variability introduced by the uniform distribution is somehow compensated for by the fact that only a limited number of parameters are varied and the remaining parameters are fixed at their mean values in the simulation. Thus, the coefficients of variation are similar in TABLES 2a and 2b. The variability of TCDD concentrations after one week was investigated for the same dose for four types of distribution. Their variability is shown in TABLE 2c. Obviously the variability of the endpoint increases with increasing parameter variability in these four settings. TABLE 2d shows the results for a simulation of a 30-weeks study with the same dose design used previously. A striking difference in the uncertainty of the endpoint is observed when only a few model parameters are assumed to be uncertain.

UNCERTAINTY FROM CHOICE OF STATISTICAL ANALYSIS METHOD

In this section we address uncertainty arising from the statistical analysis of kinetic data. The first example is provided by the kinetics of induction of the biomarkers CYP1A1 and CYP1A2 through dioxin in female SD rat livers and this is concerned with large uncertainty.[38] Model uncertainty was described in Portier et al.,[39] where an additive and independent action models were applied. Both models fitted well but yielded risk estimates that differed by several orders of magnitude. The dose response model of the type of a Hill kinetic was analyzed by using standard nonlinear regression. The fit of the nonlinear regression is given by the solid line in FIGURE 5. Recently, we reanalyzed these data with a more general statistical model in which the error term is weighted by a power function and by transforming both sides of the equation.[40] The model equations of the additive and the multiplicative models become

$$C_i^{(\lambda)} = \left(\frac{v_a (D_i + D_I)^n}{k_\alpha + (D_i + D_I)^n} \right)^{(\lambda)} + D_i^\theta \varepsilon_i$$

TABLE 3. Model parameters of the additive and the independent action model for the induction of CYP1A1 and CYP1A2 after exposure to TCDD in the experiment of Tritscher et al. (see Ref. 38)[a]

	v_α	k_α	n	D_I	λ	θ
CYP1A1	4.50	30.91	2.06	0.48		
Additiv	4.64	14.01	1.57	0.12	0.20	−0.09

	v_β	k_β	n	r_β	λ	θ
CYP1A1	4.52	19.15	1.86	1.19		
Independent	4.67	12.25	1.49	0.19	0.18	−0.12

	v_α	k_α	n	D_I	λ	θ
CYP1A2	28.36	21.10	0.39	0.04		
Additiv	7.25	6.24	0.64	0.286	0.36	0.16

	v_β	k_β	n	r_β	λ	θ
CYP1A2	24.57	19.95	0.41	2.94		
Independent	6.64	7.64	0.74	3.39	0.36	0.16

[a]Parameters obtained by standard nonlinear regression (upper value) and weighted transform-both-sides regression (lower value) of a Hill type saturation kinetic with structural parameters (v_α, k_α, n, D_I) and (v_β, k_β, n, r_β), respectively, and the nuisance parameters (λ, θ).

and

$$C_i^{(\lambda)} = \left(\frac{r_\beta + v_\beta D_i^n}{k_\beta + D_i^n}\right)^{(\lambda)} + D_i^\theta \varepsilon_i.$$

For the model parameters see Reference 39. The models have two additional parameters (λ, θ) which describe skewness of the distribution and heterogeneity of the variability of the data. When comparing the parameter estimates of the two statistical models (see TABLE 3) one can observe considerable differences between nonlinear regression and the weighted TBS regression (upper and lower line). Although the more flexible and larger class of the TBS model is preferable from a statistical point of view in terms of the distribution of the residuals (FIGS 5b and 5c), the fit of both models is almost identical. That means there are a broad class of models and, additionally, a large range of model parameters that are compatible with the observed data.

In contrast, small uncertainty was been found by Frei et al.[41] in a similar approach when investigating N-nitrodimethylamine (NTDMA), and N-nitrososdimethylamine (NDMA). Demethylation of NTDMA and of NDMA in liver microsomes was investigated under various conditions. The statistical methods used for data analysis were ordinary least squares (OLS), weighted least squares (WLS) with variance weights $x_i^\theta \varepsilon$, and transform-both-sides (TBS). By varying the values of the nuisance parameters, λ and θ, these three models were compared (weighted TBS failed). The ranges of estimates for λ and θ were small across all experiments that indicated a homogeneity of the experimental conditions. In the case of NTDMA, only marginal differences between the three methods were noted. (For numerical results see Ref. 41.) In sharp contrast to the 31-week experiments the rats in this experiment were treated for only one day, which may have reduced the biological variability to the point where uncertainty played almost no role.

REFERENCES

1. ENVIRONMENTAL PROTECTION AGENCY. 1996. Proposed guidelines for carcinogenic risk assessment. Notice, Tuesday April 23, 1996. Federal Register **61:** 17960–18011.
2. GERLOWSKI, L.E. & R.H. JAIN. 1983. Physiologically based pharmacokinetic modeling: principles and applications. J. Pharm. Sci. **72:** 1103–1127.
3. BISCHOFF, K.B. 1986. Physiological pharmacokinetics. Bull. Math. Biol. **48:** 309–322.
4. ANDERSEN, M.E. 1989. Tissue dosimetry, physiologically-based pharmacokinetic modeling and cancer risk assessment. Cell Biol. Toxicol. **5:** 405–416.
5. ANDERSEN, M.E., D. KREWSKI & J.R.WITHEY. 1993. Physiological pharmacokinetics and cancer risk assessment. Cancer Lett. **69:** 1–14.
6. CARRIER, G., R.C. BRUNERT & J. BRODEUR. 1995. Modeling of the toxicokinetics of polychlorinated dibenzo-*p*-dioxins and dibenzofurans in mammalians, including humans. Toxicol. and Pharmacol. **131:** 253–276.
7. VAN DER MOLEN, G.W., S.A.L.M. KOOIJMAN & W. SLOB. 1997. A generic toxicokinetic model for persistent lipophilic compounds in humans: An application to TCDD. Fundam. and Appl. Toxicol. **31:** 83–94.
8. LEUNG, H.W., D.J. PAUSTENBACH, F.J. MURRAY & M.E. ANDERSEN. 1990. A physiological pharmacokinetic description of the tissue distribution and enzyme-inducing properties of 2,3,7,8-tetrachlorodibenzo-*p*-dioxin in the rat. Toxicol. Appl. Pharmacol. **103:** 399–410.

9. EDLER, L. 1992. Computational aspects in uncertainty analyses of physiologically based pharmacokinetics models. *In* Computational Statistics. Y. Dodge & J. Whittaker, Eds.: 539–544. Physica, Heidelberg.
10. KOHN, M.C., G.W. LUCIER, G.C. CLARK, S. SEWALL, A.M. TRITSCHER & C.J. PORTIER. 1993. A mechanistic model of effects of dioxin on gene expression in the rat liver. Toxicol. Appl. Pharmacol. **120:** 138–154.
11. HODGES, J.S. 1987. Uncertainty, policy analysis and statistics. Statist. Sci. **2:** 259–291.
12. EDLER, L. & C. PORTIER. 1992. Uncertainty in physiological pharmacokinetic modeling and its impact on statistical risk estimation of 2,3,7,8-TCDD. Chemosphere **25:** 239–242.
13. CHATFIELD, C. 1995. Model uncertainty, data mining and statistical inference. J. Roy. Statist. Soc. A **158:** 419–466.
14. DRAPER, D. 1995. Assessment and propagation of model uncertainty. J. Roy. Statist. Soc. B **57:** 45–97.
15. KREWSKI, D., Y. WANG, S. BARTLETT & K. KRISHNAN. 1995. Uncertainty, variability, and sensitivity analysis in physiological pharmacokinetic models. J. Biopharm. Statist. **5:** 245–271.
16. HUFF, J., G. LUCIER & A. TRITSCHER. 1994, Carcinogenicity of TCDD: experimental, mechanistic, and epidemiologic evidence. Annu. Rev. Pharmacol. Toxicol. **34:** 343–372.
17. KOCIBA, R.J., P.A. KEELER, C.N. PARK & P.J. GEHRING. 1976. 2,3,7,8 Tetrachlorodibenzo-*p*-dioxin (TCDD): results of a 13-week oral toxicity study in rats. Toxicol. Appl. Pharmacol. **35:** 553–574.
18. KOCIBA, R.J., D.G. KEYES, J.E. BEYER, R.M. CARREON, C.E. WADE, D.A. DITTENBER, R.P. KALNINS, L.E. FRAUSON, C.N. PARK, S.D. BARNARD, R.A. HUMMEL & C.G. HUMISTON. 1978. Results of a two-year chronic toxicity and oncogenicity study of 2,3,7,8 tetrachlorodibenzo-*p*-dioxin in rats. Toxicol. Appl. Pharmacol. **46:** 279–303.
19. MANZ, A., J. BERGER, J.H. DWYER, D. FLESCH-JANYS, S. NAGEL & H. WALTSGOTT. 1991. Cancer mortality among workers in a chemical plant contaminated with dioxin. Lancet **338:** 959–964.
20. FINGERHUT, M.A., W.E. HALPERIN, D.A MARLOW, L.A. PIACITELLI, P.A. HONCHAR & M.H. SWEENEY, A.L. GREIFE, P.A. DILL, K. STEENLORD & A.J. SARODA. 1991. Cancer mortality in workers exposed to 2,3,7,8-tetrachlorodibenzo-*p*-dioxin. New Engl. J. Med. **199:** 212–218.
21. ZOBER, A., P. MESSERER & P. HUBER. 1990. Thirty-four year mortality follow-up of BASF employees exposed to 2,3,7,8-TCDD after the 1953 accident. Int. Arch. Occ. Environ. Health **62:** 139–157.
22. BENNER, A., L. EDLER, K. MAYER & A. ZOBER. 1993. Polychlorinated dibenzodioxin (PCDD) and dibenzofuran (PCDF) levels and morbidity data of employees occupationally exposed in the chemical industry—Dioxin Investigation Program—Part II by the Employment Accident Insurance Fund (Berufsgenossenschaft) of the Chemical Industry in Germany. Berufsgenossenschaft der Chemischen Industrie, Heidelberg.
23. FLESCH-YANYS, D.H., H. BECHER, P. GURN, D. JUNG, J., KONJETZKO, A. MANZ & O. PÄPKE. 1996. Elimination of polychlorinated dibenzo-p-dioxins and dibenzofurans (PCDD/F) in occupationally exposed persons. J. Toxicol. Environ. Health **47:** 363–378.
24. JUNG, D., P.A. BERG, L. EDLER, W. EHRENTHAL, D. FENNER, D. FLESCH-JANYS, C. HUBER, R. KLEIN, C. KOITKA, G. LUCIER, A. MANZ, A. MUTTRAY, L. NEEDHAM, P. PÄPKE, M. PIETSCH, C. PORTIER, D. PATTERSON, W. PRELLWITZ, D.-M. ROSE, A. THEWS & J. KONIETZKO. 1998. Immunologische Befunde bei ehemals gegenüber 2,3,7,8-Tetra-chlorodibenzodioxin (TCDD) und seinen Kongeneren exponierten Arbeitern in der Pestizidherstellung. Arbeitsmedizin Sonderheft **24:** 38–43.
25. EDLER, L., D. JUNG, D. FLESCH-JANYS, C. PORTIER, L. PILZ, G. CLARK, G. LUCIER & J. KONIETZKO. 1998. Herz-Kreislauf-Erkrankungen und ihre Risikofaktoren nachberuflicher Exposition gegenüber Dioxinen und Furanen. Arbeitsmedizin Sonderheft **24:** 48–53.

26. KING, F.G., R.L. DEDRICK, J.M. COLLINS, H.B. MATTHEWS & L.S. BIRNBAUM. 1983. Physiological model for the pharmacokinetics of 2,3,7,8 tetrachlorodibenzo-*p*-dioxin in several species. Toxicol. Appl. Pharmacol. **67:** 390–400.
27. TUEY, D.B. & H.B. MATTHEWS. 1980. Use of a physiological compartmental model for the rat to describe the pharmacokinetics of several chlorinated biphenyls in the mouse. Drug. Metabol. Dispos. **8:** 397–403.
28. LUTZ, R.J., R.L. DEDRICK, H.B. MATTHEWS, T.E. ELING & M.E. ANDERSON. 1977. A preliminary pharmacokinetic model for several chlorinated biphenyls in the rat. Drug Metab. Dispos. **5:** 386–396.
29. KISSEL, J.C. & G.M. ROBARGE. 1988. Assessing the elimination of 2,3,7,8 TCDD from humans with a physiologically based pharmacokinetic model. Chemosphere **17:** 2017–2027.
30. ANDERSEN, M.E., J.J. MILLS, M.L. GARGAS, L. KEDDERIS, L.S. BIRNBAUM, D. NEUBERT & W.F. GREENLEE. 1993. Modeling receptor-mediated protein induction by dioxin: Implications for pharmacokinetics and risk assessment. Risk Analysis **13:** 25–36.
31. RAMSEY, J.C. & M.E. ANDERSEN. 1984. A physiologically based description of the inhalation pharmacokinetics of styrene in rats and humans. Toxicol. Appl. Pharmacol. **73:** 159–175.
32. BOIS, F.Y., L. ZEISE & T.N. TOZER. 1990. Precision and sensitivity of pharmacokinetic models for cancer risk assessment: Tetrachloroethylene in mice, rats, and humans. Toxicol. Appl. Pharmacol. **102:** 300–315.
33. FARRAR, D.B., B. ALLEN, K. CRUMP & A. SHIPP. 1989. Evaluation of uncertainty in input parameters to pharmacokinetic models and the resulting uncertainties in output. Toxicol. Lett. **49:** 371–385.
34. HETRICK, D.M., A.M. JARABEK & C.C. TRAVIS. 1991: Sensitivity analysis for physiologically based pharmacokinetic models. J. Pharm. Biopharm. **19:** 1–20.
35. PORTIER, C.J. & N.L. KAPLAN. 1989. Variability of safe dose estimates when using complicated models of the carcinogenic process. Fundam. Appl. Toxicol. **13:** 533–544.
36. HATTIS, D.P. WHITE, L. MARMORSTEIN & P. KOCH. 1990. Uncertainty in pharmacokinetic modeling for perchloroethylene. I. Comparison of model structure, parameters, and predictions for low-dose metabolism rates for models derived by different authors. Risk. Anal. **10:** 449–458.
37. EDLER. L. 1992. Physiologically-based pharmacokinetic models and their applications in cancer risk assessment. *In* Data Analysis and Statistical Inference. S. Schach & G. Trenkler, Eds.: 349–376. Eul-Verlag, Bergisch-Gladbach.
38. TRITSCHER, A.M., J.A. GOLDSTEIN, C.J. PORTIER, Z. MCCOY, G.C. CLARK & G.W. LUCIER. 1992. Dose-response relationships for chronic exposure to 2,3,7,8-tetra-chlorodibenzo-*p*-dioxin in a rat tumor promotion model: quantification and immunolocalization of CYP1A1 and CYP1A2 in the liver. Cancer Research **52:** 3436–4332.
39. PORTIER, J., A. TRITSCHER, M. KOHN, C. SEWALL, G. CLARK, L. EDLER, D. HOEL & G. LUCIER. 1993. Ligand/Receptor binding of 2,3,7,8 TCDD: Implications for risk assessment. Fund. Appl. Toxicol. **20:** 48–56.
40. EDLER, L., F. GILBERG, C. PORTIER & W. URFER. 1997. Statistische Verfahren zur Auswertung von Enzyminduktionskinetiken in der Risikoabschätzung. Inform., Biom. und Epidem. in Med. und Biol. **28:** 213–226.
41. FREI, E., F. GILBERG, M. SCHRÖDER, A. BREUER, L. EDLER & M. WIESSLER. 1999. Analysis of the inhibition of N-nitroso-dimethylamine activation in the liver by N-nitrodimethylamine using a new nonlinear statistical method. Carcinogenesis. **20:** 459–464.

Using Molecular Epidemiology in Assessing Exposure for Risk Assessment

P.A. SCHULTE[a] AND M. WATERS

National Institute for Occupational Safety and Health (NIOSH), Education and Information Division, Robert A. Taft Laboratories, Cincinnati, Ohio, USA

ABSTRACT: Quantitative estimation of health risks depends on exposure characterization, the nature of the dose response relationships, and the toxicity of the agents involved. The greatest uncertainties in risk assessment almost always arise from sparse or inadequate exposure data, inadequate understanding of exposure mechanisms, and insufficient understanding of the exposure-dose-response pathway. Additional sources of uncertainty arise when mixed or multiple exposures are implicated in the disease pathway, and as a result of variability in both exposures and responses within and between individuals. Here we consider the role of exposure assessment in the risk assessment process, the use of biological markers or molecular epidemiology to contribute to improvements in exposure assessment for risk assessment, and uncertainties associated with the use of biological markers.

INTRODUCTION

The classic risk assessment paradigm includes hazard identification, dose-response assessment, exposure assessment, and risk characterization.[1] Using molecular epidemiology for exposure measurement may contribute in various ways to these stages in the risk assessment process. The hazard identification stage involves the determination of any threat to human health any an agent might pose. Here there is a need to link an exposure with an outcome. In the exposure and dose-response assessment stages there is need to understand the specific effects that result from different exposures, particularly lower exposures. In the exposure assessment stage, the extent of exposure depends strongly on the agent and environment. This stage builds on the specific source-path-receiver model used during hazard identification. The source-path-receiver model is the common thread in linking source chemicals, the pathway of movement in the environment, and the route or routes of exposure of various receptors—in this case individuals or groups of individuals.[3] Critical issues in exposure assessment include characterization of the magnitude, frequency, and duration of exposure; the basis for the assessment; and the identification of highly exposed subgroups. The risk characterization stage eventually results in identification of *acceptable* and *unacceptable* levels of exposures. This requires an explanation of any assumptions and models used, together with discussion of uncertainty.

---

[a]Address for correspondence: Paul A. Schulte, Ph.D., National Institute for Occupational Safety and Health (NIOSH), Education and Information Division, Robert A. Taft Laboratories, 4676 Columbia Parkway, Cincinnati, OH 45226, USA. 513/533-8481 (voice); 513/533-8588 (fax).
e-mail:pas4@cdc.gov

What role can molecular epidemiology play in the process of evaluating exposure and attendant uncertainties? This is the question that will be addressed in this paper. Molecular epidemiology is a term used for the incorporation of molecular, cellular, and physiologic biological markers (biomarkers) as dependent and independent variables in epidemiologic explorations of relationships between markers with either health outcomes or other markers within populations.[5] However, some commentators inappropriately apply these terms to a range of endeavors that use molecular measurements on people, rather than limiting the term to studies of the distribution of determinants of health effects within populations. In this discussion, we also consider using molecular and other biomarkers to serve as indicators of exposure. There is a growing body of literature to suggest that these exposure biomarkers can supplement traditional exposure assessment methods, and thus possibly make a contribution to the risk assessment process by reducing uncertainty in exposure assessment.[5–10]

HAZARD IDENTIFICATION

The role of molecular biomarkers and molecular epidemiology in hazard identification can be illustrated by the following examples. To determine whether a xenobiotic is hazardous or not, biomarkers may be used to increase the accuracy of approaches based on less sensitive measures of exposure; for example, the use of job titles as exposure proxies. Similarly, in situations where exposures occur that are variable or intermittent, and the effect of exposure is integrated, cumulative exposure biomarkers might be useful. A molecular epidemiology approach may clarify the exposure-outcome relationship better than classical methods, as a result of reduced exposure measurement error. For example, the role of aflatoxin exposure and liver cancer was not clear when studied by using a dietary questionnaire to assess intake of foods, that were potentially contaminated with aflatoxin. However, a strong association was observed by means of urinary biomarkers (metabolites and DNA adducts) of aflatoxin exposure[6,11] (see TABLE 1). In this example the molecular biomarker is useful because it is quite specific. It provides a better indicator of exposure than can be inferred from use of a questionnaire, since respondents are not aware of how much aflatoxin they consume. One might think that direct measurement of the aflatoxin component of all foodstuffs ingested, and measurement of amounts of food intake per day, could also lead to a better measure of exposure than the questionnaire surrogate. In the case of aflatoxin, this is probably not true due to the difficulty of measuring food intake, the possible variability of aflatoxin levels within food, the difficulty of extracting aflatoxin from foods, and analytical detection limits for such methods. However, for some other agents, external direct measures of exposure may be feasible, as cost effective as biological measures, and also provide improved estimates over such surrogates as questionnaire data. Qualitative tests may be used to determine whether external exposure or an exposure biomarker would offer the best predictor for disease.[12] One test is to determine if the biomarker is more highly correlated with the disease than external exposure. A second conditional test is to determine if, given the same level of exposure, those with higher levels of the biomarkers are more likely to develop the disease.

TABLE 1. Comparison between exposure data derived from questionnaires and data obtained by using biomarkers[a]

A. Relative risks based on dietary intake of aflatoxin		
Dietary aflatoxin B_1 exposure (µg/yr)	Relative risk	95% Confidence interval
<71	1.0	
71–113	1.6	0.8, 3.1
113+	0.9	0.4, 1.9
B. Relative risks based on urinary biomarkers of aflatoxin		
Biomarker	Relative risk (present/absent)	95% Confidence interval
metabolites or adducts	5.0	2.1, 11.8
aflatoxin M_1 with adduct	16.1	3.6, 72.5

[a]Study of aflatoxin and risk of liver cancer in Shanghai, China from 1986 to 1992 (55 cases).
SOURCE: Qian et al., 1994; adapted from Howe, 1998.

The basic rationale for using biomarkers is that, in some cases, they can provide a more accurate method for assessing exposure and, ultimately, risk (see FIGURE 1). This is accomplished by reducing exposure misclassification by markers for biologically effective dose, and also by incorporation of exposure and host factors (e.g., metabolic capabilities) to the same marker. Although use of biomarkers can reduce misclassification, it is also possible that measurement error in the biomarker may contribute to bias in the measure of association.[7,9] Such errors can be evaluated and their impact adjusted for, but on balance they are better avoided or, at least, minimized by good laboratory and epidemiologic practices.

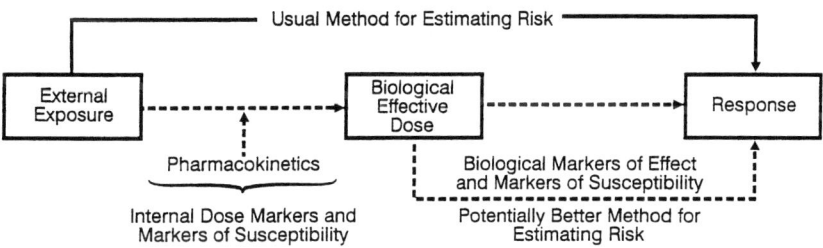

FIGURE 1. Rationale for using biomarkers to assess risk. (Adapted from numerous presentations at EPA and FDA in the 1980s.)

DOSE RESPONSE

In risk assessment the ascertainment of a dose-response relationship is crucial in ultimately determining the shape of the curve and for selecting a no-observed-adverse-effect level (NOAEL). Biomarkers for exposure can be used as indicators for dose, which can then be assessed against classical measures of morbidity or mortality. Another use of biomarkers is as outcome measures that correlate with exposure. In this case exposure markers are not what are needed; rather, the need is for effect markers. Effect markers are markers that relate to or predict disease. A marker that has been validated to predict disease can be applied to a surrogate for disease. For example, specific types of chromosomal aberrations that appear to predict cancer risk on a group basis can be used as the outcome variables in a dose-response analysis, as in the case of ionizing radiation exposure.[13]

Before a biomarker is useful in risk assessment it needs to be validated, that is, the relationship between the biomarker and what it represents needs to be established. Biomarkers can depict exposure, effect, or susceptibility. The process of biomarker validation of has been described, and it includes a laboratory phase and a population phase.[14] Molecular epidemiology is practiced in the field phase.

EXPOSURE ASSESSMENT FOR RISK ASSESSMENT

The exposure assessment component of risk assessment includes the consideration of such issues as representativeness of exposure measurements for a population, differences in exposures within and between individuals, individual differences in uptake and biotransformation, identification of factors that control or modify exposures, exposure estimation methods that are applicable in the absence of direct measurements, and identification of the most relevant dose metric for the agent under consideration. Biomarkers are most broadly defined to include markers for exposure, intermediate endpoints, host susceptibility to disease, and early clinical effects. The use of biomarkers in assessing exposure for risk assessment is usually limited to the first two of these, but increasingly may include the consideration of susceptibility factors in conjunction with exposure factors, for example, the presence of a specific genetic polymorphism for a metabolic enzyme.[15]

Quite often epidemiologic studies employ exposure surrogates rather than direct measurement of exposure. For environmental studies, surrogates might include geographic location, such as residence for a drinking water or air pollution study, age of housing in studies of lead-based paint exposures, or proximity of residence to electrical power lines. When direct measurements are not available or are limited, occupational studies use surrogates such as job title, job group, years worked at a plant, pounds of pesticide applied per week, and tasks performed.[16,17] The use of quantified direct measurements of personal exposure can lower uncertainty in the risk assessment process considerably in comparison with the use of such exposure surrogates.

EXPOSURE BIOMARKERS

The validation of biomarkers for exposure requires equal attention in assessing both the exposure and the biomarkers so that a fair comparison can be made. However, the relationship between the biomarkers and exposure varies due to host factors, as the biomarkers are further removed from the exposure depending on the number of steps in the absorption, metabolism, and clearance pathways between uptake and the specific biomarker. This applies to any form of exposure, due to intervening host factors that vary between individuals, such as breathing rate and capacity, activation, detoxification, elimination, and DNA repair. A high correlation between exposure and marker may not always be observed and an exposure-response relationship may vary between people. Therefore, it is important to identify and adjust for factors that can influence an exposure-response relationship. For example, to validate hydroxy-ethyl hemoglobin adducts as exposure biomarkers for ethylene oxide at low dose, we adjusted for age, smoking, and education in a linear regression model.[18] It may also be useful to adjust for genetic effect modifying factors.

EFFECT BIOMARKERS

Biomarkers for intermediate effects, that is, effects that are observed between exposure and disease, can be validated in case-control studies and cohort studies.[6,19,20] Once validated, these markers can serve as surrogates for disease, albeit on a probabilistic basis since generally not all people with a given biomarker will develop the disease, but the groups with high levels will generally be at greatest risk. This has been observed for both chromosomal aberrations and cancer.[21]

Other potentially useful effect markers are found in the spectra of mutations, such as in p53, since these show a unique fingerprint with a given exposure.[22,23] Most of the epidemiology studies of workers involving p53 mutations, although purporting to identify a predominant mutational spectrum, do not include one that occurred in more than 50% of the cases with purported common exposures.[22,23] This may be due to exposure misclassification but also may be due the failure to account for other important pathways not involving p53.

SUSCEPTIBILITY BIOMARKERS

Perhaps the greatest potential contributions of molecular epidemiology to risk assessment and risk management can be found in the inclusion of inherited susceptibility biomarkers.[15] Susceptibility biomarkers can influence exposure effects and are, therefore, important to consider in risk assessments. These biomarkers, offer both promises and perils for individual and population risk estimation. The promises are for a more refined assessment of risk through the identification of gene-gene and gene-environment interactions, and also for focusing prevention and control programs on high risk individuals. The perils include ethical and social issues, including stigmatization, discrimination, and the misconception that removing a susceptible person from the exposure scenario without reducing exposure opportunities reduces risk whereas this may not be so, on a comparative basis.[25] There are also issues in using susceptibility markers as effect modifiers in epidemiology studies. These include misclassification of a genotype due to various technical flaws, such as the failure to recognize a variant that contributes to the genotype.[26]

One of the most widely known examples of how a susceptibility biomarker, combined with an exposure measure, can give information about risk assessment is the metabolic polymorphism for N-acetyltransferase in the case of bladder cancer where arylamine-exposed slow acetylators have a much higher risk of bladder cancer than fast acetylators.[27–29]

Calabrese demonstrated that genetically-determined biochemical differences between people for a range of phenotypes could exceed 10-fold.[30] In a pioneering study, Bois *et al.*, by modeling of DNA adducts in the bladder of people exposed to 4-aminobiphenyl, illustrated that the adduct levels of the most susceptible individuals are 10,000 times higher than those for the least susceptible and that the 5th and 95th percentiles differ by a factor of 160.[29] Therefore, accounting for genetic variability may have important implications for risk assessment.

When these genetic polymorphic pathways represent major routes of elimination it is important that this fact be included in risk assessments.[31] Determination of the population prevalence of alleles for metabolic polymorphisms involves molecular epidemiologic approaches and this is even more true when assessing gene-environment interactions.

LOW LEVELS OF EXPOSURE

The target area in the risk assessment process is usually the risk at low levels of exposure. This is where there is a lack of data and where projections of effects and risks are most needed. The capability exists to measure extremely low levels of exposure in many contemporary situations but not necessarily in historical cases. Futhermore, it is particularly important, in the case of low exposure levels, to understand the linkages between markers of exposure, metabolites or conjugation products, subclinical effects and frank disease, and the role of mediating or buffering factors on these markers.

When using biomarkers to assess exposure at low levels it is important to account for all sources of exposure. A dose marker generally integrates all routes and sources of exposure. Thus, for example, in the study of hemoglobin adducts and ethylene oxide, we had to account for smoking as a source of hydroxy-ethyl hemoglobin adducts, and also to account for endogenous sources.[18]

ADVANTAGES OF BIOMARKERS IN ASSESSING EXPOSURE FOR RISK ASSESSMENT

One advantage to using a biomarker for exposure instead of an environmental measure is that it accounts for individual differences in uptake. These differences may arise due either to actual differences in environmental exposure levels that are not easily identified among groups of people, or to differences in uptake and biotransformation between individuals. For example, since air concentrations of chemicals are known to vary widely in many indoor and outdoor environments, individuals presumed to have the same exposure potential, may actually have different exposures. If this environmental variability is not characterized, as is often the case due to the cost associated with a greater number of environmental measurements, the contribution of this source of variability to uncertainty in assessing levels of exposure remains unknown. Uptake and metabolism of xenobiotic chemical agents may also differ widely between individuals. The kinetics and efficiency associated with each step in the relevant pathway from absorption across a dermal, inhalation, or ingestion barrier to dose at the target organ and hence to measurable response in a molecule or tissue, may vary widely between individuals and again lead to uncertainty in the estimated exposure. Measuring the biologically effective dose at the target tissue or receptor for each individual, when this is possible, minimizes these sources of uncertainty.

Biomarkers also obviate the need to estimate the effects of exposure-modifying external factors, such as the use of personal protective equipment or personal hygiene, on environmental exposure levels. Typically, environmental characterization of exposures does not incorporate these factors directly, and thus their efficacy must be estimated. This estimation process is often not validated and, therefore, makes an unknown contribution to the risk assessment process.

When multiple agents may lead to changes in the same biomarker level, the use of a biomarker may be more useful than an external measure of exposure, since the biomarker is a summary measure of exposure to all agents that are biologically processed in a similar manner. For example, trichloroacetic acid is a measurable intermediate in the biotransformation of trichloroethane, trichloroethylene, and tetrachloroethylene exposures.

When variations of biomarker levels within and between individuals are less than the variability of environmental measurements, biomarkers offer the advantage of requiring fewer measurements to estimate exposures than external measures. This dampening of variability has been demonstrated for blood lead levels.[32]

LIMITATIONS OF BIOMARKERS IN ASSESSING EXPOSURE FOR RISK ASSESSMENT

Biomarkers are most useful in assessing exposures when there is a high correlation between environmental measures of individual exposures and the biomarker, and when the variability of the biomarker is less than that of environmental exposure measures.[33,34] The data requirements to demonstrate this are not trivial, however.

The relevant time frame must be identified when using biomarkers for exposure assessment. This requires an understanding of the uptake and absorption, distribution, biotransformation, repair and clearance processes, and of the target receptors. Long-lived xenobiotics or their metabolic products may accumulate in a tissue compartment and provide a measure of long-term exposure. Examples include PCBs and DDT in adipose tissue. Similarly, certain types of chromosomal aberrations due to ionizing radiation are persistent and cumulative; they are measured years after exposure.[35] The kinetics of uptake, biotransformation, distribution, and clearance must be understood in order to identify the relevant time period for biomarker collection and to interpret biomarker data. The time between exposure and sample collection is of greater importance in cases where repair or clearance processes dominate, such as n-hexane in alveolar air, or radiation exposure and certain types of DNA damage.

When variations in biomarker levels exceed variations in environmental exposure levels, due to interindividual differences in uptake, biotransformation, distribution of chemicals, or in efficiency of repair processes, biomarker data may be less useful than environmental levels in assessing exposure. In the case of styrene exposures and sister chromatid exchanges, the increased variability of SCEs between workers compared with the variability of full-shift personal exposures, indicates that the external measures require fewer samples to assess the exposure distributions.[32]

Specificity is a desirable characteristic for a biomarker. In the simplest case the biomarker is unique to the exposure. For example, metals in blood or urine, or a unique chemical-hemoglobin, or a chemical-DNA adduct in the case of electrophilic carcinogens, are unique to the causative agent just as the TB-tubercule is to tuberculosis infection. More commonly, multiple agents may produce the biomarker, and the possibility of confounding exposures, or a mixed exposure pattern, must be accounted for. The protein adduct of benzo(a)pyrene may be indicative of either smoking or foundry work exposures, among others. In the case of chromosomal aberrations, the effects of benzene, arsenic, or ionizing radiation on elevated levels of long-lived chromosomal aberrations may be confounded with concomitant exposures to cigarette smoke, or to dietary factors such as the use of diet sweeteners.[36]

Background levels of biomarkers in unexposed groups must be available in order to properly interpret biomarker levels in exposed individuals. Often, such background data are not available and then characterization of the baseline level distribution must be a component of the study.

FUTURE APPROACHES

On the horizon for use in epidemiology studies and risk assessments are high throughput DNA chip technologies to study gene functions and expression under various conditions.[37] These technologies will allow for evaluation of temporal and spatial patterns of gene expression under various exposure conditions. It will be possible to determine which genes are up- and which are down-regulated in response to exposures. The difficulties in using DNA chips include issues of data reduction, multiple comparisons, complex interaction assessments, and interpretation of results. Ideally, if these problems can be solved, it may be possible for the first time in history to evaluate changes in expression of many genes of an individual at the same time.[37] Cross-species comparison could be enhanced. This technology could lead to better characterization and understanding of disease processes and exposure-disease relationships, which would be of great assistance to risk assessors.

CONCLUSION

Molecular epidemiology approaches may be useful in assessing exposure in the various steps in risk assessment. These approaches, however, should be viewed only as another tool available for researchers and risk assessors, not as a replacement for traditional measures such as environmental exposure assessment, job exposure matrices, questionnaires, and record reviews.

Molecular epidemiology data implies an understanding of the mechanism, and incorporation of mechanistic data into risk assessment methods is currently a laudable goal. However, risk assessments and regulations should not wait the development of mechanistic data,[1] nor should uncertainty about mechanism be used to block public health action. Conversely, if there is sufficient uncertainty about whether an agent truly causes disease, then imposing regulations may lead to inappropriate utilization of resources. This resource issue needs to be taken into account, but it should not be the deciding factor.

We have discussed how biological markers may have a use in risk assessment. We have not addressed the ethical, legal, or social implications of this use; they have been discussed elsewhere.[38] Generally, biomarkers for exposure generate fewer of these issues than biomarkers for effect or susceptibility, because an acquired effect indicating disease risk may, in some ways, be considered similar to an inherited one. Nevertheless, the distinction between these categories is subjective and is often blurry. Care needs to be taken to guard against stigmatization, discrimination, and loss of opportunity that can result from use of biomarkers in research or practice.

REFERENCES

1. BECKING, G.C. 1995 Use of mechanistic information in risk assessment for toxic chemicals. Toxicol. Lett. **77**: 15–24.
2. MCCLELLAN, R.O. 1995. Risk assessment and biological mechanisms: lessons learned, future applications. Toxicology **102**: 239–258.
3. NELSON, D.I. 1997. Risk assessment in the workplace. *In* The Occupational Environment—Its Evaluation and Control, S. DiNardi, Ed.: 328–359. American Industrial Hygiene Association Press.
4. US NATIONAL RESEARCH COUNCIL (NRC). 1983.. Risk assessment in the Federal Government: Managing the Process. National Academy Press, Washington, D.C.
5. SCHULTE, P.A. & F.P. PERERA. 1993. Molecular epidemiology: Principles and practices. Academic Press, San Diego.
6. HOWE, G.R. 1998. Practical uses of biomarkers in population studies. *In* Biomarkers: Medical and Workplace Applications. M.L. Mendelsohn, L.C. Mohr & J.P. Peeters, Eds.: 41–49. John Henry Press, Washington, DC.
7. WHITE, E. 1997. Effects of biomarker measurement error on epidemiological studies. *In* Application of Biomarkers in Cancer Epidemiology. P. Toniolo *et al.*, Eds.: 73–93. IARC Scientific Publication No. 142, Lyon.
8. HATTIS, D. & K. SILVER. 1993. Use of biomarkers in Risk assessment. *In* Molecular Epidemiology: Principles and Practices. P.A. Schulte & F.P. Perera, Eds.: 257–273. Academic Press, San Diego.
9. SARACCI, R. 1997. Comparing measurements if biomarkers with other measurements of exposure. *In* Application of Biomarkers in Cancer Epidemiology. P. Toniolo *et al.*, Eds.: 303–312. IARC Scientific Publication No 142, Lyon.
10. TIMBRELL, J.A. 1998. Biomarkers in toxicology. Toxicology **129**: 1–12.
11. QIAN, G.S., R.K. ROSS, M.C. YU, J.M. YUAN, Y.T. GAO, B.E. HENDERSON, G.N. WOGAN & J.D. GROOPMAN. 1994. A follow-up study of urinary markers of aflatoxin exposure and liver cancer risk in Shanghai, People's Republic of China. Cancer Epidemiol. Biomarkers Prev. **3**: 3–10.
12. STEENLAND, K., J. TUCKER, & A. SALVAN. 1993. Problems in assessing the relative predictive value of internal markers versus external exposure in chronic disease epidemiology. Cancer Epidemiol. Biomarkers Prev. **2**: 487–491.

13. JOKSIC, G., & V. SPASOJEVIC-TISMA. 1998. Chromosome analysis of lymphocytes from radiation workers in the tritium-applying industry. Int. Arch. Occup. Environ. Health **71**: 213–220.
14. PERERA, F.P & L.A. MOONEY. 1993. The role of molecular epidemiology in cancer prevention. *In* Cancer Prevention. V.T. DeVita, S. Hellman & S.A. Rosenberg, Eds.: 1–15. J.B. Lippincott, Philadelphia.
15. YANG, Q. & M.J. KHOURY. 1997. Evolving methods in genetic epidemiology: III. Gene-environment interaction in epidemiologic research. Epidemiologic Reviews **19**: 33–43.
16. GOLDBERG, M. & D. HEMON. 1993. Occupational epidemiology and assessment of exposure. Int. J. Epidemiol. **22**(Suppl. 2): s5–s9.
17. STEWART, P.A., A. BLAIR, M. DOSEMICI *et al.* 1991. Collection of exposure data for retrospective occupational epidemiologic studies. Appl. Occup. Environ. Hygiene **6**: 280–289.
18. SCHULTE, P.A., M. BOENIGER, J.T. WALKER, S. SCHOBER, S.E. PERERA, D.K. GULATI, J.P. WOJCIECHOWSKI, A. GARZA, R. FROELICH, G. STRAUSS, W.E. HALPERIN, R. HERRICK & J. GRIFFITH. 1992. Biological markers in hospital workers exposed to low levels of ethylene oxide. Mutat. Res. **278**: 237–151.
19. MUNOZ, A. & S.J. GANGE. 1998. Methodological issues for biomarkers and intermediate outcomes in cohort studies. Epidemiologic Rev. **20**: 29–42.
20. ROTHMAN, N., W.F. STEWART & P.A.SCHULTE. 1995 Incorporating biomarkers into cancer epidemiology: a matrix of biomarker and study design categories. Cancer Epidemiol. Biomarkers Prev. **4**: 301–311.
21. HAGMAR, L., L. BROGGER, I.L. HANSTEEN, S. HEIM, B. HOGSTEDT, L. KNUDSEN, B. LAMBERT, K. LINNAINMAA, F. MITELMAN, I. NORDENSON, C. REUTERWALL, S. SALOMAA, S. SKERFVING & M. SORSA. 1994. Cancer risk in humans predicted by increased levels of chromosomal aberrations in lymphocytes: Nordic Study Group on the Health Risk of Chromosome Damage. Cancer Res. **54**: 2919–2922.
22. NIGRO, J.M. & S.J. BAKER. 1989. Mutations in the p53 gene occur in diverse human tumour types. Nature **342**: 705–708.
23. HERNANDEZ-BOUSSARD, T.M. & P. HAINART. 1998. A specific spectrum of p53 mutations in lung cancer from smokers: review of mutations compiled in the IARC p 53 database. Env. Health Perspect. **106**: 385–391.
24. GREENBLATT, M., W. BENNETT, M. HOLLSTEIN & C. HARRIS. 1994. Mutations in the p53 tumor suppressor gene: clues to cancer etiology and molecular pathegenesis. Cancer Res. **54**: 4855–4878.
25. VINEIS, P. & P.A. SCHULTE. 1995. Scientific and ethical aspects of genetic screening of workers: the case of the N-acetyltranferase phenotype. J. Clin. Epidemiol. **48**: 189–197.
26. ROTHMAN, N., W.F. STEWART, N.E. CAPORASO & R.B. HAYES. 1993. Misclassification of genetic susceptibility biomarkers: implication for case-control studies and cross population comparisons. Cancer Epidemiol. Biomarkers Prev. **2**: 299–303.
27. CARTWRIGHT, R.A., R.W. GLASHAN, H.J. ROGERS *et al.* 1982. Role of N-acetyltransferase phenotype in bladder carcinogenesis: a pharmacogenetic epidemiological approach to bladder cancer. Lancet **11**: 842–846.
28. TAYLOR, J.A., D.M. UMBACH, E. STEPHENS *et al.* 1998. The role of N-acetylation polymorphisms in smoking–associated bladder cancer: evidence of a gene–gene-exposure three-way interaction. Cancer Res. **58**: 3403–3610.
29. BOIS, F.Y., G. KROWECH & L. ZEISE. 1995. Modeling human interindividual variability in metabolism and risk: The example of 4-aminobiphenyl. Risk Analysis **15**: 205–213.

30. CALABRESE, E.J. 1997 Role of genetic factors in environmentally induced toxic response: historical consideration, present status and future directions. University of Massachusetts, Amherst.
31. RENWICK, A.G. & N.R. LAZARUS. 1998. Human variability and noncancer risk assessment-an analysis of the default uncertainty factor. Reg. Tox. Pharmacol. **27:** 3–20.
32. RAPPAPORT, S.M. 1985. Smoothing of exposure variability at the receptor: implications for health standards. Ann. Occup. Hyg. **29:** 201–214.
33. RAPPAPORT, S.M., E. SYMANSKI, J.W. YAGER & L.L. KUPPER. 1995. The relationship between environmental monitoring and biologic markers in exposure assessment. Env Health Perspectives **103**(Suppl. 3): 49–53.
34. BRUNEKREEF, B., D. NOY & P. CLAUSING. 1987. Variability of exposure measurements in environmental epidemiology. Am. J. Epidemiology **125:** 892–898.
35. TUCKER, J.D., E.J. TAWN, D. HOLDSWORTH, S. MORRIS *et al.* 1997 Biological dosimetry of radiation workers at the Sellafield nuclear facility. Radiation Res. **148:** 216–26.
36. RAMSEY, M.J., D.H. MOORE, J.F. BRINER *et al.* 1995. The effects of age and lifestyle factors on the accumulation of cytogenetic damage as measured by chromosomal painting. Mutation Research **338:** 95–106.
37. WOYCHIK, R.R., M.L. KLEBIG, M.J. JUSTICE, T.R. MAGNUSON & E.D. AVNER. 1998. Functional genomics in the post-genome era. Mut. Res. **400:** 3–14.
38. SCHULTE, P.A., D. HUNTER, N. ROTHMAN. 1997. Ethical and social issues in the use of biomarkers in epidemiological research. *In* Application of Biomarkers in Cancer Epidemiology. P. Toniolo, P. Boffetta, D.E.G. Shuker *et al.,* Eds.: 313–318. IARC Scientific Publications No. 142, Lyon.

Kaplan-Meier Tumor Probability as a Starting Point for Dose-Response Modeling Provides Accurate Lifetime Risk Estimates from Rodent Carcinogenicity Studies

WIL F. TEN BERGE[a]

DSM, Department Environment and Product Safety,
P.O. Box 6500, 6401 JH Heerlen, The Netherlands

ABSTRACT: In rodent carcinogenicity studies the linearized multistage model for modelling the dose-response for specific tumor incidence has limitations in accuracy. This note provides an alternative basic method for analyzing the dose-response relationship. It is based on an actuarial analysis of mortality and specific tumor incidence. The survival and the Kaplan-Meier specific tumor probability are fitted to a Weibull model, in which exposure level, exposure period, and observation period are independent variables. The mortality from specific cancers at a certain time is simulated by means of the product of survival and specific tumor rate (derivative of Kaplan-Meier tumor probability) as function of exposure level, exposure duration, and observation period, integrated over the observation period. The model is demonstrated by means of fitting the mortality and tumor incidence data from the second NTP mice study on butadiene to a Weibull model and to the linear, so-called, one-hit model. It will be shown that, in the experimental exposure range, the Weibull model is far superior to the one-hit model and predicts the specific tumor incidence with a high accuracy over the total dose range. The Kaplan-Meier probability model for a specific tumor is also useful for regulatory risk estimation. It is proposed that to develop a specific tumor a risk level of 1 in 1,000 over a lifetime is about equal to 5 in 10,000 at 50% survival of the population. The Kaplan-Meier probability may be estimated at the time of 50% survival of the exposed population, which can be deduced from the all mortality data. This estimation method provides meaningful data, using exposure level, exposure duration, and observation period properly. The advantage of the actuarial analysis method for interpreting rodent studies is that allowance is made for competition between death causes, which is essential in case of considerable difference in mortality and specific mortality between dose groups. Integrating the product of survival and specific tumor rate is the proper way to predict, comparatively, mortality and specific mortality in exposed and unexposed rodent populations.

INTRODUCTION

This paper aims to improve the dose-response relationships for carcinogenic endpoints in rodent studies. The basis of this improvement is to completely remove the

[a]Address for correspondence: 31-45-5787128 (voice); 31-45-5787112 (fax).
e-mail: wtberge@wxs.nl

influence of survival in establishing a dose response relationship for a specific tumor incidence over the whole lifespan. This is achieved by calculating the Kaplan-Meier probability for bearing a specific tumor at the time of death. If the tumor of interest is a malignant tumor, it is assumed that the tumor is the cause of death. The advantage of the Kaplan-Meier tumor probability for dose response modelling is that it depends only on the observation period and the applied dose levels of the study, but not on the survival of the specific dose groups. The Kaplan-Meier tumor probability is therefore the appropriate starting point for estimating a relationship between dose and specific tumor response, independent of mortality by other death causes.

A further advantage to deriving the Kaplan-Meier tumor probability is that the derivative with respect to time of this parameter is equivalent to the specific rate of the tumor of interest, depending only on dose and observation period in the experimental animal study. The specific tumor rate and the dose- and time-dependent survival control the tumor incidence actually observed. The product of survival and specific tumor rate, integrated over the observation period provides an excellent estimate of the observed incidence of the tumor of interest in the study.

Finally, the Kaplan-Meier probability for a specific tumor can also be used to estimate the dose causing an additional risk that is equal to the regulatory risk limit values. The dose level estimated is that for which the increase in Kaplan-Meier probability at 50% survival is set equal to half of the acceptable regulatory risk limit values over a lifetime (0% survival, 100% death). This is a fair assumption, because the dose level, causing an additional risk equal to the acceptable regulatory risk limit values for additional tumor mortality (10^{-4} or 10^{-6}) over a lifetime, is so small that this will not influence the average survival time at all.

This new method was applied to the second NTP mice inhalation study on butadiene, also making use of the data obtained from animals that were exposed for only a short period of time to increased levels of butadiene. The concept of effective dose was explored. The effective dose was assumed to be related to the concentration C, to C^N, to $C \cdot T$ and to $C^N \cdot T^M$. The effective dose concept was fitted to the specific tumor response according to a Weibull model. A plot of estimated and actual specific tumor incidence made it possible to determine the appropriateness of the different effective dose concepts.

METHODS

Evaluation of Data

All mice (exposed continuously and for limited periods) of the second NTP butadiene inhalation study[1] were included in the dose response analysis for mortality. The Kaplan-Meier probability for having a tumor at death was estimated until the time of termination. Tumors found at termination were not used in estimating the Kaplan-Meier tumor probability.

Furthermore, the data of male and female mice were pooled. The reason for this is mitigating the influence of random fluctuations of specific tumor incidence data in small groups on the dose response estimates. The incidence of the malignant tumors of interest were not overtly different between exposed male and female animals.

The following data were recorded for each mouse:

- sex
- dose level
- duration of exposure
- day of mortality
- type of mortality (spontaneous or termination)
- presence of the tumor of interest (lung carcinoma, heart angiosarcoma, or malignant lymphoma).

From these data the cumulative mortality per dose group and the Kaplan-Meier tumor probability for bearing the tumor of interest at death was estimated. Animals dying before day 100 of the study were not taken into account.

Estimation of the Kaplan-Meier Tumor Probability

Estimation of the K-M-probability for having a tumor is shown in TABLE 1 for an example, in which a group of 10 experimental animals were followed.[2] The first two mortalities without a tumor occurred in week 61 and 62. In week 63 eight animals remained and one died with a tumor. Thus, in week 63 the probability to remain tumor free is 7/8, and the probability to have a tumor is $1 - 7/8 = 1/8$ or 0.125. In week 66 again a tumor was found in five surviving animals. The probability to remain tumor free in week 66 is $7/8 \times 4/5 = 0.7$. Thus, the probability to have a tumor is $1 - 0.7 = 0.3$ in week 66. Note that the observed approximate incidence rate of 2/10, or 0.2, is quite different from 0.3 and does not reflect the real tumor probability in week 66.

TABLE 1. Example calculation of Kaplan-Meier (K-M) probability for a population of 10 animals

Week	Death	Death with tumor	Crude tumor incidence	K-M probability tumor free	K-M probability tumor	K-M probability tumor
61	1		0	1	0	0
62	1		0	1	0	0
63	1	1	0.1	7/8	1 − 7/8	0.125
64	1		0.1	7/8	1 − 7/8	0.125
65	1		0.1	7/8	1 − 7/8	0.125
66	1	1	0.2	7/8	1 − 7/8	0.300
67	1		0.2	7/8 · 4/5	1 − 7/8 · 4/5	0.300
68	1	1	0.3	7/8 · 4/5 · 2/3	1 − 7/8 · 4/5 · 2/3	0.533
69	1		0.3	7/8 · 4/5 · 2/3	1 − 7/8 · 4/5 · 2/3	0.533
70	1		0.3	7/8 · 4/5 · 2/3	1 − 7/8 · 4/5 · 2/3	0.533

It is interesting to note the great difference between the crude observed tumor incidence and the Kaplan-Meier cumulative probability of having a tumor at death. The K-M cumulative probability is equal to the mortality incidence if the tumor in the table is the only cause of death in of the population. The tumor and other diseases cause 100% mortality at day 70. If the tumor was the only cause of death, only 53% of the population would have died from the tumor. It is not possible to construct a dose-response estimate for specific tumor incidence by using the crude specific tumor incidence, this should always be carried out with the Kaplan-Meier specific tumor incidence.

Modeling Survival

$$Survival(C, T_{exp}, T_{obs}) = \exp[-(B_0 + B_1 \times D_{eff}) \times T_{obs}^N]$$

$$D_{eff} = C, \quad D_{eff} = C^P, \quad D_{eff} = C \cdot T_{exp}, \quad \text{and} \quad D_{eff} = C^P T_{exp}^Q,$$

where C is the exposure level in ppm, T_{exp} is the exposure period in days, T_{obs} is the observation period in days, and D_{eff} is the effective dose.

The survival data were fitted to these models by means of the method of the *maximum likelihood*.[2,3]

Modeling Kaplan-Meier Tumor probability

$$(K\text{-}M\,prob(C, T_{exp}, T_{obs}) = 1 - \exp[-(A_0 + A_1 \times D_{eff}) \times T_{obs}^M]),$$

$$Q = \exp[-(A_0 + A_1 \times D_{eff}) \times T_{obs}^M],$$

$$D_{eff} = C, \quad D_{eff} = C^R, \quad D_{eff} = C \cdot T_{exp}, \quad D_{eff} = C^R T_{exp}^S, \quad \text{and}$$

$$Specific\ Tumor\ Rate(C, T_{exp}, T_{obs}) = \frac{d[K\text{-}M\,prob(C, T_{exp}, T_{obs})]}{Q dT_{obs}}.$$

The estimated K-M tumor probability data were fitted to these models by using iterative nonlinear regression analysis.

Modeling the Actual Tumor Incidence

The actual observed tumor incidence is controlled by survival and the specific tumor rate according to the following model:

$$Actual\ Tumor\ Incidence(C, T_{exp}, T_{obs})$$
$$= \int_0^X Survival(C, T_{exp}, T_{obs}) \times Spec.Tum.Rate(C, T_{exp}, T_{obs}) dT_{obs}$$

The specific tumor incidence was estimated by means of the above equations, using different concepts for the effective dose.

Dose Level at a Regulatory Risk Limit Value

The dose level estimated is that for which the increase of the Kaplan-Meier probability (95% upper confidence limit) at a 50% survival is equal to the half of the acceptable regulatory risk limit values over a lifetime (0% survival, 100% death).

RESULTS

Observed/Estimated Tumor Incidence Against Effective Dose

The estimated (smooth lines) and the observed (markers) specific tumor incidence at day 730 of the study (termination) were plotted against the exposure level or the exposure period, using different concepts for the effective dose.

FIGURES 1, 3, and 5 show plots of the observed and estimated specific tumor incidence against exposure level or exposure period, on the basis of the assumption that the effective dose is linearly related to the exposure concentration C (FIG. 1) or linearly related to the product of concentration C and exposure period T_{exp} (FIGS. 3 and 5).

FIGURES 2, 4, and 6 show plots of the observed and estimated specific tumor incidence against exposure level or exposure period, under the assumption that the effective dose is exponentially related to the exposure concentrations, C^P and C^R, (FIG. 2) or related to products of concentration and exposure period, $C^P \cdot T_{exp}^Q$ and $C^R \cdot T_{exp}^S$, (FIGS. 4 and 6).

The plots that assume the effective dose is exponentially related to concentration and exposure period, provide a closer fit between observed and estimated specific tumor incidence than the plots that assume effective dose is linearly related to concentration and exposure period.

Dose Levels Related to Specified Risk Limits

Dose levels were estimated (see METHODS) from the derived model for Kaplan-Meier tumor probability, causing no more additional life time risk than 10^{-3}, 10^{-4}, or 10^{-6} as the 95% upper confidence limit (95% UCL). These dose levels are presented in TABLES 2 through 4 for different concepts of the effective dose. In case of an exponential dose concept, the estimated exponent of the concentration is presented in the column headed *effective dose.*

In order to provide meaningful data for acceptable exposure levels in relation to occupational exposure that agree with the effective dose concept of $C^R \cdot T_{exp}^S$, it is assumed that mice are exposed for 500 days to butadiene, that is 60% of their life span. In case of an exponential dose concept, the estimated exponent of the exposure concentration and of the exposure period is presented in the column headed *effective dose* in TABLES 5 through 7.

It can be seen that the estimated exposure levels related to a specified limit risk value are several orders of magnitude higher in the case of an effective dose concept that assumes an exponential relation with concentration (and exposure period) than in the case of an effective dose concept that assumes a linear relation.

It is appropriate to emphasize the fact, that the fit between observed and estimated incidence on the basis of an exponential effective dose concept is superior to the fit

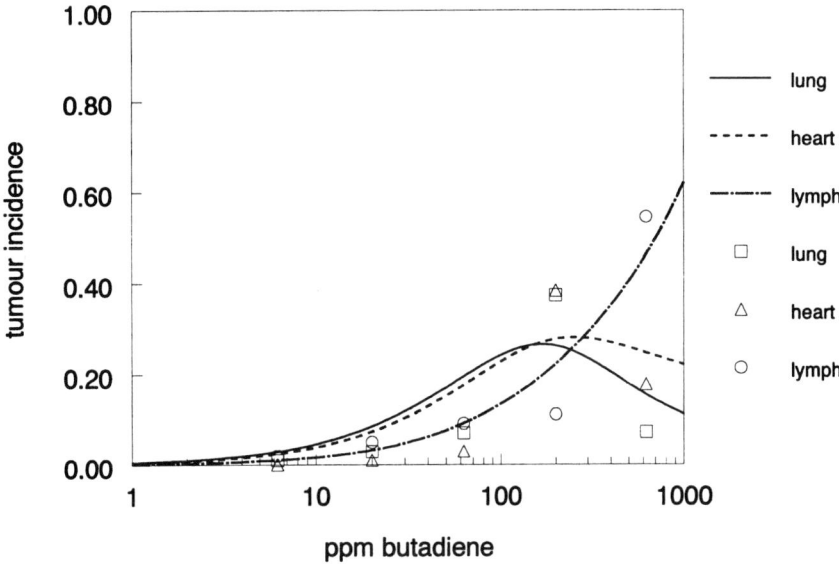

FIGURE 1. Butadiene exposure of mice. Specific tumor incidence (C linear one-hit).

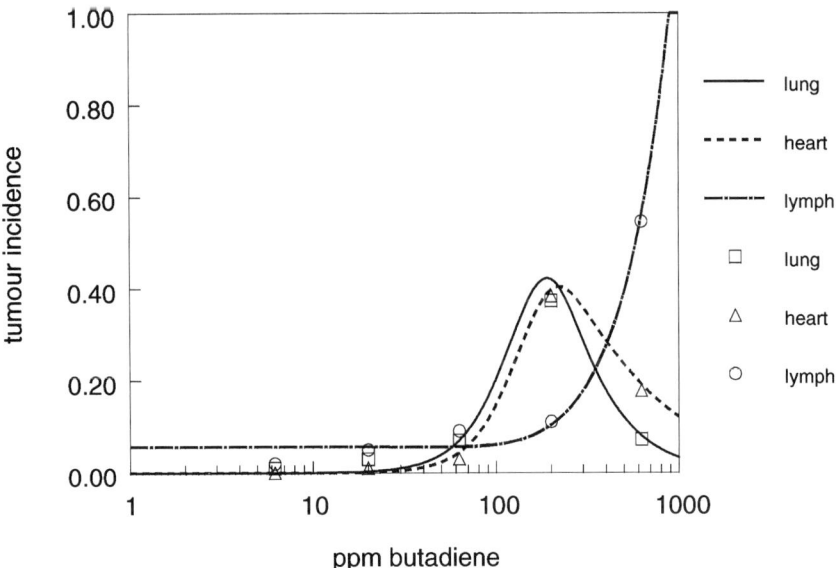

FIGURE 2. Butadiene exposure of mice. Specific tumor incidence (C exponent).

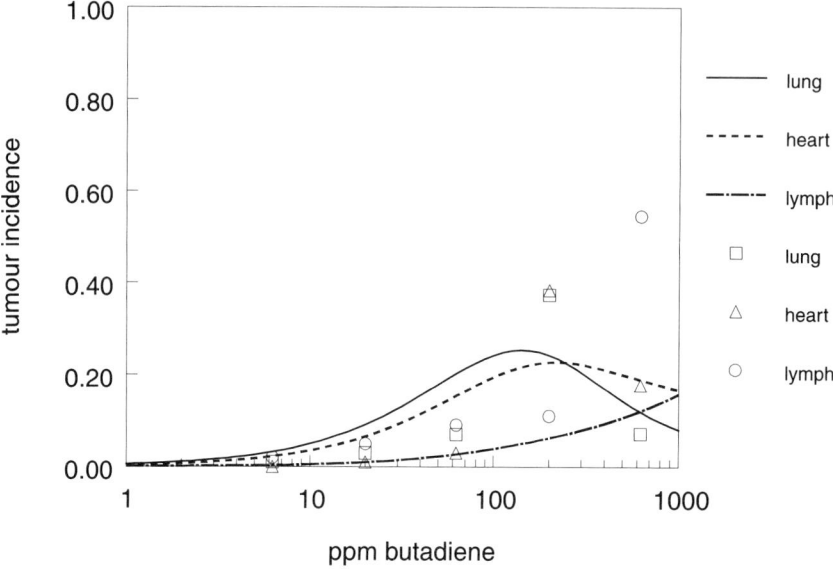

FIGURE 3. Butadiene exposure of mice. Specific tumor incidence (C and T linear one-hit).

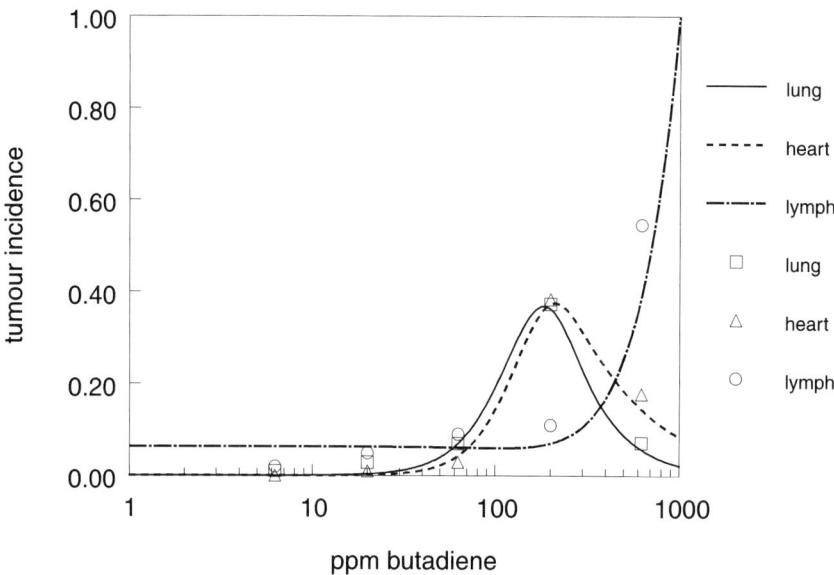

FIGURE 4. Butadiene exposure of mice. Specific tumor incidence (C and T exponent).

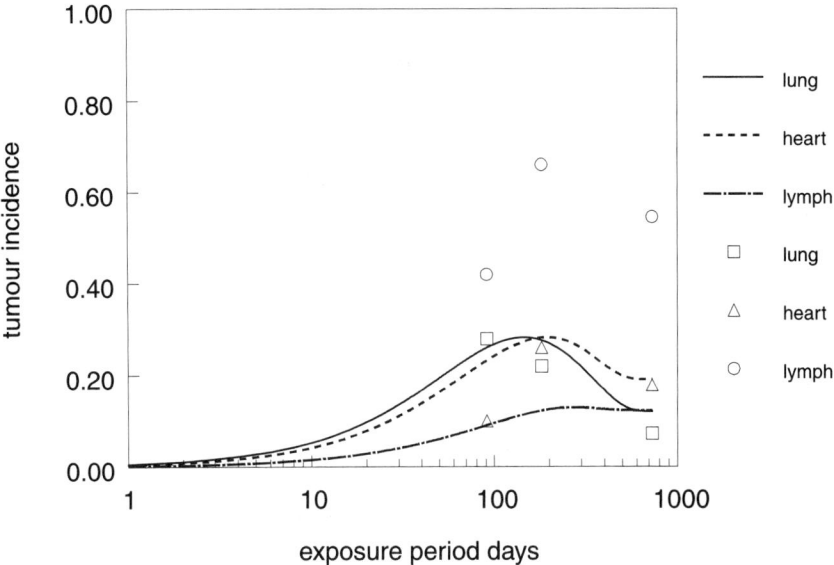

FIGURE 5. Butadiene exposure of mice to 625 ppm. Specific tumor incidence (C and T linear one-hit).

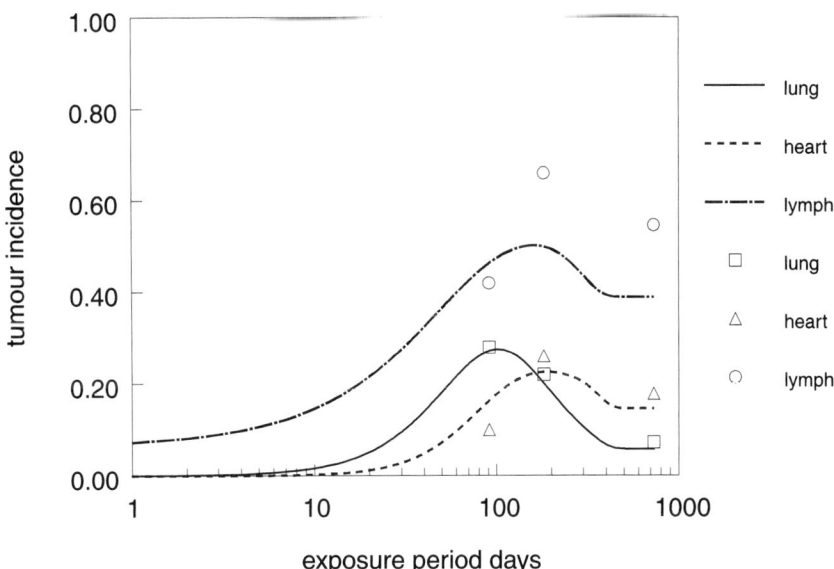

FIGURE 6. Butadiene exposure of mice to 625 ppm. Specific tumor incidence (C and T exponent).

TABLE 2.

Continuous exposure effective dose	Estimated concentration of butadiene in ppm related to the 95% UCL of risk for lung carcinoma		
	10^{-3}	10^{-4}	10^{-5}
C	0.0253	0.00253	0.0000253
$C^{2.78}$	6.596	2.814	0.515

TABLE 3.

Continuous exposure effective dose	Estimated concentration of butadiene in ppm related to the 95% UCL of risk for heart angiosarcoma		
	10^{-3}	10^{-4}	10^{-5}
C	0.0369	0.00369	0.0000369
$C^{3.06}$	9.847	4.532	0.962

TABLE 4.

Continuous exposure effective dose	Estimated concentration of butadiene in ppm related to the 95% UCL of risk for malignant lymphoma		
	10^{-3}	10^{-4}	10^{-5}
C	0.211	0.0192	0.000169
$C^{3.14}$	27.0	12.8	2.86

TABLE 5.

Exposure for 500 days effective dose	Estimated concentration of butadiene in ppm related to the 95% UCL of risk for lung carcinoma		
	10^{-3}	10^{-4}	10^{-5}
$C \cdot T_{exp}$	0.0481	0.00481	0.0000481
$C^{2.61} \cdot T_{exp}^{1.81}$	5.76	2.32	0.377

TABLE 6.

Exposure for 500 days effective dose	Estimated concentration of butadiene in ppm related to the 95% UCL of risk for heart angiosarcoma		
	10^{-3}	10^{-4}	10^{-5}
$C \cdot T_{exp}$	0.0786	0.00786	0.0000786
$C^{2.97} \cdot T_{exp}^{2.36}$	10.1	4.564	0.930

TABLE 7.

Exposure for 500 days effective dose	Estimated concentration of butadiene in ppm related to the 95% UCL of risk for malignant lymphoma		
	10^{-3}	10^{-4}	10^{-5}
$C \cdot T_{exp}$	0.211	0.0192	0.000169
$C^{2.97} \cdot T_{exp}^{2.36}$	27.0	12.8	2.86

based on a linear effective dose concept, and that the estimated exposure levels related to a specified risk on the basis of an exponential effective dose concept are very close to, or within, the experimental range.

DISCUSSION

Evaluation of the Simulation of the Observed Specific Tumor Incidence

This paper shows that it is well possible to reliably simulate the observed specific tumor incidence over time of a chronic rodent inhalation study with a high variation in mortality between the dose groups. This was mainly possible because:

- A separate analysis was made for general mortality and specific tumor mortality that was independent of survival (Kaplan-Meier tumor probability) as a function of the effective dose.
- The effective dose was assumed to be related to an exponential function of exposure concentration and exposure period.
- The specific tumor rate was estimated as the derivative of the Kaplan-Meier tumor probability, divided by the probability of being tumor free, to the observation time.
- The observed specific tumor incidence was simulated by integrating the product of survival and specific tumor rate over the observation period.

The model estimate did not fit very well in the case of a linear effective dose concept related to the product of just the exposure concentration and exposure period. This is easy to observe by comparing FIGURES 1, 3, and 5 (effective dose C or $C \cdot T$) with FIGURES 2, 4, and 6 (effective dose C^X or $C^X \cdot T^Y$). In the case of an effective dose on the basis of C or $C \cdot T$, the specific observed tumor incidence estimate was generally too high at lower dose levels, and too low at higher dose levels, in comparison with the observed specific tumor incidence. In the case of an effective dose on the basis of C^X or $C^X \cdot T^Y$, the estimate of the specific tumor incidence showed an excellent fit with the actual data. Thus, the exponential model of the effective dose is to be preferred for an appropriate model description.

Influence of the Effective Dose Concept on the Estimated Concentration Related to Regulatory Risk Limit Values

The choice of model for the effective dose is quite important for interpolation or extrapolation of the experimental data to dose levels related to regulatory risk-limit values, such as permissible lifetime risks of 10^{-3}, 10^{-4} or 10^{-6}. In the section *Dose Levels Related to Specified Risk Limits*, the tables provide estimated dose levels related to permissible lifetime risks as upper 95% confidence limits on the basis of linear and exponential models for the effective dose. In the case of the exponential model, the dose level estimates are within or close to one order of magnitude of the experimental dose range. In the case of the linear model of the effective dose, however, the estimated dose levels are all far below the experimental dose rate. Because of the better fit of the exponential model for the effective dose, it is to be preferred for estimating dose levels in relation to regulatory limit values.

The estimated butadiene levels in relation to specified risk limits in this paper differ from the estimates of Dankovic *et al.*[4] Dankovic *et al.* did not include dose groups above 200 ppm, because of saturation of the metabolism of butadiene at higher dose levels. Because the incidence of malignant lymphoma was strongly increased at 625 ppm, and because it was the main cause of death at 625 ppm, the higher dose levels were also included in this paper.

The Effective Dose Concept in Mice as a Model for Epidemiology Studies

In epidemiology studies, generally the cumulative dose $C \cdot T$ is used as the effective dose concept. The specific tumor response, at a cumulative butadiene dose of 20,000 ppm × days was estimated for the NTP-mice. In order to make a comparison with general epidemiology studies feasible, specific tumor incidence was simulated for an observation period of 676 days, at which 30% mortality occurred in the mice cohort. The cumulative dose of 20,000 ppm × days involved of the following exposure scenarios:

- 800 ppm, 25 exposure days.
- 400 ppm, 50 exposure days.
- 200 ppm, 100 exposure days.
- 100 ppm, 200 exposure days.
- 50 ppm, 400 exposure days.

TABLE 8. Simulation of malignant lymphoma incidence following the exponential dose concept $C^{3.5} \cdot T^{0.96}$

	Malignant lymphoma in B6C3F1 mice			
Butadiene exposure ppm	Exposure duration days	Total tumor incidence	Additional tumor incidence	Relative risk
800	25	0.4373	0.3745	6.97
400	50	0.1406	0.07788	2.24
200	100	0.07646	0.01372	1.22
100	200	0.06509	0.002348	1.04
50	400	0.06314	0.0003996	1.006
0	0	0.06274	0	1

The total and additional specific tumor incidence and the relative risk for malignant lymphoma in mice with these exposure scenarios after an observation period of 676 days was simulated on the basis of the exponential effective dose concept (see TABLE 8).

From this table it is easy to see that, at the same cumulative butadiene exposure dose, the response for the different tumor endpoints may be quite different. High exposures of short duration seem to be more effective in causing malignant lymphoma in the case of butadiene exposure, than long-term low-level exposure.

This is a very important observation with respect to epidemiologic studies. Epidemiologists are accustomed to use exposure level times and exposure duration as a general effective dose measure. In case of butadiene exposure of mice it is obvious that cumulative dose (linear effective dose concept) is not the appropriate measure for effective dose, especially for the malignant lymphoma endpoint.

Using cumulative dose $C \cdot T$ as a linear effective dose concept resulted in the second NTP butadiene inhalation study into:

- a severe flattening of the dose response relationship, and
- conservative extrapolation to extremely low safe exposure levels at regulatory risk limit values,

in comparison with an exponential effective dose concept. A flat dose response relationship (incidence related to square root of cumulative exposure) was estimated for leukemia death in butadiene exposed workers.[5]

Recommendation for Effective Dose

The observed specific tumor incidence in mice exposed to butadiene could be well simulated by means of the following effective dose concept:

$$\text{Effective Dose} = C^N T^M,$$

with C in mg/m^3, $N > 1$, $M \geq 1$, and I in days.

In the experimental exposure of mice to butadiene the concentration was kept constant during the exposure period. However, in epidemiologic studies workers are exposed to variable TWA eight hour levels of exposure during their working life. In this connection it might be worthwhile to use the following general equation for estimation of the effective dose in industrial cohort mortality studies:

$$Effective\ Dose = \int_0^X C(T)^N dT^M$$

$$Effective\ Dose = \int_0^X M \times C(T)^N T^{M-1} dT.$$

It might not be easy to estimate the exponents N and M, but it should be possible to explore which values for these exponents provide an optimum fit to a regression analysis of specific tumor mortality on effective dose by means of the multiplicative hazard model in a cohort mortality study.[6]

REFERENCES

1. NTP. 1993. Toxicology and carcinogenesis studies of 1,3-butadiene (CAS NO. 106-99-0) in B6C3F1 mice (inhalation studies). National Toxicology Program, Technical Report Series No. 434.
2. GART, J.J., D. KREWSKI, P.N. LEE, R.E. TARONE & J. WAHRENDORF. 1986. Chapter 6. Model fitting. In Statistical Methods in Cancer Research Volume III. The design and analysis of long term animal experiments. 107–145. IARC Scientific Publications No. 79.
3. DEWANJI, A., D. KREWSKI & M.J. GODDARD, 1993. A Weibull model for the estimation of tumorigenic potency. Biometrics 49: 367–377.
4. DANKOVIC, D.A., R.J. SMITH, L.T. STAYNER & A.J. BAILER. 1993. Time-to-tumour risk assessment for 1,3-butadiene based on exposure of mice to low doses by inhalation. In Butadiene and Styrene: Assessment of Health Hazards. 335–344. IARC Scientific Publications No. 127
5. SATHIAKUMAR, N., E. DELZELL, M. HOVINGA, M. MACALUSO, J.A. JULIAN, R. LARSON, P. COLE & D.C.F. MUIR. 1998. Mortality from cancer and other causes of death among synthetic rubber workers. Occupational Environmental Medicine 55, 230–235.
6. BRESLOW, N.E. & N.E. DAY. 1987. Fitting models to grouped data.Statistical In Methods in Cancer Research Volume II, The design and the analysis of cohort studies, Chapter 4. 119–176. IARC Scientific Publications No. 82.

Uncertainty in Estimating Exposure Using a Toxicokinetic Model

The Example of 2,3,7,8-Tetrachlorodibenzo-*p*-Dioxin

ALBERTO SALVAN,[a,b] KARL THOMASETH,[b] PAOLA BORTOT,[c] AND NICOLA SARTORI[c]

[b]*Institute of Systems Science and Biomedical Engineering (LADSEB-CNR), National Research Council, Corso Stati Uniti 4, 35127 Padova, Italy*

[c]*Department of Statistics, University of Padova, via San Fracesco 33, 35121 Padova, Italy*

ABSTRACT: This paper deals with sources of uncertainty in the use of a minimal physiological toxicokinetic model to obtain dose estimates for a dose-response analysis of cancer in an occupational cohort. Toxicokinetic models make it possible to construct exposure parameters that are more closely related to the individual dose than traditional measures of exposures to toxic agents. However, the process introduces a wide array of sources of uncertainty. Selecting a model structure to describe the kinetics of a toxic agent implies necessarily making simplifications and assumptions that influence the range of applicability of the model. Once a model has been selected, the value of certain model parameters (constants) must be assigned, for example, from anthropometric data. The question then arises of how sensitive the model predictions are to variations in the values of these constants. Other model parameters, typically those describing the kinetics of the agent, are next estimated from actual data. There may be limitations in the data concerning, for example, sparseness (too few observations per subject) or missing values. The methods used for parameter estimation carry their own set of assumptions that need to be appropriate to the situation at hand. In summary, the dioxin example is used to characterize the sources of uncertainty at different levels, such as model structure, methods and data used for parameter estimation, estimation of occupational exposure, and imputation of missing values in exposure indices derived from the kinetic model.

INTRODUCTION

This papers deals with sources of uncertainty in the use of a kinetic model for 2,3,7,8-tetrachlorodibenzo-*p*-dioxin (TCDD) for dose-response analyses in an occupational cohort. Attention is restricted to a minimal physiological toxicokinetic (MPTK) model. The scope of the model is the construction of individual exposure indices in the presence of arbitrarily complex temporal patterns of TCDD intake. *Minimal* models can be contrasted with statistical models on one hand and with physiological models on the other.

[a]Address for correspondence: Alberto Salvan, Ph.D., LADSEB-CNR, Corso Stati Uniti 4, 35127 Padova, Italy. +39-049-829-5771 (voice); +39-049-829-5763 (fax).
e-mail: salvan@ladseb.pd.cnr.it

Statistical regression models provide a black-box description of TCDD kinetics, generally assuming a fixed halflife for TCDD. Additional covariates account for deviations from the fixed halflife model.[1–3]

Physiological models provide a mechanistic description of the network of biochemical and biophysical processes related to TCDD and characteristically require a large number of parameters.[4–6] Animal experimental data are often used to identify these models since adequate data from humans are generally difficult to obtain.

Minimal models provide a concise and selective description of underlying physiological processes and contain a small number of parameters that can be estimated from human data. A minimal physiological toxicokinetic model for TCDD has been recently proposed for the estimation of occupational exposure.[7,8] This model permits the reconstruction of long-term variations in TCDD serum concentrations from which exposure indices can be derived. The modeling procedure is based on the following steps: (1) estimation of TCDD kinetic parameters, (2) estimation of the rate of occupational intake of TCDD, and (3) application of the kinetic model to obtain TCDD dose estimates for dose-response analyses.

In this paper we focus on evaluating sources of uncertainty that can be identified in the overall process of model selection, parameter estimation, estimation of occupational exposure, and calculation of exposure indices for dose-response analyses. For each source of uncertainty we discuss its potential impact and possible ways to account for it.

BACKGROUND

We begin by briefly reviewing the MPTK model for TCDD and our previous work on parameter estimation, estimation of occupational exposure and calculation of exposure indices (for a detailed account see Ref. 8).

Subjects

Estimation of TCDD kinetic parameters was carried out on a set of observations with repeated measures of serum TCDD taken in Vietnam Veterans (Ranch Hand data[9] and data from an unexposed reference group).

Estimation of the rate of occupational intake of TCDD was carried out on a subsample of 253 male workers at chemical plants from the NIOSH cohort[10,11] for whom a single measure of serum TCDD was available, usually taken long after termination of employment.

The MPTK model was then applied to the full NIOSH cohort to obtain TCDD dose estimates. The cohort consists of 5172 male workers employed at 12 chemical plants in the United States. In this cohort there are missing values for work histories, body heights, or for body weights. All of these pieces of information are required to run the MPTK model.

MPTK Modeling of TCDD

The toxicokinetic model of TCDD in humans proposed in Reference 7, and developed in Reference 8 is based on minimal physiological assumptions that allow direct estimation of most model parameters. In particular, the model is based on the assumption of a dynamic equilibrium in TCDD concentration between various body lipid compartments (blood, liver, and adipose tissue), with a fixed fractional clearance rate due to hepatic TCDD degradation. Estimates for total lipid compartment volumes and fractional liver lipid content are obtained by means of anthropometric formulæ. These involve fixed constants, as well as body mass (modeled as a time-varying process depending on age), to account for long-term variations that affect TCDD elimination from the body. Daily TCDD intake is assumed to be proportional to body weight and is described as the sum of a fixed basal exposure due to background sources such as food intake, and a time-varying occupational exposure depending on the work history in TCDD exposed jobs.

We review the simplified version of the model[8] that describes TCDD kinetics in adults. Assuming a constant body height, the model equations depend only on the body mass index (BMI) and on its time variation. All quantities are normalized with respect to body weight. In particular, the average weight (in grams) of adipose tissue per Kg BW are calculated from $v_{adipose}(t) = 1000(f_{pf1} BMI(t) - f_{pf2})$, where $BMI(t)$ is expressed in Kg/m^2 and $f_{pf1} = 0.01264$, $f_{pf2} = 0.13305$ represent constants for calculating the fraction of percent body fat.[12] Liver weight (v_{liver}, g/Kg) is calculated from: $v_{liver} = f_{vl}(1000 - v_{adipose})$, with $f_{vl} = 0.0311$ representing the fraction of lean body mass.[13] Finally, the mass of other tissues (v_{other}, g/Kg) is calculated from: $v_{other} = 1000 - v_{adipose} - v_{liver}$.

The actual total distribution volume per Kg BW (tlv, g/Kg) of TCDD is represented by lipids, and is calculated for the above tissue compartments according to Man,[13] $tlv = f_{la} v_{adipose} + f_{ll} v_{liver} + f_{lo} v_{other}$, where $f_{la} = 0.8$, $f_{ll} = 0.069$, and $f_{lo} = 0.022$ represent the fraction of lipid content in the above tissues. The distribution volume of the liver is, $lv_{liver} = f_{ll} v_{liver}$.

Elimination of TCDD due to liver degradation is assumed proportional to the amount present in the liver with proportionality factor k_f.

Daily intake per Kg BW of TCDD is represented as the sum of background exposure, characterized by a parameter *input* (pg/Kg/day), and by a term proportional to the exposure time curve derived from the individual work history:

$$intake(t) = input + exposure \, u_{exp}(t, \mathbf{p}_w), \qquad (1)$$

where *exposure* (pg/Kg/day) is the occupational exposure level (assumed to be identical for all exposed jobs) and $u_{exp}(t, \mathbf{p}_w)$ is the piecewise constant exposure function, with values of 1 if the job at time t was exposed to TCDD and 0 otherwise. The vector $\mathbf{p}_w$ represents the information relating to individual work history.

Defining $x(t)$ as the average TCDD amount per Kg BW (pg/Kg), the TCDD kinetic model is described by the dynamic equations

$$\frac{dx(t)}{dt} = -\left(k_f \frac{lv_{liver}(t)}{tlv(t)} + \frac{dBMI(t)/dt}{BMI(t)} \right) x(t) + intake(t) \qquad (2)$$

$$x(t_0) = ladj(t_0) tlv(t_0) \qquad (3)$$

$$ladj(t) = x(t)/tlv(t), \qquad (4)$$

where (3) represents the initial condition at time of hire t_0, with $ladj(t_0)$ (ppt) the lipid-adjusted serum TCDD concentration; and (4) represents the predicted lipid-adjusted serum TCDD concentration, $ladj(t)$ (ppt), at time t.

It can be observed from (2) that relative variations of body mass over time contribute to TCDD kinetics and determine variations in TCDD concentrations independently of liver elimination. Moreover, differences in adipose tissue become the major source of variation in TCDD kinetics among individuals and within an individual over time, since adipose tissue in humans displays a much larger variation than liver volume.

The TCDD kinetic model is completed by describing the time course of *BMI*, which was found to be suitably expressed as a function of age.[8] In particular, time variations of *BMI* were expressed as a linear function of age according to the model

$$\frac{dBMI}{dt} = \alpha_{BMI} t + \beta_{BMI}. \qquad (5)$$

This yields the time course

$$BMI(t) = BMI(t_0) + \frac{\alpha_{BMI}}{2}(t^2 - t_0^2) + \beta_{BMI}(t - t_0), \qquad (6)$$

where $BMI(t_0)$ is the individual body mass index measured at the time of hire, and $\alpha_{BMI} = -3.76 \times 10^{-3} \pm 0.9 \times 10^{-3}$ ($\pm$SE) (Kg/m^2/year^2), and $\beta_{BMI} = 0.269 \pm 0.04$ (Kg/m^2/year) were estimated from the subgroup of chemical plant workers with more than one *BMI* measure available.

In summary, the complete list of model parameters and constants is: $\theta = [k_f,$ *input*, *exposure*, $ladj(t_0), BMI(t_0), \mathbf{p}_w, \alpha_{BMI}, \beta_{BMI}, f_{pf1}, f_{pf2}, f_{vl}, f_{la}, f_{ll}, f_{lo}]$. Numerical values for these parameters were obtained as follows: k_f was estimated by using the Ranch Hand Veterans data; α_{BMI} and β_{BMI} were estimated from the NIOSH subcohort *BMI* data; *input* and *exposure* were estimated from the NIOSH subcohort serum TCDD concentrations data; $ladj(t_0)$ was set to the mean value among an unexposed group;[11] $BMI(t_0)$ was measured (or imputed if missing) for a single individual with known work history, $\mathbf{p}_w$; and the parameters of the anthropometric formulæ $f_{pf1}, f_{pf2}, f_{vl}, f_{la}, f_{ll}$, and f_{lo} were taken from other studies.[12,13] A summary of the MPTK model parameters is provided in TABLE 1. Individualization of the above parameters to the *i*th subject are denoted by using superscript *i*, for example, θ^i.

Computation of Exposure Indices

Given an individual work history for the *i*th subject, the corresponding simulated time course of TCDD serum lipids concentration, $ladj(t|\theta^i)$, is obtained. A cumulative exposure index for the *i*th subject computed at T (time at risk), $D_i(T; \pi)$, is computed as a weighted integral of the TCDD plasma concentration profile[14]

$$D_i(T;\pi) = \int_{t_0}^{T} f(T - t, \pi) ladj(t|\theta^i) dt \qquad (7)$$

where $f(T - t, \pi)$ is a weighting function parameterized by π: for example, (1) the unweighted cumulative exposure with $f(\tau, \pi) = 1$, and (2) the lagged cumulative exposure with $f(\tau, \pi) = 1$ if $\tau \geq \pi$, and $f(\tau, \pi) = 0$ if $\tau < \pi$.

Sensitivities of Exposure Indices

Sensitivity analysis is an important component of the evaluation of uncertainty. For this purpose we quantify variations in computed indices with respect to variations of a specific assigned model parameter θ_j as:

TABLE 1. Summary of parameters used in the MPTK model for TCDD

Parameter	Description	Source
		Estimated from
k_f	liver elimination constant	Ranch Hand
input	background exposure	Ranch Hand
exposure	occupational exposure	NIOSH subcohort
α_{BMI}	quadratic coefficient in BMI model	NIOSH subcohort
β_{BMI}	linear coefficient in BMI model	NIOSH subcohort
		Input Data
$BMI(t_0)$	BMI at hire	NIOSH cohort
$\mathbf{p}_w$	work history	NIOSH cohort
		Assigned
$ladj(t_0)$	serum TCDD at hire	7 ppt (Ref. 11)
f_{pf1}	constant in fraction of percent body fat	0.01264 (Ref. 12)
f_{pf2}	constant in fraction of percent body fat	0.13305 (Ref. 12)
f_{vl}	fraction of lean body mass for liver	0.0311 (Ref. 13)
f_{la}	fraction of lipids in adipose tissue	0.8 (Ref. 13)
f_{ll}	fraction of lipids in liver	0.069 (Ref. 13)
f_{lo}	fraction of lipids in other tissues	0.022 (Ref. 13)

$$\frac{\partial D_i(T;\pi)}{\partial \theta_j^i} = \int_{t_0}^{T} f(T-t,\pi)\frac{\partial ladj(t|\theta^i)}{\partial \theta_j^i}dt. \quad (8)$$

To compare the sensitivities of the exposure index to several parameters it is convenient to use the logarithmic derivative defined by

$$\frac{\partial \log D_i(T;\pi)}{\partial \log \theta_j^i} = \frac{\partial D_i(T;\pi)}{\partial \theta_j^i}\frac{\theta_j^i}{D_i(T;\pi)}, \quad (9)$$

which quantifies the percentage variation in the exposure index relative to percentage variation in the parameters.

DEALING WITH SOURCES OF UNCERTAINTY

Model Structure

The purpose of a model is to provide a simplified description of reality, one with useful predictive abilities however. Oversimplification may negatively affect the predictive abilities of a model. In the MPTK model, the choice of the time scale that describes the TCDD dynamics is such that short-term phenomena are not considered, thereby restricting the use of the model for long-term predictions. However,

TABLE 2. Comparison of apparent halflife of TCDD with results of Michalek *et al.* (see Ref. 9) for different body weights (height = 170 cm)

Body weight (Kg)	Percent body fat[a]	Serum TCDD halflife (years)	
		Reference 9	this study
70	17.3	7.78	7.68
80	21.7	8.87	9.85
90	26.1	10.03	12.3

[a]Percent body fat, $1.264 \times BMI - 13.305$ (Ref. 12).

phenomena such as liver sequestration or TCDD binding, which are not accounted for by the MPTK model, may be relevant to long-term kinetics.[15] Their omission from the model might produce biased predictions, although we did not observe this.[8]

One way to account for uncertainty in the model structure is to compare the model predictions with those obtained with different models. For this purpose we used the statistical mixed-effects model due to Michalek *et al.*, which describes TCDD elimination rate in the Ranch Hand data as a linear function of individual percent body fat, change in percent body fat, and age.[9] Under certain conditions (constant percent body fat over time and zero TCDD *intake*) one can compare the apparent TCDD halflives for the two models. TABLE 2 shows that, within the conditions defined above, there is good agreement between the two approaches.

Liver accumulation of TCDD may be less relevant in the range of concentrations encountered in the Ranch Hand group. However, it may be of importance for a sizable portion of the NIOSH data that display higher levels of TCDD.[8] There is, nevertheless, some evidence that human hepatocytes may be less sensitive than rat hepatocytes to the protein-inducing effect of TCDD.[16]

Anthropometric formulæ were used to compute TCDD distribution volumes in the kinetic model.[12] These formulæ were derived for young adults and their use in older age groups (represented in the NIOSH cohort) may be affected by error. One way to deal with the arbitrariness of these formulæ is to evaluate the sensitivity of the quantities of interest derived from the model (such as TCDD dose estimates) to variations in the parameter values of the anthropometric formulæ (see below).

Estimation of Kinetic Parameters (Ranch Hand Data)

Estimation Methods

In classical pharmacokinetic studies, parameters are estimated at the individual level after administering a known test dose and on the basis of several repeated measurements on the compound of interest. These conditions are not met by the Ranch Hand data for TCDD, both because there is lack of information on intake due to exposure and because the complexity and cost of dioxin assays preclude the availability of data with frequent repeated measures of TCDD. Model parameters were estimated at the population level using different approaches.

Nonlinear Weighted Least Squares. We first ignored all interindividual variability (naive pooled data approach) assuming that model parameters k_f and *input* were the same for all individuals. Interindividual variability of TCDD clearance is, therefore, attributed to changes in body mass index alone. We applied nonlinear weighted-least-squares (NWLS) with several weighting schemes, and a log-transformation of the data. The results proved to be sensitive to these choices. There was no significant information on measurement error to provide guidance in choosing a weighting scheme. However, based on model predictions and distribution of residuals, a log-transformation of the data was preferable.

Nonlinear Mixed Effects Approach. To assess possible interindividual variability of TCDD kinetics, we considered a nonlinear mixed-effects (NLME) model. Parameter estimation was carried out only with log-transformed data and was based on linearization of the model predictions (model output) for propagating the variability of the random effects as considered elsewhere.[17] In particular, we assumed the following model for the fractional clearance parameter

$$k_f(i) = k_f + e_{k_f}(i), \qquad e_{k_f}(i) \sim \mathcal{N}(0, \sigma_{k_f}^2), \tag{10}$$

where i represents the ith subject, k_f is the population mean, and $\sigma_{k_f}^2$ is the unknown variance of the random effect. For measurement noise, the following model was assumed for the log-transformed data

$$z_{ij} = \log ladj(t_j|\theta^j) + \varepsilon_i(t_j), \qquad \varepsilon_i(t_j) \sim \mathcal{N}(0, \sigma_\varepsilon^2), \tag{11}$$

where $z_{i,j}$ represents the jth observation of the logarithm of the concentration for subject i. The fixed effects parameters k_f and *input*, and the variance of the random effects, $\sigma_{k_f}^2$ and σ_ε^2, were obtained by maximum likelihood estimation.

Bayesian Approach and Markov Chain Monte Carlo Methods. An alternative inference procedure for the TCDD kinetic model can be derived by adopting a Bayesian approach.[18] From a Bayesian perspective, all unknown quantities are random variables that are assigned a prior distribution to synthesize the *a priori* information available on the data. The prior distribution is then combined with the likelihood function through Bayes' theorem to produce a posterior distribution from which inferences are drawn about the unknown parameters. The complete hierarchical model for TCDD kinetics is specified by:

Stage 1. The intraindividual error model is given by (11).

Stage 2. The model adopted to define the interindividual variation differs from the NLME approach, and is based on the bidimensional parameter $\psi_i = [\log k_f(i), \log ladj_i(t_{i0})]$

$$\psi_i = \mu + \delta_i, \qquad \delta_i \sim \mathcal{N}(0, \Sigma), \tag{12}$$

where μ is the population mean, and δ_i represents the random effect for the ith subject. Logarithmic transformations of the parameters are used in ψ_i and for the *input* parameter, due to positivity restrictions.

Stage 3. In the third stage the prior distribution for the population parameters, $[\mu, \phi, \sigma_\varepsilon^2, \Sigma]$, is assigned, where $\phi = \log input$. We assume that parameters are independent, *a priori*, and that $\mu \sim \mathcal{N}(\eta, C)$, $\phi \sim \mathcal{N}(\alpha, \beta^2)$, $\sigma_\varepsilon^{-2} \sim \Gamma(p,q)$, where p and q are shape and scale parameters, respectively. $\Sigma^{-1} \sim W_{ishart}(\rho, R)$ where ρ is the number of degrees of freedom, and R is the dispersion matrix. Since no prior information is available on the parameters, we use flat priors. Specifically, we set $p = q = a = 0$, $\rho = 2$, $\eta = 0$, $\beta = 10$, $C = \text{diag}[100,100]$, and $R = \text{diag}[25,25]$, where diag indicates a diagonal matrix.

For the model defined by Stages 1–3, the posterior distribution cannot be written in closed form, since it is known only up to a proportionality constant. To overcome this difficulty we employ Markov chain Monte Carlo (MCMC) techniques.[19,20] The basic idea of these Monte Carlo methods is to simulate a Markov chain whose stationary distribution is the target distribution, in our case the posterior distribution of the model parameters.

Results

Parameter estimates obtained by the three estimation methods outlined above are reported in TABLE 3. All estimates were obtained by log-transformation of the data. An additional log-transformation of the parameters was used in the Bayesian MCMC analysis (preliminary results). The estimates obtained with the NWLS and NLME approaches are very similar. Those obtained by using the MCMC appear to be shifted towards smaller values, more so for the background *input* parameter. Nevertheless, the estimation of the parameter k_f appears to be only slightly sensitive to the choice of the estimation method.

Mechanisms for Selection of Observations

Some selection criteria were operating in the data used to estimate parameters of the MPTK model for TCDD: follow-up data for the exposed Ranch Hand observations were available only if the 1987 serum TCDD level was greater than 10 ppt. A sample of RH veterans with 1987 serum TCDD less than 10 ppt (the unexposed reference group) was offered an additional measure in 1992, however this was not based on additional selection criteria. Within our analysis, based on the MPTK model, it was not possible to account for the complex sampling mechanism that had generated the data. Thus, the possibility of bias arises. We have already shown (TABLE 2) that the apparent TCDD halflife predicted by our model agrees closely with values obtained from the statistical model by Michalek *et al.*[9] It is interesting to note that Michalek *et al.*, were able to account for the selection criteria in the exposed group through a data-conditioning approach. It is, therefore, possible that the bias in our analysis due to omitting the sampling mechanism may be small.

Undetectable Values

A few observations (12) with undetectable levels of serum TCDD were excluded from our analysis. These interval-censored observations with low levels of serum TCDD would have provided additional information on the background input parameter. However, the detection limit for the lipid-adjusted serum TCDD varies across measurements. Given the size of the problem, we simply chose to discard these 12 observations.

TABLE 3. Parameter estimates for k_f (days^{-1}) and *input* (pg/Kg/day) obtained from various methods

Method	k_f	95% CI	input	95% CI
NWLS	0.0218	0.020–0.024	0.1139	0.050–0.178
NLME	0.0220	0.020–0.024	0.1251	0.071–0.179
MCMC	0.0203	0.019–0.023	0.0077	0–0.067

Estimation of Occupational Exposure (NIOSH Subcohort)

The occupational intake rate for TCDD was estimated by applying the MPTK model to the NIOSH subcohort of 253 workers with a single measure of TCDD. In the model we fixed k_f to the value estimated from the Ranch Hand data based on the nonlinear mixed-effects model and log-transformed data. We estimated the occupational *exposure* and background *input* by means of linear regression. To account for *BMI* changes over time we used the model described in (5) and (6). The resulting parameter estimates were sensitive to data transformation and the model fit showed a higher dispersion than with the Ranch Hand data.[8] On the basis of model predictions and residual plots, we selected those estimates that, based on log-transformed data, yielded an occupational exposure rate of 232.7 pg/Kg/day (95% CI 192, 273). The estimate of background *input* at 0.45 pg/Kg/day had to be adjusted to maintain a prediction of 7 ppt,[11] the average value observed in a group of unexposed workers (*input* = 0.293 pg/Kg/day). The need for this adjustment may indicate that the single available data point may not have provided sufficient information. However, the need to estimate background input precisely is obviated by the results of sensitivity analysis (see below). The main source of uncertainty in estimating occupational exposure is the assumption that the occupational exposure intake of TCDD was identical across exposed jobs, given that a job-exposure matrix was not available. This results in nondifferential (independent of disease status) misclassification of exposure. Overall, the uncertainty about the occupational exposure estimate is high, as several concurring sources of uncertainty can be identified. The kinetic parameters of the model were estimated in an overall younger population (Ranch Hand) than the NIOSH subcohort, in which TCDD measurements were taken long after termination of employment. Age differences may be related to differences in TCDD kinetics. The model anthropometric constants had also been obtained for young adults and their use in older age groups may be questionable. Sensitivity analysis, as shown below, may partially help in sorting out some of the sources of uncertainty in order to identify the more critical model parameters for the dose-response analysis.

Occupational Exposure Indices (NIOSH Cohort)

Calculation of the cumulative exposure index (7) was carried out by using the MPTK model with fixed values of the occupational *exposure*, background *input*, k_f parameters, and of the assumed TCDD concentration at hire. This step also requires knowledge of *BMI* at hire and of the complete work history for each subject.

Missing Values

The NIOSH cohort consists of 5172 male workers.[10] Some observations without a detailed work history were excluded from analysis, thus leaving 4935 individuals. Furthermore, this set includes some units with missing $BMI(t_0)$, so we can think the data set as partitioned in two blocks: one with 4049 completely observed units and another with 886 partially missing units. For this second subset we cannot obtain dose estimates since $BMI(t_0)$ is an essential input for the MPTK model. On the other hand, an analysis using only complete units can be inefficient because of the amount of information discarded. Furthermore, omitting incomplete units could bias the results, to the extent that the incompletely observed cases differ systematically from the completely observed cases. Therefore, we looked into ways to impute the missing $BMI(t_0)$ values. Multiple imputation techniques are suggested in the literature as the approach of choice, since it is then possible to take into account the uncertainty associated with the imputation itself. Traditional methods rely on simple imputation, for example, regression on available covariates (conditional means method), and do not take this uncertainty into account. The main drawback of simple imputation, besides the possibility of bias, is the artificially reduced variance of the imputed values. Multiple imputation[21,22] is a Monte Carlo approach to the analysis of incomplete data. Every missing value is replaced with $m > 1$ simulated values. Eventually, m augmented data sets are generated. Each data set consists of observed and simulated data. Standard analysis methods are then used on each of the m data sets. Estimates obtained from these analyses are then combined in order to obtain a pooled estimate that takes into account the uncertainty due to inclusion of missing data. A *missing at random* (MAR) mechanism was assumed.[21] To create imputations we use a data augmentation technique, a particular type of Gibbs sampling, that is an iterative simulation based procedure.[22] For valid inference, it is not necessary to use large values for m. The main difference between multiple imputation and the more commonly used conditional mean method is that the imputed values obtained under multiple imputation are random draws from the hypothesized distribution, whereas those obtained with the conditional means are mean values. Under multiple imputation it is therefore expected that the variability associated with the imputation process is not underestimated. For each of the m data sets, individual time-dependent exposure indices to TCDD were calculated based on the MPTK model. Relative-risk regression (Cox proportional hazard) models were used on each of the completed data sets.[23] The m estimates of Cox regression coefficients were combined by taking into account the within-imputation and the between-imputation variance, as shown in Reference 21.

An Application Example

In the NIOSH data set we imputed $BMI(t_0)$ with normal regression and with a multiple imputation multivariate normal model. The best results were obtained with the log-transformed data and the uninformative prior. First, we used a model with just the variable, *age at first employment*, that represents the age at which the *BMI* measurement was made. Then, we added other variables found to be related to the absence of $BMI(t_0)$ data: *age at last employment, duration of exposure, race, plant*, and the response variable of the proportional hazard model (*race* and *plant* are indicator variables representing, respectively, white/nonwhite race and two sets of plants that differ in fraction of missing values). Using the MPTK model with each of the imputed data sets we obtained the variable dose $D(T)$, see (**7**), for all 4935 units. The logarithm of this variable, $ldose(T)$, was then used as a time-dependent covariate in a multiplicative Cox model. Results are shown in TABLE 4 for the outcome *all cancer*. Exposure was delayed by 10 years and model terms were $ldose(T)$, *age at entry, year of entry*, and *duration of employment*.

The results show substantial differences between complete and imputed cases. Imputed values of $BMI(t_0)$ are not systematically different from the observed values. However, the work history shows a lower exposure for the group of units with missing $BMI(t_0)$. These facts lead to lower values of $D(T)$, as output from the MPTK model, for subjects of the missing group. These results may be due to an increase in risk among short-term workers.

The results show a similarity between various types and models of imputation. This is due mainly to the low fraction of missing values (lower than 18% and just on one variable), to the large sample size and to the appropriateness of the normality assumption. In this situation, normal regression imputation may perform nearly as well as multiple imputation. Furthermore, the two different models for multiple imputation give quite similar results (see footnotes b and c to TABLE 4). This means that results were not affected by predictors for absence other than age at first employment.

As a final remark, we note that there are direct methods to correct estimators for the Cox model in presence of missing covariates.[24–26] The use of these methods does, however, imply that available information about the work history of the missing units were discarded, whereas they are taken into account by the MPTK model.

Model Sensitivity Analysis

The sensitivity equations defined above can be used to evaluate the relative importance, over time, of model parameters and constants for determining the value of TCDD serum level and of its time integral (cumulative exposure). FIGURE 1 shows the time course of serum TCDD and of the cumulative exposure corresponding to a continuous occupational exposure starting at age 20 and lasting for 20 years.

TABLE 4. Estimates of the coefficient of log cumulative dose in a multiplicative Cox model with added covariates[a]

Case	Estimate	95% CI
C	0.1539	0.0387–0.2691
RI[b]	0.1736	0.0673–0.2798
RI[c]	0.1751	0.0688–0.2814
MI[b] $m = 2$	0.1740	0.0678–0.2803
MI[b] $m = 3$	0.1727	0.0666–0.2789
MI[b] $m = 5$	0.1729	0.0667–0.2790
MI[b] $m = 10$	0.1731	0.0669–0.2792
MI[c] $m = 2$	0.1736	0.0674–0.2799
MI[c] $m = 3$	0.1756	0.0693–0.2820
MI[c] $m = 5$	0.1755	0.0693–0.2818
MI[c] $m = 10$	0.1752	0.0689–0.2815

[a]*Age at entry*, *year of entry*, and *duration of employment*. 95% limits for the complete case (C), the regression imputation case (RI), and the multiple imputation case (MI), where m is the number of imputed data sets.

[b]Imputation with just *age at first employment*.

[c]Imputation with *age at first employment* and *age at last employment, duration of exposure, race, plant*, and the response variable of the proportional hazard model.

FIGURE 2 shows the corresponding logarithmic sensitivities from age 20 to age 80 for the cumulative exposure. This index seems to strongly depend on *exposure* throughout the age interval. Other parameters have an initial influence that decreases with increasing age. This is true for $BMI(t_0)$ at hire, and for the fraction $BMI(t)$, f_{pf1}, and the constant coefficient f_{pf2} used to convert to average grams of adipose tissue per Kg of body weight. Certain parameters do not initially affect the index, but they do so increasingly over time; for example, the fraction of lipid volume in the liver, f_{vl}, the fraction of lean body mass, f_{ll}, and the elimination parameter, k_f. Little or no dependence characterizes the parameters of the *BMI* model, α_{BMI} and β_{BMI}, the fraction of lipids in other tissues, f_{lo}, and the serum TCDD at hire, $ladj(t_0)$. Similar results were obtained for a short (six months) continuous exposure. These results are

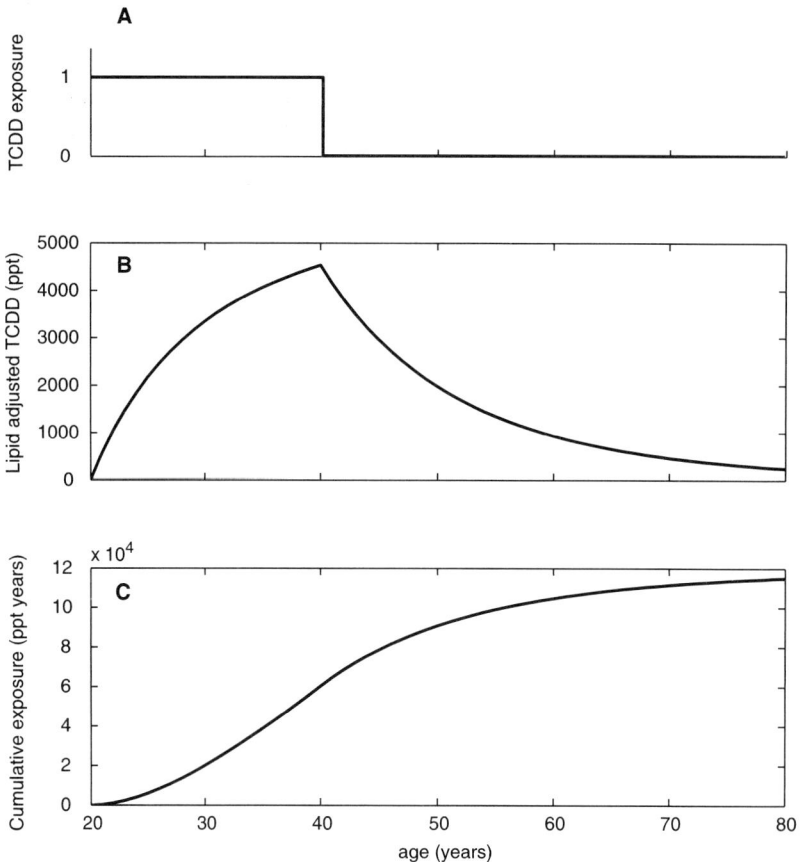

FIGURE 1. Model prediction of the time course of serum TCDD and the cumulative exposure corresponding to continuous occupational exposure starting at age 20 and lasting for 20 years. (**A**) TCDD exposure function, (**B**) lipid adjusted TCDD concentration, (**C**) cumulative exposure.

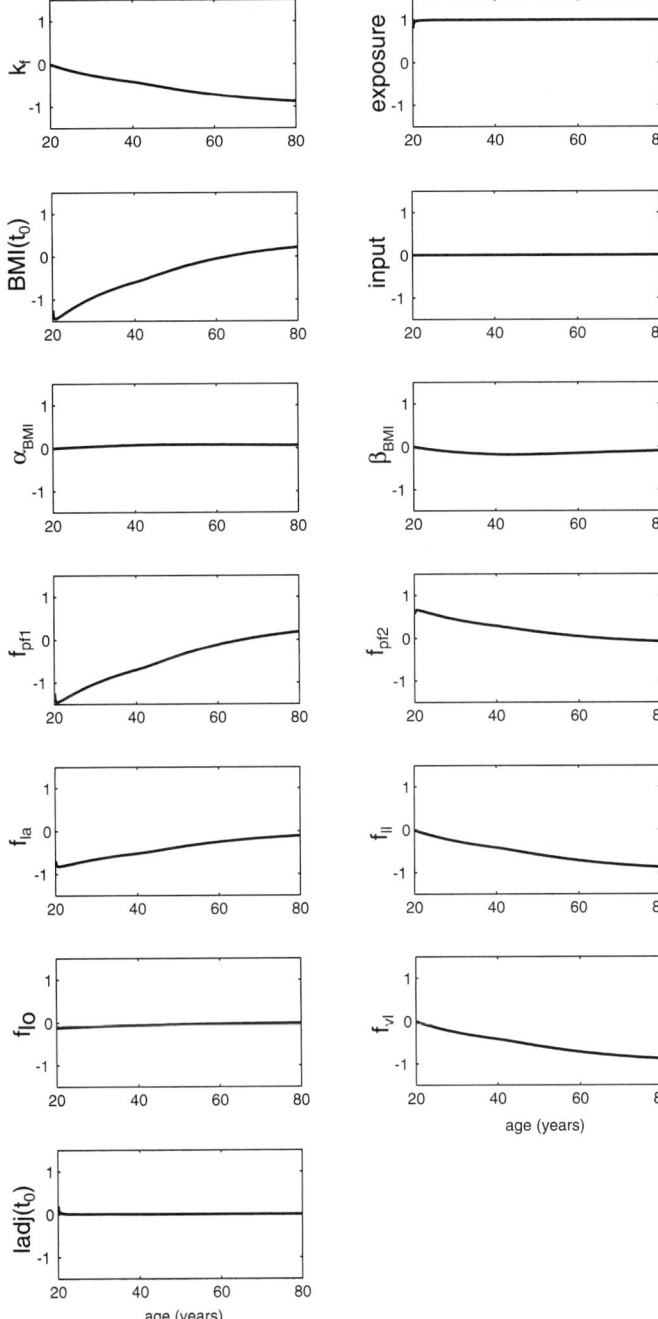

FIGURE 2. Time-dependent percentage variations in the cumulative exposure index (FIG. 1C) relative to percentage variations in the model parameters (logarithmic sensitivities, dimensionless).

useful in indicating which sources of uncertainty should receive more attention and which can actually be disregarded. For example, the occupational exposure is certainly the most important determinant of the time integral of the serum TCDD curve. For long follow up times, an increasingly important role over time is also played by k_f and some of the anthropometric constants related to the liver (f_{vl}, f_{ll}). For relatively short follow up times f_{pf1} and, less so f_{pf2}, are influential. It is clear that it seems useful to invest effort in characterizing the occupational exposure rate, in the anthropometric model, and in estimating k_f, whereas it is not necessary to try to estimate background input or the concentration of TCDD at hire more accurately. It should be noted that the results of the sensitivity analysis depend on the given model, the assigned exposure function, and the parameter values.

DISCUSSION

We have reviewed the sources of uncertainty in several aspects of toxicokinetic modeling of TCDD for occupational dose-response analysis. Uncertainty about model structure is certainly a critical step. The minimal physiological toxicokinetic model approach provides the advantage of a concise and manageable description of long-term TCDD kinetics. However, this is at the expense of lumping or disregarding processes that may be of relevance. Appropriateness of structure may also depend on the domain of use of the model: kinetic parameters were estimated from data that display a lower concentration range than that observed with occupational exposures, to which the model is applied. A comparison between model predictions and data and predictions from other models, provides a guidance on the need, if any, to further complicate the model.

Parameter estimation needs to address the limited amount of data often available (sparse data, with very few repeated measures per subject). This requires that estimation be made at the population level and not at the individual level. Comparing the results obtained from different estimation methods provides an idea of the robustness of the parameter estimates. Results obtained with NLWS, NLME, and MCMC were found to be comparable for the k_f parameter but less so for the background input parameter. (The sensitivity analysis results do, however, indicate that k_f is the more important parameter.)

Estimation of occupational exposure involved the estimation of one additional parameter (*exposure*) from the NIOSH subcohort data. Several sources of uncertainty were identified at this stage: model structure (possibly); lack of repeated measures of TCDD in the subcohort; assumption of a unique exposure level for all exposed jobs, due to the unavailability of an exposure matrix; a value for the k_f parameter, estimated on a population (Ranch Hand) that might have differed in TCDD kinetics, perhaps due to lower exposure levels than observed in the NIOSH subcohort.

Whereas nondifferential misclassification of exposure has traditionally been associated with a downward bias in risk estimates,[27] no assumptions can be made here on the direction of that bias. This is because the predicted serum TCDD is a continuous function of several variables and because of the multivariate structure of the risk estimation models in which the TCDD exposure indexes are used.[28]

The construction of time-dependent exposure indices (e.g., area under the curve of serum TCDD over time) is a straightforward step with the MPTK model, in the presence of any arbitrarily complex pattern of work histories (as a series of exposed and unexposed jobs). We discussed a missing value problem that originated because some of the data did not have information on *BMI* at hire, a requirement for obtaining exposure indices from the MPTK model. We have provided evidence on the impact of missing values on risk estimates, thus showing that imputation of missing values is an additional tool in evaluating uncertainty.

ACKNOWLEDGMENTS

This research was partially supported by NIOSH/CDC, Cincinnati, USA, and by a grant from the Italian Ministero del Lavoro e della Previdenza Sociale.

REFERENCES

1. WOLFE, W.H. *et al.* 1994. Determinants of TCDD halflife in veterans of operation Ranch Hand. J. Toxicol. Environ. Health **41:** 481–488.
2. FLESCH-JANYS, D. *et al.* 1996. Elimination of polychlorinated dibenzo-*p*-dioxins and dibenzofurans in occupationally exposed persons. J. Toxicol. Environ. Health **47:** 363–378.
3. OTT, M.G. & A. ZOBER. 1996. Cause specific mortality and cancer incidence among employees exposed to 2,3,7,8-TCDD after a 1953 reactor accident. Occup. Environ. Med. **53:** 606–612.
4. PORTIER, C. *et al.* 1993. Ligand/receptor binding for 2,3,7,8-TCDD: Implications for risk assessment. Fundam. Appl. Toxicol. **20:** 48–56.
5. ANDERSEN, M.E. *et al.* 1993. Modeling receptor-mediated processes with dioxin: implications for pharmacokinetics and risk assessment. Risk Analysis **13:** 25–36.
6. KOHN, M.C. *et al.* 1993. A mechanistic model of the effects of dioxin on gene expression in the rat liver. Toxicol. Appl. Pharmacol. **120:** 138–154.
7. DANKOVIC, D.A. *et al.* 1995. A simplified model describing the kinetics of TCDD in humans. (Abstract). Toxicologist **15:** 272.
8. THOMASETH, K. & A. SALVAN. 1998. Estimation of occupational exposure to 2,3,7,8-tetrachlorodibenzo-*p*-dioxin (TCDD) using a minimal physiological toxicokinetic model. Environ. Health Persp. **106**(S2): 743–753. Erratum. Health Persp. 1998 **106**(S4): CP2.
9. MICHALEK, J.E. *et al.* 1996. Pharmacokinetics of TCDD in veterans of operation Ranch Hand: 10-year follow-up. J. Toxicol. Environ. Health **47:** 209–220. Erratum. J. Toxicol. Environ. Health 1997 **52:** 557–558.
10. FINGERHUT, M.A. *et al.* 1991. Cancer mortality in workers exposed to 2,3,7,8-tetrachlorodibenzo-p-dioxin. N. Engl. J. Med. **324:** 212–218.
11. PIACITELLI, L.A. et al. 1992. Serum levels of PCDDs and PCDFs among workers exposed to 2,3,7,8-TCDD contaminated chemicals. Chemosphere **25:** 251–254.
12. KNAPIK, J.J., R.L. BURSE & J.A. VOGEL. 1983. Height, weight, percent body fat, and indices of adiposity for young men and women entering the U.S. army. Aviation Space and Environ. Med. **54:** 223–231.
13. ICRP—INTERNATIONAL COMMISSION ON RADIOLOGICAL PROTECTION. 1975. The Reference Man. Report No.23. Pergamon Press, Oxford.
14. THOMAS, D.C. 1983. Statistical methods for analyzing effects of temporal patterns of exposure on cancer risks. Scand. J. Work Environ. Health **9:** 353–366.

15. CARRIER, G., R.C. BRUNET & J. BRODEUR. 1995. Modeling of the toxicokinetics of polychlorinated dibenzo-p-dioxins and dibenzofurans in mammalians, including humans. I Nonlinear distribution of PCDD/PCDF body burden between liver and adipose tissues. Toxicol. Appl. Pharmacol. **131:** 253–266.
16. SCHRENK, D. *et al.* 1995. Induction of Cyp1A and glutathione S-transferase activities by 2,3,7,8-tetrachlorodibenzo-*p*-dioxin in human hepatocyte cultures. Carcinogenesis **16:** 943–946.
17. SHEINER, L.B. 1984. The population approach to pharmacokinetic data analysis: rationale and standard data analysis methods. Drug Metab. Rev. **15:** 153–171.
18. WAKEFIELD, J.C. 1996. The Bayesian Analysis of Population Pharmacokinetic Models. J. Am. Statist. Assoc. **91:** 62–75.
19. SMITH, A.F.M. & G.O. ROBERTS. 1993. Bayesian Computation via the Gibbs Sampler and Related Markov Chain Monte Carlo. J. Roy. Statist. Soc. B **55**: 39–52.
20. GILKS, W.R., S. RICHARDSON & D.J. SPIEGELHALTER. 1995. Markov Chain Monte Carlo in Practice. Chapman and Hall, London.
21. RUBIN, D.B. 1987. Multiple Imputation for Nonresponse in Survey. Wiley, New York.
22. SCHAFER, J.L. 1997. Analysis of Incomplete Multivariate Data. Chapman and Hall, London.
23. COX, D.R. 1972. Regression models and life tables (with discussion). J. Roy. Statist. Soc. B **34:** 187–220.
24. LING, D.Y. & Z. YING. 1993. Cox regression with incomplete covariate measurements. J. Am. Statist. Assoc. **88:** 1341–1349.
25. PAIK, M.C. 1997. Multiple imputation for the Cox proportional hazard model with missing covariates. Lifetime Data Analysis **3:** 289–298.
26. PAIK, M.C. & W.-Y. TSAI. 1997. On using the Cox proportional hazard model with missing covariates. Biometrika **84:** 579–593.
27. COPELAND, K.T. *et al.* 1977. Bias due to misclassification in the estimation of relative risk. Am. J. Epidemiol. **105:** 488–495.
28. CARROLL, R.J., D. RUPPERT & L.A. STEFANSKI. 1995. Measurement Error in Nonlinear Models. Chapman and Hall, London.

Uncertainty in the Relation between Exposure to Magnetic Fields and Brain Cancer due to Assessment and Assignment of Exposure and Analytical Methods in Dose-Response Modeling

HANS KROMHOUT,[a] DANA P. LOOMIS,[b] AND ROBERT C. KLECKNER[b]

[a]*Environmental and Occupational Health Group, Department of Environmental Sciences, Wageningen University, Wageningen, The Netherlands*

[b]*Department of Epidemiology, School of Public Health, University of North Carolina, Chapel Hill, North Carolina, USA*

ABSTRACT: **Incomplete scientific knowledge ensures that, in every study, uncertainty will enter the processes of exposure estimation and exposure-response modeling. In the light of the heated debate about the health effects of magnetic fields resulting from power production and usage, we undertook a sensitivity analysis to evaluate uncertainty related to key decisions in a previous study of brain cancer and occupational exposure to magnetic fields. The findings appeared to be relatively insensitive to most variations in the methods of exposure assessment, exposure assignment, and data analysis. The results can be visualized by defining bands of uncertainty about a best-bet estimate of the association based on our original study. These bands of methodological uncertainties were similar in magnitude to the conventional 95% confidence interval, but they provide a measure of the potential range of systematic bias in the results, rather than reflecting statistical variability alone. The methodology employed here can be applied to other studies, and other researchers are encouraged to conduct sensitivity analysis in order to estimate methodological uncertainty as an alternative to statistical confidence intervals.**

INTRODUCTION

Some degree of uncertainty surrounds the three crucial phases of exposure assessment, exposure assignment, and exposure-response modeling in every epidemiologic study. The handling of these uncertainties in any phase of research can affect the study results obtained. For example, the use of different proxy measures of exposure, or different methods of applying data to estimate individual exposure can affect the assigned exposure level and its observed relationship to a biological response. Divergent strategies for building regression models can have similar consequences,

---

[a]Address for correspondence: Environmental and Occupational Health Group, Department of Environmental Sciences, Wageningen University, PO Box 238, 6700 AE Wageningen, The Netherlands. + 31 317 484147 (voice); + 31 317 485278 (fax).
   e-mail: Hans.Kromhout@staff.eoh.wau.nl

with the selection of different model forms or specification of different sets of covariates potentially giving qualitatively and quantitatively different dose-response functions.

The fact that scientific knowledge is always incomplete ensures that uncertainty will always enter the processes of exposure estimation and exposure-response modeling. Nevertheless, relatively little research has been done to identify the specific sources of these uncertainties in occupational and environmental epidemiologic studies, to describe their magnitude and effects on study findings, or to develop methods for assessing those effects. Characterization of uncertainty is generally limited to the presentation of statistical confidence intervals that reflect only the hypothetical uncertainty related to random sampling error.

Analysis of methodological uncertainty, in addition to statistical precision, can improve researchers' understanding of and ability to interpret study results. Furthermore, the ability to disentangle and predict the effects of errors in exposure assessment and data handling can aid decisions both about the allocation of resources when planning studies and about procedures for obtaining, handling, and analyzing exposure data once a study is underway. The relative importance of uncertainties in the three essential stages; exposure assessment, exposure assignment, and data analysis; is largely unknown and analyses that investigate their influence are rarely published as part of the research. Here we present a brief review of the literature on the problem and an empirical illustration using data from a recent, large study of electric utility workers.

BACKGROUND

The use of quantitative exposure data in epidemiology studies can be thought of as involving three principal phases: exposure assessment, exposure assignment, and data analysis.

Exposure assessment is the process of estimating exposure levels through measurement, modeling, and other procedures. For simplicity we refer to studies in which the units of observation are individual people, but the same concepts apply to other designs in which the units are aggregates, such as occupational groups, work areas, or communities.

The results of an exposure assessment may be used directly in dose-response analysis, if complete, relevant data are available for every person in the study. However, it is often the case that exposures cannot be measured for some individuals (as in a historical mortality study, where some workers have died by the time the study takes place). Furthermore, the assessment of exposures often does not provide complete information (as when a worker has held a series of jobs, but only the current job is measured). In these situations, and in others, procedures for exposure assignment are necessary.

By means of the process of *exposure assignment*, the results of an *exposure assessment* are used to construct a derived exposure score that is assigned to the individuals (or other types of analytical units) in an epidemiologic study.

An exposure assignment procedure may also be used to modify the assessed exposure value in order to derive a more theoretically meaningful index of risk. For example, estimates of cumulative exposure in occupational studies are usually derived by first assessing exposure intensity from environmental measurements, and then combining this information with estimates of exposure duration to assign a measure that approximates dose.

Data analysis involves the use of exposure scores and health outcome data, in combination, to estimate the association between exposure and biological responses, typically through the use of statistical models.

Clearly, the boundaries between these three phases of research are somewhat arbitrary, but the concepts are distinct and readily understood.

Uncertainty in Exposure Assessment and Assignment

Large temporal variability is intrinsic to occupational and environmental exposures and must be handled appropriately. Although large variability in exposure concentrations can lead to measurement error, with its attendant bias and imprecision, it also enables the researcher to optimize exposure assessment and consequently exposure assignment. Understanding the components of variability in exposure concentrations and knowledge of factors affecting exposure levels is crucial to this process.

The effects of random error in exposure assessment have become of interest only recently. Simple dichotomous treatment of the exposure entity (exposed or unexposed) and lack of quantitative exposure data has resulted in lack of attention to this issue. Recent work in the field of occupational exposure assessment has made the notion of an *homogeneous exposed group*[1] questionable, for instance. Data show that workers sharing the same environment and performing similar tasks were not experiencing the same exposure,[2,3] as was assumed *a priori*. This fact together with a large day-to-day variability in exposure concentrations has complicated the life of the present-day epidemiologist considerably. It has long been known that grouping strategies reduce bias, but it seems to be accompanied by decreased precision. Equations were derived that enable evaluation of different strategies to group exposure measurement data.[4-6] In recent years a few studies have been performed with prospective exposure assessment components, in which large amounts of quantitative exposure data were collected.[7,8] These studies enable simultaneous application of different strategies for exposure assessment and assignment, and they will provide insight in the uncertainty inherent in the treatment of occupational exposure data.[9,10]

As noted previously, the results of an exposure assessment may be used to derive and assign other exposure indices in order to improve the prediction of risk. Ideally, the selection of a measure for exposure should be based on scientific understanding of the toxicokinetics of the agent and the pathophysiologic processes of the health outcome under study.[11] Cumulative exposure is a derived measure of exposure with particular interest, because it is used frequently in studies of chronic diseases. The intensity, I, of an exposure multiplied by its duration, d, yields cumulative exposure. This measure can be considered a surrogate for total dose, which also depends on exposure intensity and duration. Cumulative exposure is generally an adequate predictor of risk if the metabolism of the agent and the disease process behave linearly.[11,12] To estimate cumulative exposure (CE) in occupational studies, the product of intensity and duration in a series of jobs or work environments is often summed over the career of a worker, using the equation $CE = \sum_{x} I_x d_x$.

Cumulative exposure is usually considered preferable to exposure duration alone, if information on exposure intensity is also available.[13] Nevertheless, several limitations of cumulative exposure have been pointed out, with most criticism focussing on biological assumptions that may not always be satisfied.[12,14–17] Less attention has been paid to the statistical aspects of cumulative exposure and the quality and characteristics of the intensity and duration components that constitute the input data.[18]

An often overlooked feature of cumulative exposure is that intensity and duration are given equal weight, although duration, being measured in years, is usually numerically larger than intensity, and it often has greater contrast as well. Consequently, the duration component of cumulative exposure may be dominant. This may be one explanation for the observation that disease is associated with both duration and cumulative exposure in many studies (see e.g., Refs. 7, 18, and 19). In addition, different errors may be associated with the intensity and duration components. The possibility for both random and systematic errors in measuring exposure intensity is generally acknowledged, whereas duration is assumed to be measured without error by job history records. Finkelstein[19] demonstrated, by means of simulations, that cumulative exposure could still predict risk when random, simulated intensity estimates are combined with actual, measured durations. However, it is likely that duration is also measured with error because of inaccurate or incomplete job history records.

Uncertainty in Analytical Methods

The statistical and epidemiologic literature on analytical methods is far too extensive to review here. We focus on just two issues in modeling with exposure-response data: the selection of cutpoints for categorical exposure variables, and the use of data analysis to elucidate temporal relationships between exposure and disease, as in analyses of cancer latency.

Despite criticism of the practice,[20] exposure data that are measured on a continuous scale are often analyzed in categorical form for convenience. Differences in the cutpoints used to define exposure categories are a potential source of uncertainty in comparing studies and conducting meta-analyses. Moreover, within a study, the choice of cutpoints can affect the results by influencing the probability and direction of misclassification between exposure categories.[21,22] Both attenuation and exaggeration of exposure-response relations can result from such misclassification.

Analyses that describe temporal links between exposure and disease have become a standard part of the analysis of longitudinal occupational studies of cancer and other chronic diseases. The principal purpose of these analyses is to enhance the prediction of risk by excluding exposures hypothesized to be biologically irrelevant, such as those occurring after a latent tumor is already present. However, the relevant time period is never known with certainty, consequently latent intervals are often approximated empirically, by trial and error.[23] The standard approach involves fitting an array of models in which the exposure is lagged by a varying amount or considered within moving *windows*.[23–25] This process can generate considerable uncertainty because of its ability to produce a range of results that are different, yet compatible with the data. However, whereas methods for selecting the best lag period have been considered,[26] little attention has been given to the overall contribution of exposure periods to the total uncertainty in epidemiologic studies.

ILLUSTRATION USING A STUDY OF BRAIN CANCER AND OCCUPATIONAL EXPOSURE TO MAGNETIC FIELDS

Sensitivity analyses and simulations provide a useful means for disentangling the uncertainties in exposure assessment, exposure assignment, and data analysis and for gauging their effects on study results. We applied these methods to assess the results of a large historical cohort study of electric power workers that is described in detail elsewhere.[7,27,28]

METHODS

The original study was based on a cohort of 139,000 men employed at five electric companies in the United States and followed for mortality from 1950 to 1988. About 2,800 personal measurements of work shift magnetic-field exposure were obtained on randomly selected workers[27,28] and combined with full work histories to estimate cumulative magnetic field exposures.[7]

Details of the procedures used to investigate the effects of applications of different job exposure matrices, and different ways of calculating cumulative exposure using the empirical data have already been described.[9,29] Briefly, we used Poisson regression models to describe the relationship between brain cancer and cumulative magnetic field exposure, applying an array of different methods to estimate the intensity of exposures, and to assign exposure scores to individual workers using those intensity estimates.

We first examined the effect on the exposure-response relationship of estimating intensity using six different groupings of the personal monitoring results, while using full, observed work histories to estimate individual cumulative exposure and applying the same analytical methods for each set of exposure estimates.[9] A continuous variable for magnetic field exposure was used, and regression coefficients were adjusted for age, race, social class, calendar time, and active work status.

We then fitted a second series of models, holding the job exposure matrix constant and varying the methods used to estimate individual cumulative exposure or to handle the derived cumulative exposure estimates during data analysis.[29] Cumulative exposure was estimated using all jobs, the longest-held, and the last job. We also considered exposures with four different lag periods and five time-windows, as well as five different sets of cutpoints for categorizing the exposure variable.

In this paper, we examine the combined effects of variations in exposure assessment, exposure assignment, and analytical methods by fitting models for those combinations of these elements that gave the most extreme results in the preceding analyses. A categorical magnetic field variable was used for these analyses, and covariates for age, race, social class, calendar time, and active work status were included. In previous publications,[7,29] variables for occupational chemical exposures were also included in the models, but since they did not change the association of brain cancer with magnetic fields, we omitted this adjustment for simplicity and comparability with other results.

The effects of contrast and measurement error in the intensity and duration components of cumulative exposure were simulated using a case-control design. Workers who died of brain cancer were matched to four men who survived to the same calendar year. The actually measured exposure intensity and duration were manipulated to introduce measurement error and modify the contrast in both components. We began with the best-performing job-exposure matrix and the duration of exposure data obtained from work history records, which for this exercise were assumed to be without error. We then considered extreme situations in which all workers were assigned the same artificial exposure intensity but their observed (i.e., variable) exposure duration, and another where the observed (variable) intensity was used but an invariant duration was assigned. For each scenario, we also added simulated random errors with geometric standard deviations of 0.4, 0.9, and 1.1 and a mean of 0 to each component. We considered 10 error configurations that resulted from combining these procedures (one with no error, six with error in only one component, and three with equal, simultaneous errors in both components). For each configuration of random error, 1,000 data sets were generated and analyzed and the results averaged to estimate the odds ratio and its 95% confidence interval.

RESULTS

Detailed results of our previous analyses of the effects of varying the treatment of the exposure data and the methods of analyzing the assigned (derived) exposure estimates were presented previously.[9,29] Briefly, we found that, when considered separately, the way the exposure data were treated prior to assignment to individual workers generally had a greater impact on the estimated dose-relationship than subsequent treatment of the exposure measures or variations in the methods of dose-response analyses (see TABLE 1). The exceptions to this pattern were analyses that took into account only very recent exposures (0–5 year time window) and very early exposures (10-20 year window, 20 year lag). They appeared to be unrelated to brain cancer mortality.

Cumulative Exposure Simulations

FIGURES 1a and 1b show the most important findings of the cumulative exposure simulations. The odds ratios of groups with lower cumulative exposure appeared to be related primarily to the duration component. The odds ratios in the group with the highest cumulative exposure were related to both the intensity and duration components (FIG. 1a). FIGURE 1b shows that some random error would still allow an exposure-response trend to be seen, but the odds ratios are somewhat biased towards the null.

Combined Effects

The combined effects of varying the job exposure matrices, the exposure cut-points and the exposure periods are shown in FIGURES 2a–2d. Specifying the longest exposure lag (20 years) or the most recent time window (0–5 years) resulted in no consistent exposure-response relations regardless of the job-exposure matrix or exposure cutpoints. Categorization of cumulative exposures at quintiles of the distribution resulted in a more distinct exposure-response relation, but only for the original (optimal) job exposure matrix with the two-year lag (FIG. 2b). The two job exposure matrixes generally yielded similar RRs in this analysis, except in the highest exposed group where the original job exposure matrix yielded higher rate ratios (compare FIGS. 2a and 2c).

TABLE 1. Sensitivity of the rate ratios of the highest exposed group to various ways of exposure data treatment and analytical methods

Exposure Index	RR for highest exposure level[a]	Relative RR[b]
Job used to assign exposure		
complete work history	2.47*	1.00
last job	2.98	1.21
usual job	2.88	1.17
Cutpoints		
original	2.47*	1.00
tertiles	1.93	0.78
quintiles	3.34	1.35
Exposure periods		
2–10 year window	2.54*	1.00
0-year lag	2.49	0.98
10-year lag	2.47	0.97
20-year lag	1.36	0.54
0–5 year window	0.67	0.26
10–20 year window	0.83	0.33
Groupings and zero-year lag		
optimal	1.51*	1.00
occupational category	1.22	0.81
expert judgment	1.19	0.79
Groupings and 2–10 year window		
optimal	2.27*	1.00
occupational category	1.56	0.69
expert judgment	1.53	0.67

[a]Original data presented in References 9 and 29; adjusted for age, race, calendar decade, social class, and active work status (adjustment for chemical exposure omitted). For analyses with continuous exposure variables (Ref. 9), rate ratios were calculated at the median cumulative exposure in the highest category of the corresponding categorical analysis.

[b]Ratio of RR in highest exposure group for each model relative to corresponding referent RR in the preferred model (indicated by *).

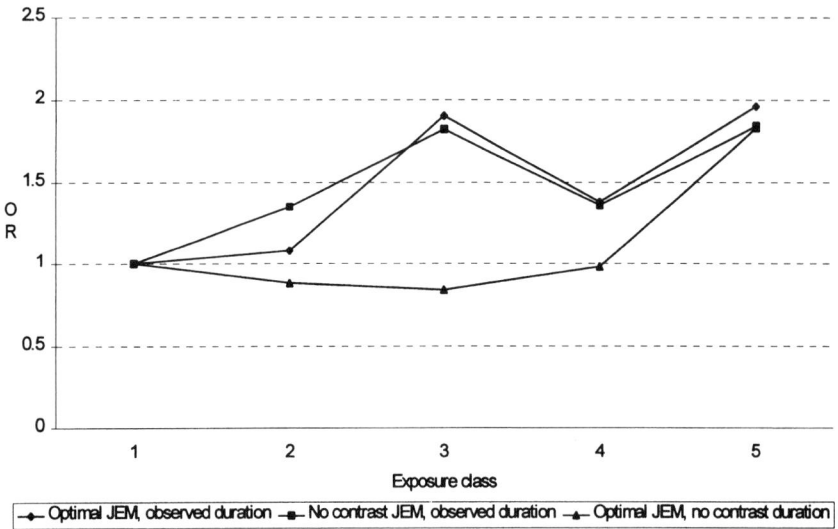

FIGURE 1a. Dose-response relations for cumulative exposure estimates based on two contrast scenarios for intensity and duration.

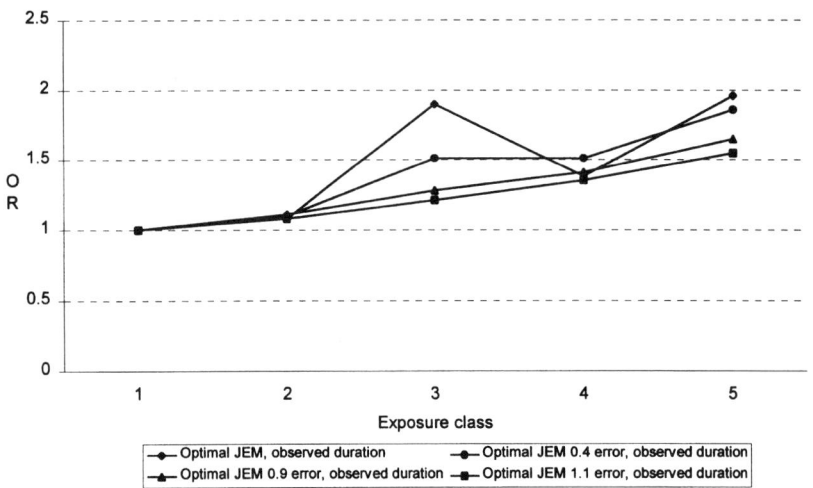

FIGURE 1b. Dose-response relations for cumulative exposure estimates based on the optimal job exposure matrix, observed duration, and three increasing random error scenarios.

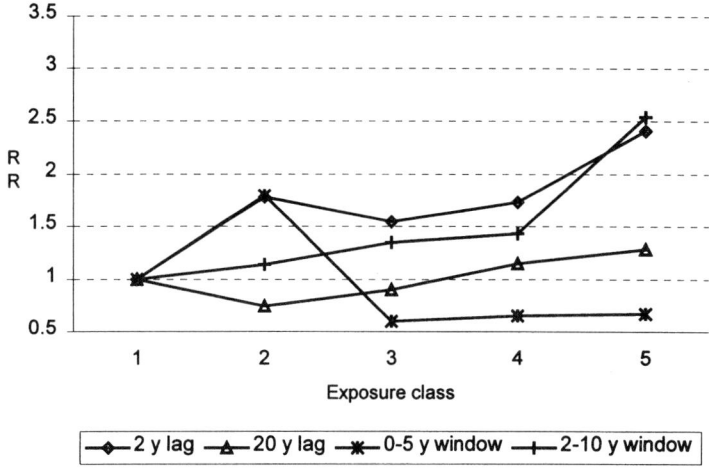

FIGURE 2a. Relation between magnetic field exposure class and brain cancer using the optimal job exposure matrix, original cutpoints, and different time periods.

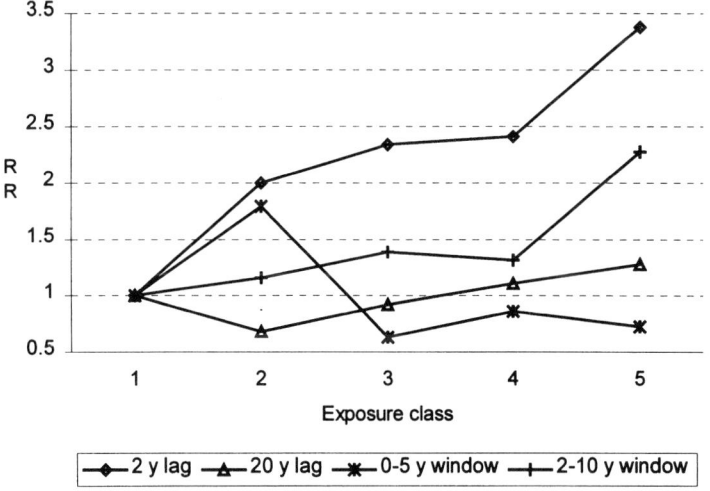

FIGURE 2b. Relation between magnetic field exposure class and brain cancer using the optimal job exposure matrix, quintile cutpoints, and different time periods.

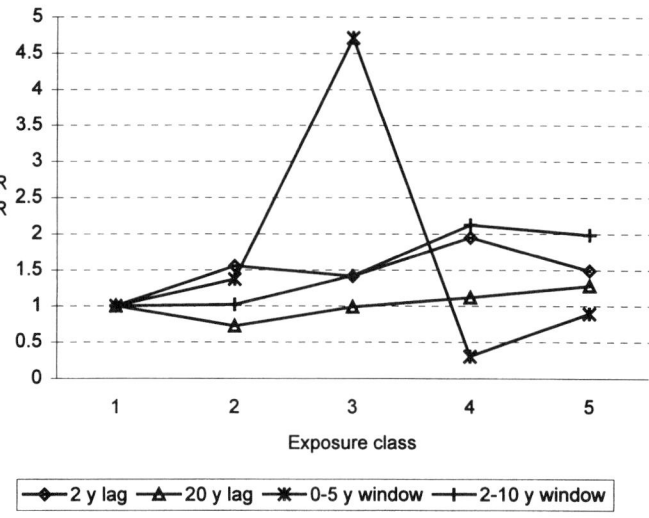

FIGURE 2c. Relation between magnetic field exposure class and brain cancer using the expert judgement job exposure matrix, original cutpoints and different time periods.

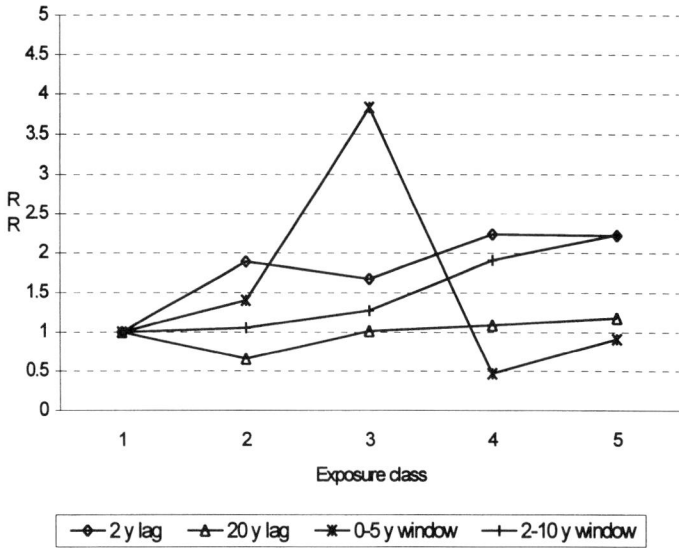

FIGURE 2d. Relation between magnetic field exposure class and brain cancer using the expert judgement job exposure matrix, quintile cutpoints, and different time periods.

To depict the overall methodological uncertainty associated with exposure assessment, exposure assignment, and exposure-response analysis, we plotted the most extreme results of the combined analyses as bands of uncertainty about the results of our original analysis (see FIGURE 3). In that original study[7] we optimized all three steps based on criteria established in advance and therefore considered our reported exposure-response relation to be our *best-bet* estimate (FIG. 3). The combination of the original job-exposure matrix, quintile cutpoints, and a two-year lag gave the strongest exposure-response relation (FIG. 2b), whereas the expert-judgement matrix, original cutpoints and 20-year lag yielded the associations that were consistently the lowest. We therefore judged these configurations to represent the plausible range of methodological uncertainty due to the factors that we examined. For the most exposed men, this approach suggests a rate ratio for brain cancer between 1.28 and 3.34, with 2.54 as the most likely value (FIG. 3).

The range of methodological uncertainty based on our sensitivity analyses was broadly similar to the range of statistical precision based on conventional 95% confidence intervals around our *best-bet* estimate (FIG. 3). However, the confidence interval was compatible with notably higher values of the RR for the most exposed workers, and with notably lower values for the next-most exposed group. Consideration of the statistical precision associated with our estimates of methodological uncertainty would further expand the potential range of uncertainty (FIG. 3).

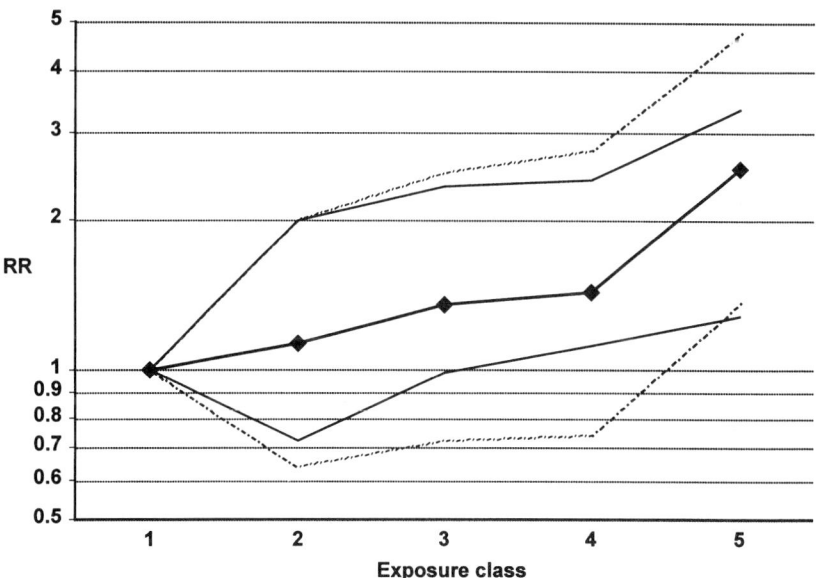

FIGURE 3. Bands of uncertainty (*solid lines*) and 95% confidence intervals (*dotted line*) around best-bet exposure-response relationship.

DISCUSSION AND CONCLUSIONS

In light of the heated debate around the health effects of magnetic fields resulting from power production and usage, we undertook a sensitivity analysis to examine the robustness of our previously published finding of a positive exposure-response relation with brain cancer.[7] In our original study, we tried to base key decisions about the crucial steps of exposure assessment, exposure assignment, and analytical methods on *a priori* criteria. Nevertheless, such decisions are always uncertain because of subjective elements and incomplete information. To gauge the importance of uncertainty in these three areas of study methods, we revisited several key decisions in the original study.

When these aspects of the study methods were considered separately, the findings appeared to be relatively insensitive to most variations in the methods of exposure assignment and data analysis.[29] Methods of exposure assessment had greater impact when considered separately: the dose-response relation obtained with exposure estimates based on a grouping scheme that was optimized by using objective criteria was notably stronger than relations produced with standard grouping approaches.[9]

The cumulative exposure simulations showed that the duration component of the cumulative exposure had a larger effect on the exposure-response relation for the groups with lower cumulative exposure than the intensity component. This was not a surprise, given the much larger contrast in duration of employment than in intensity of exposure to magnetic fields. However, for the group with the highest cumulative exposure, both components played an important role. The finding of a steeper exposure-response relation was, therefore, largely determined by accurate exposure assignment for the highest exposed group. It was also shown that some random error would still have allowed the exposure-response trend to be recognized.

Combined analyses of sensitivity related to exposure assessment, exposure assignment, and data analysis methods suggest a more complex picture than consideration of each in isolation. These results can be interpreted by visualizing the most divergent results of our sensitivity analyses as bands of uncertainty about the *best-bet* estimates that we published originally. Variations in the study methods generally tended to weaken, rather than strengthen, the evidence of an association between brain cancer and exposure to magnetic fields. Only categorizing the exposure data with cutpoints at quintiles of the distribution consistently produced a steeper exposure-response relation than our preferred model. The differences in the results that would have been obtained if we had used quintile cutpoints would not, however, have been sufficient to change our overall interpretation of the study. These cutpoints might have led to a conclusion that lagging cumulative exposure by two years provided the best estimate of the relevant exposure, since the two-year lag generally yielded stronger associations with these cutpoints than the 2–10 year window that we preferred *a priori*. Because a two-year lag period includes all exposures but those in the last two years, a conclusion favoring that lag interval over the 2–10 year window, would provide less specific support for the hypothesis that magnetic fields act at a late stage of carcinogenesis.

Several combinations of factors did, however, yield weaker, or less consistent, relationships relative to our preferred model. In particular, limiting the analysis to either exposure in the five most recent years or more than 20 years in the past produced exposure-response relationships that were notably weaker and less stable. Exposures in these time intervals have limited biological plausibility, however. Long-previous exposures may not be relevant because, if magnetic fields have any effect on cancer risk, they are more likely to promote than to initiate tumors, whereas exposures immediately prior to a death from brain cancer may not be relevant because a tumor may have already been present for several years by the time of death.

Exposure grouping methods continued to have an important effect on the results when other aspects of the methods were considered simultaneously. The optimized job-exposure matrix consistently gave the strongest associations and results obtained with the job-exposure matrix based on expert assessment of exposure defined the lower range of associations. Nevertheless, the relative impact of the grouping approach on the overall results depended on other aspects of the study methods: with some combinations of exposure periods and cutpoints, the expert-judgement job-exposure matrix gave results in the range we obtained with the preferred, optimized matrix.

It is noteworthy that the magnitude of methodological uncertainty from our sensitivity analyses and the statistical precision expressed by 95% confidence intervals were quite similar. Despite this quantitative similarity, methodological uncertainty is likely to be a more meaningful indicator of the range of possible study results. Although confidence intervals are often used as a guide to the range of results that are compatible with the data, their intended meaning is far more limited. Conventional confidence intervals express only statistical uncertainty related to random sampling error, and then only under assumptions that are violated in most observational epidemiologic studies.[30]

Sensitivity analyses of methodological uncertainty can be a useful alternative to confidence intervals for gauging the range of results that might be obtained from a study in the light of the potential for uncontrolled and unmeasured bias from such sources as measurement error, confounding, and subject selection.[31] Nevertheless, sensitivity analysis is limited by its dependence on the existing data and the analyst's ability to develop and evaluate scenarios that are informative about the uncertainties most likely to affect a study and their characteristics. Sensitivity analysis is, itself, an inherently uncertain exercise because it can generate many possible results but does not directly provide a way to assess which of these results are most likely to represent the truth.

For this research, we evaluated a range of scenarios that were selected either to represent plausible alternative situations for our particular study (for example, alternative schemes for grouping exposure measurements) or to reflect common practices in epidemiologic research (such as evaluating an array of exposure periods, ranging from long-previous to recent). The true range of methodological uncertainty in our study of brain cancer and magnetic field exposure might nevertheless be larger than we have shown here; we considered only a limited number of issues in closely related areas of study methods. An exploration of uncertainty in other aspects of the study could produce a broader range of possible results.

Sensitivity analyses suggested that the use of a range of different approaches to exposure assessment, exposure assignment, and data analysis would generally have produced study results that fell within a rather narrow range. The results were more sensitive, however, to the choice of grouping factors for the exposure data, and to specific choices of exposure period and analytical cutpoints. These findings are helpful both for interpreting the epidemiologic results of our earlier study and for assessing the relative importance of uncertainties in several aspects of the study methods. However, our empirical findings may not be generalized to other studies since the questions we examined reflected concerns that arose from our own research, and the methods we used depended heavily on existing data. Current data and theory are not developed enough to judge whether similar findings can be expected if other studies are evaluated using similar methods.

Although our empirical findings may or may not have general implications, the methodology we employed clearly can apply to other studies. We encourage researchers to explore their own findings via sensitivity analysis, and to attempt to construct bounds of uncertainty as an alternative to conventional confidence intervals.

ACKNOWLEDGMENTS

Supported by Contract RP-2964-05 from the Electric Power Research Institute, Palo Alto, California.

REFERENCES

1. HAWKINS, N.C., S.K. NORWOOD & J.C. ROCK, Eds. 1991. A Strategy for Occupational Exposure Assessment. American Industrial Hygiene Association, Akron, Ohio, USA.
2. KROMHOUT, H., E. SYMANSKI & S.M. RAPPAPORT. 1993. A comprehensive evaluation of within- and between-worker components of occupational exposure to chemical agents. Ann. Occup. Hyg. **37:** 253–270.
3. RAPPAPORT, S.M., H. KROMHOUT & E. SYMANSKI. 1993. Variation of exposure between workers in homogeneous exposure groups. Am. Ind. Hyg. Assoc. J. **54:** 654–662.
4. KROMHOUT, H. & D. HEEDERIK. 1995. Occupational epidemiology in the rubber industry. Implications of exposure variability. Am. J. Ind. Med. **27:** 171–185.
5. KROMHOUT, H., E. TIELEMANS, L. PRELLER & D. HEEDERIK. 1996. Estimates of individual dose from current measurements of exposure. Occup. Hyg. **3:** 23–29.
6. TIELEMANS, E., L.L. KUPPER, H. KROMHOUT, D. HEEDERIK & R. HOUBA. 1998. Individual-based and group-based occupational exposure assessment: some equations to evaluate different strategies. Ann. Occup. Hyg. **42:** 115–119.
7. SAVITZ, D.A. & D.P. LOOMIS. 1995. Magnetic field exposure in relation to leukemia and brain cancer mortality among electric utility workers. Am. J. Epidemiol. **141:** 123–134.
8. GARDINER, K., N.W. TRETHOWAN, J.M. HARRINGTON, C.E. ROSSITER & I.A. CALVERT. 1993. Respiratory health effects of carbon black: a survey of European carbon black workers. Br. J. Ind. Med. **50:** 1082–1096.
9. KROMHOUT, H., D.P. LOOMIS, R.C. R.C. KLECKNER & D.A. SAVITZ. 1997. Sensitivity of the relationship between cumulative magnetic field exposure and brain cancer mortality to choice of grouping scheme. Epidemiology **8:** 442–445.
10. VAN TONGEREN, M., K. GARDINER, I. CALVERT, H. KROMHOUT & J.M. HARRINGTON. 1997. Efficiency of different grouping schemes for dust exposure in the European carbon black respiratory morbidity study. Occup. Environ. Med. **54:** 714–719.
11. RAPPAPORT, S.M. 1991. Selection of the measures of exposure for epidemiology studies. Appl. Occup. Environ. Hyg. **6:** 448–457.
12. SMITH, T.J. 1992. Occupational exposure and dose over time: limitations of cumulative exposure. Am. J. Ind. Med. **21:** 35–51.

13. JOHNSON, E.S. 1986. Duration of exposure as a surrogate for dose in the examination of dose-response relations. Br. J. Ind. Med. **43:** 427–429.
14. CHECKOWAY, H. & C. RICE. 1992. Time-weighted averages, peaks, and other indices of exposure in occupational epidemiology. Am. J. Ind. Med. **21:** 25–33.
15. KRIEBEL, D. 1994. The dosimetric model in epidemiology. Occup. Hyg. **1:** 55–68.
16. SEIXAS, N.S., T.G. ROBINS & M. BECKER. 1993. A novel approach to the characterization of cumulative exposure for the study of chronic occupational disease. Am. J. Epidemiol. **137:** 463–471.
17. VACEK, P.M. & J.C. MCDONALD. 1991. Risk assessment using exposure intensity: an application to vermiculite mining. Br. J. Ind. Med. **48:** 543–547.
18. KRIEBEL, D. 1994. Cumulative exposure: conditions for its use as a robust estimator of exposure in occupational epidemiology. Presented at the Conference on Retrospective Assessment of Occupational Exposures in Epidemiology. Lyon, France, 13–15 April, 1994.
19. FINKELSTEIN, M.M. 1995. Potential pitfall in using cumulative exposure in exposure-response relationships: demonstration and discussion. Am. J. Ind. Med. **28:** 41–47.
20. GREENLAND, S. 1995. Dose-response and trend analysis in epidemiology: alternatives to categorical analysis. Epidemiology **6:** 356–365.
21. FLEGAL, K.M., P.M. KEYL & F.J. NIETO. 1991. Differential misclassification arising from nondifferential errors in exposure measurement. Am. J. Epidemiol. **134:** 1233–1244.
22. BRENNER, H. & D.P. LOOMIS. 1994. Varied forms of bias due to nondifferential error in measuring exposure. Epidemiology **5:** 510–517.
23. ROTHMAN, K.J. 1981. Induction and latent periods. Am. J. Epidemiol.**114:** 253–259.
24. CHECKOWAY, H., N. PEARCE, J.L.S. HICKEY & J.M. DEMENT. 1990. Latency analysis in occupational epidemiology. J. Occup. Med. **45:** 95–100.
25. PEARCE, N. 1988. Multistage modelling of lung cancer mortality in asbestos textile workers. Int. J. Epidemiol. **17:** 747–752.
26. SALVAN, A., L. STAYNER, K. STEENLAND & R. SMITH. 1995. Selecting an exposure lag period. Epidemiology **6:** 387–390.
27. LOOMIS, D.P., H. KROMHOUT, L.A. PEIPINS, R.C. KLECKNER, R. IRIYE & D.A. SAVITZ. 1994. Sampling design and methods of a large, randomized, multi site survey of occupational magnetic field exposure. Appl. Occup. Environ. Hyg. **9:** 49–52.
28. KROMHOUT, H., D.P. LOOMIS, G.J. MIHLAN, L.A. PEIPINS, R.C. KLECKNER, R. IRIYE & D.A. SAVITZ. 1995. Assessment and grouping of occupational magnetic field exposure in five electric utility companies. Scand. J. Work Environ. Health **21:** 43–50.
29. LOOMIS, D.P., H. KROMHOUT, R.C. KLECKNER & D.A. SAVITZ. 1998. Effects of the analytical treatment of exposure data on associations of cancer and occupational magnetic field exposure. Am. J. Ind. Med. **34:** 49–56.
30. GREENLAND, S. 1990. Randomization, statistics, and causal inference. Epidemiology **1:** 421–429.
31. GREENLAND, S. 1996. Basic methods for sensitivity analysis of biases. Int. J. Epidemiol. **25:** 1107–1116.

Measures of Exposure to Environmental Tobacco Smoke

Validity, Precision, and Relevance

ALISTAIR WOODWARD[a] AND WAEL AL-DELAIMY

*Department of Public Health, Wellington School of Medicine,
PO Box 7343, Wellington South, New Zealand*

ABSTRACT: It is often not clear what the best measures of exposure are for a risk assessment, or even how one should answer this question. Environmental tobacco smoke (ETS) provides a good example for an exploration of uncertainty. There are a variety of methods for estimating exposure and each has shortcomings. In this paper we summarize the physical characteristics of ETS and the principal methods for assessing exposure. We review the accuracy and applicability of these methods, and explore major sources of uncertainty in the assessment of ETS.

INTRODUCTION

Environmental tobacco smoke (ETS) is a good example for any consideration of uncertainty in risk assessment. Exposure is widespread, occurring in workplaces and in general environmental settings. The topic has been closely studied, but much is still not known about the characteristics of ETS and its effects on health. Relative risks associated with ETS are modest, are certainly smaller than those related to active smoking, and they increase the importance of accuracy in exposure assessment. The potential social implications of ETS risk assessments are huge—smoke free policies may affect all work sites and enclosed public spaces. The tobacco industry regards ETS as a serious threat to its own commercial interests,[1] consequently, the industry funds and promotes its own reviews that, on the whole, emphasize the shortcomings of the scientific case against ETS.[2] For all these reasons, there is keen public interest in the nature and extent of uncertainties in ETS risk assessment.[3]

WHAT IS ENVIRONMENTAL TOBACCO SMOKE?

ETS is made up mostly of so-called sidestream smoke, which passes directly from the glowing tip of the cigarette into the environment. Small contributions stem from other sources, including exhaled mainstream smoke. The chemistry and distribution dynamics of ETS are complex. We focus on the major characteristics of ETS that are relevant to exposure assessment and calculation of health risks.

[a]Address for correspondence: +64 4 385 5999 (voice); +64 4 3895319 (fax).
e-mail: woodward@wnmeds.ac.nz

ETS includes thousands of compounds, the levels of which depend on the way the cigarette is smoked and its composition. For example, puff volume and puff frequency determine the proportions of ETS made up by glow and smoulder stream smoke. Sidestream to mainstream ratios depend on the compound that is measured, the way the cigarette is smoked, and the quantity of tobacco made available for combustion. In general, sidestream smoke is produced at lower temperatures, and in less oxygen-rich conditions, than mainstream smoke. As a consequence, the products of combustion differ. For example, sidestream smoke contains more CO and less CO_2, and higher levels of combustion products formed by nitrosation and amination. Within a short distance of a burning cigarette ETS is largely undiluted, and exposure to potentially harmful smoke components is likely to be heavier and more uniform than in the case of *distant* passive smoking.

The age of ETS influences the balance of semivolatile constituents between vapor and particulate phases. Some compounds are rapidly oxidized. Others (such as nicotine) are in equilibrium between vapor and gas phases, and are affected by dilution of the smoke and changes in temperature and humidity. In mainstream smoke (and fresh sidestream smoke) nicotine is held on the surfaces of droplets but, with air dilution, most of the nicotine evaporates.[4]

Sidestream smoke is less acidic than mainstream smoke (pH about 7, compared with pH about 6 for mainstream cigarette smoke).[4] This is due chiefly to the much higher levels of ammonia in undiluted sidestream smoke. As a result, nicotine is present in greater quantities in the unionized form, in which it is more readily absorbed by the body.

The size of particles in sidestream smoke varies with many factors, including the age of the smoke, ambient temperature, and humidity. Overall the particles tend to be smaller than those present in mainstream smoke,[4] resulting from the evaporation of semivolatile constituents. Due to their size (mostly between 0.1–0.4 µm in diameter) the particles are distributed rapidly by convection currents throughout a room or any other closed space.

The number of people in the mixing space and their level of activity influence the rate of adsorption of smoke constituents and the circulation of smoke particles, as do the physical characteristics of the indoor environment, such as the presence of furniture, drapes, and carpets.[5] The dispersion and decay of ETS occurs at different rates for different constituents. Levels of particulate matter in the atmosphere are likely to fall more quickly than do levels of gaseous smoke products. Reactive components (such as NO_2) decay more rapidly than more stable compounds (for example, CO).

The deposition of smoke particles is influenced by characteristics of the smoke (particle size most importantly) and by biological variables concerned with manner of inhalation and the configuration of the respiratory tract. The fraction of ETS particles deposited in the respiratory tract is estimated to be between 10–20%.[6] By contrast, 70–90% of particles in mainstream smoke inhaled by smokers are deposited in the respiratory tract.[7] The proportion of ETS deposited in the lungs of a child may be considerably higher than for an adult due to differences in the diameter and configuration of the airways. Studies of air flow and aerosol deposition in models of infant lungs have found that the total deposition is up to 50% greater than in adult lungs, with proportionately heavier deposits in the tracheobronchial area.[8]

WHY DO WE NEED GOOD MEASURES OF EXPOSURE TO ETS?

In etiologic studies, estimation of the risk of disease associated with ETS depends on accurate measurement of exposure. The extension of biomarker studies to measures of early biological response, such as carcinogen-hemoglobin adducts, contributes biological plausibility to epidemiological studies of cancer and ETS. This may in future add to our understanding of the mechanisms of disease.[9] The accuracy of measures of exposure is particularly important when the relative risks are modest in magnitude and the results of the studies have substantial policy implications.

At the population level, measures of exposure are necessary for estimating the burden of disease that is attributable to ETS, and to guide public health policy. For example, in many countries 30–40% of children are exposed to smoke in the home and, consequently, a substantial proportion of cases of common childhood illnesses may be attributed to ETS. In Australia, it is estimated that 2,330 hospital admissions

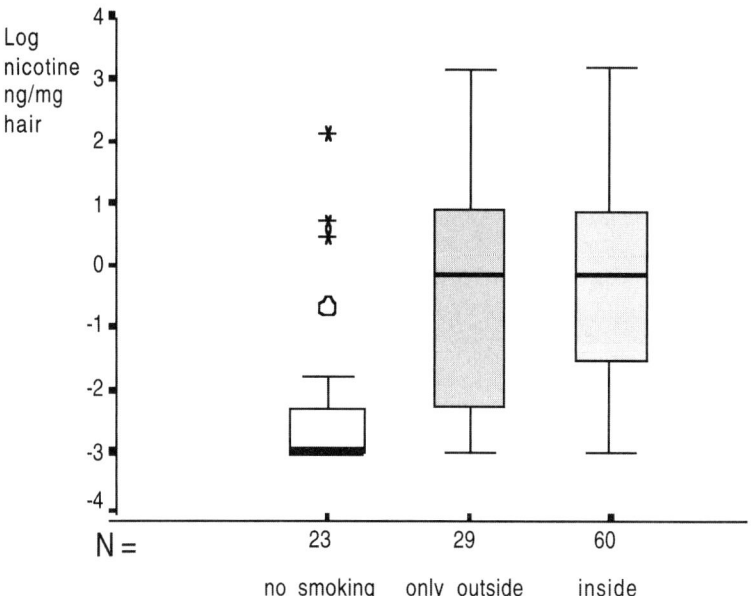

FIGURE 1. Hair nicotine levels in New Zealand children whose parents reported they were nonsmokers, smoked only outside the house, or smoked indoors. (Source: Al-Delaimy *et al.* Ref. 12.)

per year, or 13% of all admissions for lower respiratory illness in the first 18 months of life, are due to exposure to parental cigarette smoke in the home.[10]

Measures of exposure are needed to study the effect of interventions that reduce ETS. For example, questionnaires and cotinine measures have been used to assess the outcome of health education programmes that encourage parents to reduce exposure of children to ETS.[11] More than one method may be required to obtain an accurate picture of exposures. A recent study in Wellington found that children of parents who reported that their house was smoke free had similar levels of nicotine in their hair as did children whose parents reported that they smoked inside the house, suggesting that parents inaccurately report their smoking habits, either that or smoke free homes make little difference to childhood exposure to ETS in New Zealand[12] (see FIGURE 1).

Other examples of exposure assessment include physically monitoring smoking in specific workplaces,[13] and national surveys to track the effect of smoke free legislation.[14]

HOW CAN EXPOSURE TO ETS BE MEASURED?

Questionnaires

Questionnaires are the most commonly used method of exposure assessment in studies of the health effects of ETS (see TABLE 1). Advantages include the ability to provide detailed information on ETS source strength, retrospective exposure information, measures of exposure over an extended period, and simultaneous information on time-activity patterns and modifying environmental factors. Questionnaires provide information at relatively low cost, which is important for studies that require large sample sizes.[15]

The principal disadvantage of this method of assessment is the susceptibility of questionnaires to misclassification. In the case of active smoking, the number of cigarettes smoked by an individual is commonly accepted as providing a reasonable quantitative index of exposure to tobacco smoke. However, ETS exposure cannot be simply related to the number of cigarettes smoked by others.[16] Many other variables are important, such as the size of the space, amount and quality of ventilation and crowding. The breathing and smoke-puff patterns of the smoker, the proximity to the source of ETS, and the precise time spent in a room in which smoking has occurred are variables that cannot be readily accounted for in questionnaires. Low-level exposures may be overlooked: biomarker studies show that tobacco-specific substances such as nicotine and cotinine are frequently present in blood, urine, and saliva of people who report that they are not aware they have been exposed to ETS.[17] Even more troublesome is the potential for systematic errors in exposure assessment by questionnaire. For example, growing awareness of the hazards of passive smoking to health, and possibly a social stigma associated with exposing others (especially children) to ETS, may lead to differential under-reporting.[18]

TABLE 1. Methods of exposure assessment used in studies of health effects of passive smoking (see Ref. 10)

Health effect	No. of studies[a]	Exposure questionnaire	Exposure biomarker	Exposure questionnaire and biomarker
low birth weight (due to maternal exposure to ETS)	18	15	2	1
childhood asthma	68	64	1	3
lower respiratory illness in first 18 months	47	44	1	2
lung function in childhood	25	19	3	3
sudden infant death syndrome	8	8	—	—
middle ear disease in childhood	19	17	2	—
lung cancer	40	39	—	1
major coronary events	17	16	—	1

[a]Drawn from peer-reviewed literature published before July 1997.

Biological Markers

The major advantage of biomarkers is the ability to measure an absorbed dose of ETS rather than the potential dose (exposure) in the external environment. Biomarkers are said to be *objective*. This is not true, since any method of measurement requires some degree of judgement. However, biomarkers might be regarded as less subjective than questionnaires in the sense that they rely on the discretion of the investigator alone. Choices must still be made. For instance, the selection of analytic method involves a trade-off among sensitivity, specificity, cost, and acceptability. Measurement of cotinine in urine by radioimmunoassay (RIA) is cheaper than measurement by chromatography, but RIA is less specific due to cross-reactions with other nicotine metabolites.[16] Mass spectroscopy is the most accurate technique of all, but this is considerably more expensive than the alternatives. The quantitative aspect of measurement by biomarker is attractive, but the appearance of precision may be misleading. Absorption, distribution, storage, metabolism, and elimination of nicotine and cotinine in human bodies, for example, are not fully understood, adding uncertainty to the interpretation of test results, which may be compounded by inter-laboratory variation.

Most recent work on biomarkers for ETS has been based on nicotine and its metabolites (especially cotinine), because of the high degree of specificity of these substances for exposure to tobacco smoke. (Although there are other sources of nicotine, such as fruit and vegetables, the contribution is negligible except in extreme circumstances. Benowitz[16] estimates that to reach a level of cotinine typically seen following ETS exposure, a person would need to consume each day more than 4.6 Kg of cauliflower or 7.6 Kg of tomatoes.) The principal advantage of cotinine measurement over nicotine in body fluids is its greater persistence in the body—the halflife of cotinine is 20–24 hours, compared with two hours for nicotine. In addition, a range of DNA and protein adducts and other carcinogen biomarkers have been identified in nonsmokers, with levels related to self-reported exposure to ETS.[9,19] Difficulties in applying these measures to risk assessment include lack of specificity (due to environmental sources other than tobacco smoke) and the high cost of many of the analyses.

Cotinine is the major proximate metabolite of nicotine that can be measured in urine, serum, saliva, other body fluids, and hair.[16] Levels of exposure to ETS in the home, as assessed by the reported smoking habits of the family members, have been correlated with urinary cotinine levels of children[20,21] and nonsmoking adults.[22] Limitations apply chiefly to the duration of exposure that is recorded, and the uncertain relation between cotinine levels and the biologically effective dose or doses of ETS constituents that are relevant to the disease under study. Cotinine is itself biologically inert and is formed principally by oxidation of nicotine in the liver. Consequently, measures of cotinine may provide an imperfect reflection of significant *upstream* exposures, such as those impacting on the respiratory mucosa. Since the ratio of nicotine to other components of ETS varies with many factors, such as the age of the smoke, spot measures of cotinine may misrepresent the levels of other constituents that are absorbed. The half-life of cotinine means that, at most, measures refer to several days of past exposure to nicotine. Moreover, there is considerable between-individual variability in the proportion of nicotine metabolized to cotinine (ranging between approximately 50% and 90%) and the rate at which cotinine is metabolized.[16,23] Cotinine clearance varies with factors such as ethnicity, sex, and age.[16] Children tend to have higher cotinine levels in urine than adults for similar exposures to ETS. This may be due to age-related differences in nicotine metabolism, or to higher doses of ETS resulting from higher relative ventilation rates among children.

Recently, the search for more stable measures that avoid some of the disadvantages encountered with testing of body fluids has led to the investigation of hair as a biomarker for ETS. Each centimeter of hair reflects approximately one month of exposure, since hair has a fairly uniform growth rate (1.0 ± 0.3 cm per month.[24] Nicotine in hair is derived mainly from nicotine in blood, although some may be absorbed directly from the atmosphere.[25] Cotinine is present in hair, but at much lower concentrations than nicotine. Both compounds are preserved in the shaft throughout the life of the hair and, after cutting, samples can be stored at room temperature for years within a closed envelope without loss or degradation of hair nicotine.[26] Among active smokers, the centimeter-by-centimeter distribution of nicotine corresponds moderately well with average month-by-month number of cigarettes smoked.[24] Among nonsmokers, several studies have reported that the method is sufficiently sensitive to be able to detect changes in ETS exposure and to differentiate people according to their levels of exposure.[26] In one study of children, nicotine in hair correlated more closely with smoking history of parents of exposed and unexposed children than did cotinine in urine.[27]

There are many possible causes of between- and within-individual variation of uptake of nicotine into hair, including variable reporting of exposure history, differences in ventilation, exposure time, and distance from the source of exposure.[28]

Moreover there are confounding factors specific to hair, such as irregular hair growth, diffusion, and washing out of nicotine following application of bleaches and dyes. Hair color is also relevant: black hair tends to contain higher levels of nicotine than fair hair for similar exposures to ETS.[29]

Environmental Measurements

Components of ETS that may be monitored in the environment include nicotine, particulates, and a number of gases. Recently studies have examined the value of solanesol, a tobacco leaf constituent present in cigarette smoke condensate.[10] Its utility lies in its abundance, lack of volatility, and lack of any indoor sources other than tobacco.

Environmental measurements may be obtained by stationary air sampling monitors, personal sampling with pump driven nicotine or respirable suspended particulate samplers, or personal sampling with a diffusion-based nicotine sampler. Using these methods it has been shown that the number of smokers in a household has a strong effect on indoor levels of respirable suspended particulates (RSP)—a pack-a-day smoker adds approximately 15–20 $\mu g/m^3$ to typical household levels, which is similar to RSP concentrations observed in outdoor air in some cities.[30] Personal monitors provide more direct measures of ETS exposure than stationary samplers, but there are obstacles to applying this technique in large scale surveys. Generally these environmental monitors can be used for short time periods only, which may be sufficient for some purposes (such as comparisons of workplaces with and without smoking policies) but is less helpful in studies of disease etiology. However, passive monitors may be used to check the accuracy of questionnaires which are applied subsequently to measure exposure in large scale surveys.

VALIDITY, PRECISION, AND RELEVANCE IN ASSESSMENT OF ETS EXPOSURE

The validity of an exposure measure is a function of bias (average measurement error) and precision (variability in measurement error). In the absence of a "gold standard" measurement of true exposure, the extent of bias and imprecision can only be estimated by making comparisons between different measures of exposure.

Questionnaire assessments of exposure to ETS often rely on self-reported smoking (for example, parents reporting on smoking in the home during studies of ETS and children). The accuracy of self-reported smoking depends on the circumstances under which the information is elicited. Patrick *et al.*[31] reviewed 26 studies in which questionnaire responses had been compared with biochemical measures of smoking. On the whole, the different measures of smoking were consistent, but the extent of agreement varied widely. Treating the biochemical measures as a reference, sensitivity ranged from 6% to 100% (mean 87.5%) and specificity from 33% to 100% (mean 89.2%). The wording of the questionnaire and the context in which questions were asked were important: higher estimates of sensitivity and specificity were observed when the questionnaire was administered by an interviewer, for observational studies rather than interventions, when adults answered rather than adolescents, and when the biochemical assessment was by cotinine rather than other markers (such as nicotine or exhaled CO).

The reliability of ETS exposure estimates may be tested by repeating questionnaires that refer to a particular period, or repeating biochemical measures on the same sample. On retesting, questionnaires do well in terms of broad categories of *presence* or *absence* of exposure. For example, in an Australian study mothers were asked about smoking during the first year after delivery; 97.7% gave the same answer ("yes" or "no") as they did two months earlier.[32] Questions on the extent of exposure are less reproducible. A study of lifetime exposure to ETS of adult nonsmokers in New Mexico found a high degree of agreement between two interviews within six months (more than 90%) for parental smoking during childhood, but much lower figures for amount smoked or hours of exposure.[33] Similarly when Pron *et al.*[34] reinterviewed 117 subjects after six months, good agreement was found for reports of occupational and residential ETS exposure, but the reliability of reported duration of exposure was poor. Within-sample variability in biochemical measures of exposure to ETS should be low for a given laboratory; variability between laboratories is seldom reported.

Repeated tests of biomarkers and environmental measures of ETS show considerable within-individual variation. Coultas *et al.*[35] reported that indicator variables for self-reported exposure explained no more than 6–10% of the variability in atmospheric monitoring, and 18–20% of variability in urinary and salivary cotinine levels. It is difficult to know how much of this unexplained variation is due to underlying variability in the true exposure, and how much is due to measurement error. Repeated measures improve the characterization of an individual's exposure to ETS, but single measures may be sufficient to distinguish between groups that are *exposed* or *unexposed* (or, more accurately, *more exposed* or *less exposed*). Henderson *et al.*[36] reported that levels of nicotine in air and cotinine in urine fluctuated widely on retesting, but the ranking of individuals from one test to another was less variable, and both air nicotine and urine cotinine measures consistently distinguished *exposed* households (those containing smokers) from *unexposed* households (those without smokers).

Which measures of exposure to tobacco smoke best predict health outcomes? Bias aside, the most accurate measure of exposure should be associated with the strongest measure of effect (assuming that an effect does exist).

Few studies have reported risk estimates based on measures of exposure other than questionnaires. In addition to those listed in TABLE 2 (passive smoking) and TABLE 3 (active smoking), de Waard *et al.*[37] compared questionnaires and urine cotinine levels in relation to incidence of lung cancer in a cohort of women, but the data are not reported in full. In this study, after up to 15 years of followup, 23 incident cases were identified among nonsmokers. ETS exposure to the time of enrolment was compared with controls chosen from within the cohort. The odds ratio for those nonsmokers in the top tertile of cotinine compared with the bottom tertile was 2.4 (0.7–8.3). No comparable results were reported for the questionnaire results, but the paper noted, for active smokers, that "lung cancer distribution between different levels of self-reported cigarette consumption did not differ significantly from [the distribution across] corresponding cotinine categories". Wang *et al.*[38] reported a clear inverse dose-response association of cotinine in maternal urine during pregnancy

TABLE 2. Health effects of exposure to ETS from studies reporting results using both questionnaire and biomarker assessments of exposure

Reference	Study population	Health outcome	Exposure measure	Measure of effect
Ehrlich et al.[50]	72 children 3–14 years, attending emergency room with acute asthma, 121 emergency room controls	emergency room treatment for acute asthma	(1) maternal caregiver smokes: yes vs. no	odds ratio = 2.0 (1.1–3.4)
			(2) urine cotinine: $\geq$ 30 ng/mg creatinine vs. < 30 ng/mg	OR = 1.9 (1.0–3.4)
Chilmonczyk et al.[51]	199 asthmatic children aged 8 months to 13 years	acute exacerbations of asthma	(1) No. of care-givers who smoke: mother and others vs. none	ratio = 1.8 (1.4–2.2)
			(2) urine cotinine: 40+ ng/ml vs. < 10 ng/ml	ratio = 1.7 (1.4–2.1)
Rebagliato et al.[52]	710 nonsmoking pregnant women	mean birthweight	(1) h/week reported exposure to ETS: 42+ (top quintile) vs. none	deficit = 88 g
			(2) maternal serum cotinine: 1.8+ ng/ml (top quintile) vs. < 0.5 ng/ml	deficit = 98 g
Rylander et al.[53]	112 hospital cases aged 4–18 months, 196 population controls	hospital admission for wheezing bronchitis	(1) number of parents who smoke: both vs. none	OR = 2.0 (1.1–3.7)
			(2) urine cotinine: 10+ µg/L vs. < 2.5 µg/L	OR = 2.1 (1.1–4.6)
Tunstall-Pedoe et al.[54]	population sample of 986 men and 1492 women aged 40–59 years	prevalence of diagnosed coronary heart disease	(1) reported exposure to ETS: *a lot* vs. *none*	OR = 2.4 (1.1–4.8)
			(2) serum cotinine: > 4 ng/ml vs. < 0.01 ng/ml	OR = 2.7 (1.3–5.6)

TABLE 3. Health effects of active smoking from studies reporting results using both questionnaire and biomarker assessments of exposure

Reference	Study population	Health outcome	Exposure measure	Measure of effect
Haddow et al.[55]	4211 pregnant women providing a blood sample at 15–21 weeks gestation	birth weight	(1) self-reported no. of cigarettes smoked per day: top 2.7% (25+) vs. nonsmokers (2) serum cotinine: top 2.7% (284 ng/ml) vs. < 24 ng/ml	mean difference in birth weight −289g −441g
Woodward et al.[56]	79 mothers of children in top quintile of frequency of respiratory illness in first 18 months of life, compared with 72 mothers of children in bottom quintile	prone to acute respiratory illness in childhood	(1) self-reported smoking in mid-trimester of pregnancy: yes vs. no. (2) cotinine in serum collected at 16–20 weeks gestation: 57+ nmol/L vs. < 57 nmol/L	OR = 1.50 (0.73–3.08) OR = 1.72 (0.83–3.50)
Perez-Stable et al.[57]	743 adults participating in national nutrition survey	acute biochemical and physiological changes	(1) self-reported number of cigarettes smoked per day (2) serum cotinine	cotinine more strongly correlated with hematocrit, hemoglobin, white cell count and diastolic blood pressure

and infant size at birth. The relation with maternal self-reported smoking was less striking. Surveys of passive smoking and lung function in children found that salivary cotinine and questionnaire estimates of exposure were similarly associated with small decrements in most spirometric indices.[39,40]

These comparisons should be treated with caution. The definitions of exposure are to some extent arbitrary (for example, there is no fixed cut point for serum cotinine that distinguishes an active smoker from a nonsmoker heavily exposed to ETS) and may be made *post hoc*. Consequently results are susceptible to reinterpretation and, possibly, reporting bias. Questionnaire and cotinine measures of exposure do tend to be correlated,[40] indicating that to some extent the two approaches measure common events. One would expect questionnaires to have greater predictive validity when the relevant exposure occurred in the distant past (for example, in case control studies of cancer), whereas cotinine measures are likely to be more strongly related to acute outcomes, but this is not apparent in TABLE 2. Perhaps the most likely reason for these findings is that the two approaches are similarly imperfect, although the source and nature of the errors differ. Assuming that the errors in biomarkers and questionnaires are not correlated, consistency in the risk estimates supports the validity of both methods of exposure assessment.

The question of which is the *best* measure of exposure of ETS must take account of operational issues, such as acceptability and cost. The cost of the different methods of exposure assessment varies widely. For example, hair nicotine testing may add $30–100 per participant (depending on the method of analysis) to the cost of questionnaires. This means that possible gains in precision and face validity and reductions in systematic error must be weighed against the loss of statistical power that occurs if the number of study participants needs to be limited. The acceptability of collecting biological samples may also be an issue in some populations. For example, most cultures have restrictions of some kind on the cutting of hair. Some groups strictly prohibit cutting the hair of young male children: other cultures restrict the time of day at which hair may be cut.

WHAT ARE THE MAJOR SOURCES OF UNCERTAINTY IN ASSESSMENT OF ETS?

Uncertainty has many meanings and arises from multiple sources; sometimes it results from a lack of information, and on other occasions it is caused by disagreement about what is already known. Some categories of uncertainty are amenable to quantification; others defy numerical boundaries and probabilities.

Morgan and Henrion[41] proposed these sources of uncertainty in risk assessment:

- linguistic imprecision
- statistical variation
- variability
- approximation
- subjective judgement
- disagreement.

Ambiguity in language certainly contributes to confusion and misunderstanding in exposure assessment of ETS. For example, the term *ETS* may refer to undiluted smoke emitted directly from the cigarette, or to aged and diluted smoke, which has quite different characteristics. As in other areas of science, commonly-used phrases such as "the weight of the evidence" and "adequate data" mean quite different things depending on the perspective of the author; a small number of studies becomes "several" or "a few" depending on whether or not the studies are being cited as supportive evidence.

In this instance, statistical variation, which is well understood and relatively straightforward to describe and allow for, poses less of a problem for risk assessment than does the underlying variability in exposures. The nature of ETS, with intermittent releases and many factors in the chain between source and biologically effective dose, virtually ensures that uncontrolled variability will be high.

TABLE 4. Issues for which the experts disagree—uncertainty in risk assessment of ETS

	Risk-tolerant view	Risk-sensitive view
extrapolating from home exposures to work exposures	most work exposures much less than in home with one or more smokers	in high exposure settings, work exposures comparable to heavy ETS exposure at home
risk estimates	emphasize small relative risks	emphasize substantial attributable risks
confounding and bias	focus on potential for unrecognized or uncontrolled errors	focus on factors that have already been controlled
biological mechanisms	biological plausibility a high priority in determining causation	plausibility a soft criterion for causation
heterogeneity in exposures and study designs	assumed to be high	assumed to be sufficiently low to justify pooling results
what constitutes acceptable quality of evidence	more demanding—quality of the science is the only consideration	less demanding—severity of problem requires decision
variability in exposure measures	emphasize differences between individuals	emphasize differences between groups
analogy with active smoking	depending on implications for risk—differences or similarities emphasized	depending on implications for risk—similarities or differences emphasized
exposure to ETS represented as cigarette-equivalents	cite cigarette-equivalents of nicotine	cite cigarette-equivalents of substances with higher ETS: mainstream ratios than nicotine

Approximation is a cause of uncertainty when processes are complex and simplifying assumptions must be made. For example, the use of biomarkers in ETS exposure assessment is based on assumptions about the biological mechanisms of action, although it is not clear at present which components of ETS are most important in the etiology of disease. Cotinine measures are used in studies of ETS and heart disease, for example, although it is not clear whether the cardiotoxic components of ETS are gaseous or particulate, whether nicotine is directly relevant, or what period must elapse between exposure and presentation of disease.

Bridging data gaps such as these requires judgement, and differences in judgement are a common cause (although not the only one) of disagreement. We searched the literature on ETS to identify common disagreements, and characterized these in terms of *risk tolerant* (slow to concede that ETS causes health risks) and *risk sensitive* (quick to claim that ETS is a health risk) positions (see TABLE 4).

The tension between the risk tolerant and risk sensitive points of view affects exposure assessment in many ways. For example, the definition of an *acceptable quality of evidence* determines which data are included in assessments, and which are excluded.[42] Accepting or excluding studies for pooled analyses also depends on judgement, in this instance assessment of the degree of heterogeneity in study design.

When considering the use of cotinine and nicotine as measures of ETS exposure, emphasis on variations between individuals[23] leads to a higher estimate of uncertainty than is apparent from a perspective that concentrates on comparisons between groups.[16] In a similar vein, the *risk tolerant* perspective on ETS in the workplace emphasizes the low exposures that individuals receive (on average), and the small increase in personal risk that may result.[43] The *risk sensitive* perspective takes a population-wide view and emphasizes the substantial burden of illness that results from a widespread exposure.[17] Commentators who are *risk tolerant* emphasize the differences between active and passive smoking (e.g., dilution, particle size, and lung clearance) when considering the question of whether ETS is hazardous.[44] The *risk sensitive* perspective on the same question highlights similarities (e.g., the presence of proven carcinogens in both mainstream and sidestream smoke).[4] Interestingly, the positions are somewhat different with regard to risk assessment. Those who hold that there is a minimal (or nonexistent) risk sometimes support this position by linear extrapolation from the effects of active smoking, using the notion of *cigarette equivalents* of ETS exposure.[45] Those who believe that there are indeed nontrivial risks from ETS argue that ETS may differ significantly from active smoking in its mechanisms of action (in, for example, its greater than expected effect on the progression of atherosclerosis[46]). The idea of cigarette-equivalents is itself an ambiguous one, since the magnitude of the imputed exposure to ETS depends very strongly on which compound is chosen as the index.[6]

Disagreement also results from differences due to factors such as career expectations, disciplinary background, and economic interests. A study of reviews of ETS for example, found that an article produced by authors with affiliations to the tobacco industry was 88 times more likely to conclude that passive smoking is not harmful, than articles written by authors with no connections to the industry.[47] Such a divergence of views on a common data set is not peculiar to ETS. Brunk *et al.*[48] describe the different pathways taken in Canada by industry, government, and an independent inquiry to the risk assessment of the pesticide alachlor; and van Asselt et al.[49] describe how various world views affect estimates of the impact of population growth on human health. Differences among perspectives are to be expected and should not paralyze the decision-making process. Disagreement and uncertainty are not, on their own, sufficient reasons for failing to act to reduce risks to health.

CONCLUSIONS

Whether or not a measure of exposure is sufficiently accurate depends on its purpose. For public health and regulatory purposes, such as the monitoring of smoke-free policies, simple questionnaires are effective measures of exposure to ETS. Studies of disease etiology may require more discriminating measures. None of those that are presently available provide a comprehensive, long-term picture of individual exposures to ETS. However, questionnaires and cotinine measurements may provide satisfactory instruments for epidemiology studies, which aim to distinguish groups in terms of the magnitude of exposure to ETS. There are still uncertainties associated with the assessment of ETS. Some of these are due to missing data and will be overcome when more is known about ETS. However, uncertainty is also a consequence of differing values and expectations that scientists and commentators bring to the analysis and interpretation of the data.

REFERENCES

1. CHAPMAN, S. 1997. Tobacco industry memo reveals passive smoking strategy. BMJ **314:** 1569.
2. BERO, L.A., A. GALBRAITH & D. RENNIE. 1994. Sponsored symposia on environmental tobacco smoke. J.A.M.A. **271:** 612–617.
3. JAMROZIK, K., S. CHAPMAN & A. WOODWARD. 1997. How the NHMRC got its fingers burnt. Med. J. Aust. **167:** 372–374.
4. SURGEON GENERAL. 1986. The Health Consequences of Involuntary Smoking. US Department of Health and Human Services, Rockville.
5. HUGOD, C., L.H. HAWKINS & P ASTRUP. 1978. Exposure of passive smokers to tobacco smoke constituents. Int. Arch. Occup. Environ. Health **842:** 21–29.
6. ENVIRONMENTAL PROTECTION AGENCY (EPA). 1992. Respiratory health effects of passive smoking: lung cancer and other disorders. EPA Office of Research and Development, Washington, D.C.
7. DALHAMN, T., M. EDFORS & R. RYLANDER. 1968. Retention of cigarette smoke components in human lungs. Arch. Environ. Health. **17:** 746–748.
8. XU, G.B.Y.C. 1986. Effects of age on deposition of inhaled aerosols in the human lung. Aerosol Science & Tech. **5:** 349–357.
9. HAMMOND, S.K., J. COGHLIN, P.H. GANN, M. PAUL et al. 1993. Relationship between environmental tobacco smoke exposure and carcinogen-hemoglobin adduct levels in nonsmokers. J. Natl. Cancer Inst. 85: 474–478.
10. NATIONAL HEALTH AND MEDICAL RESEARCH COUNCIL. 1997. The health effects of passive smoking. A scientific information paper. Commonwealth of Australia, Canberra.
11. WOODWARD, A., N. OWEN, N. GRGURINOVICH, F. GRIFFITH & H. LINKE. 1987. Trial of an intervention to reduce passive smoking in infancy. Pediatr. Pulmonol. **3:** 173–178.

12. AL-DELAIMY, W., J. CRANE & A. WOODWARD. 1998. Measurement of exposure to environmental tobacco smoke in children by the analysis of hair (Abstract). Epidemiology **9:** S71.
13. BECKER, D.M., H.F. CONNOR & H.R. WARANCH et al. 1989. The impact of a total ban on smoking in the Johns Hopkins Children's Center. J.A.M.A. **262:** 799–802.
14. WOODWARD, A. & T. FRASER. 1997. Passive smoking in New Zealand: health risks and control measures. NZ Health Report **4:** 35–36.
15. JAAKKOLA, M.S. & J.J. JAAKKOLA. 1997. Assessment of exposure to environmental tobacco smoke. Eur. Respir. J. **10:** 2384–2397.
16. BENOWITZ, N.L. 1996. Cotinine as a biomarker of environmental tobacco smoke exposure. Epidemiol. Rev. **18:** 188–204.
17. PIRKLE, J.L., K.M. FIEGAL, J.Y. BERNERT, D.J. BRODY, R.A. ETZEL & K.R. MAURER. 1996. Exposure of the United States population to environmental tobacco smoke. J.A.M.A. **275:** 1233–1240.
18. JARVIS, M.J., A.D. MCNEILL, M.A.H. RUSSELL et al. 1987. Passive smoking in adolescents: one-year stability of exposure in the home. Lancet. **i:** 1324–1325.
19. HECHT, S.S., S.G. CARMELLA, S.E. MURPHY, A. AKERKAR, K.D. BRUNNEMANN & D. HOFFMANN. 1993. A tobacco-specific lung carcinogen in the urine of men exposed to cigarette smoke. N. Engl. J. Med. **329:** 1543–1546.
20. BAKOULA, C.G., Y.J. KAFRITSA, G.D. KAVADIAS, D.D. LAZOPOULOU, M.C. THEODORIDOU, K.P. MARAVELIAS et al. 1995. Objective passive-smoking indicators and respiratory morbidity in young children. Lancet **346:** 280–281.
21. CUMMING, K.M., S.J. MARKELLO, M. MAHONEY et al. 1990. Measurement of current exposure to environmental tobacco smoke. Arch. Environ. Health **45:** 74–79.
22. RIBOLI, E., S. PRESTON-MARTIN, R. SARACCI et al. 1990. Exposure of nonsmoking women to environmental tobacco smoke: a 10-country collaborative study. Cancer Causes & Control **1:** 243–252.
23. IDLE, J.R. 1990. Titrating exposure to tobacco smoke using cotinine—a minefield of misunderstandings. J. Clin. Epidemiol. **43:** 313–318.
24. UEMATSU, T., A. MIZUNO, M. NAGASHIMA, A. OSHIMA & M. NAKAMURA. 1995. The axial distribution of nicotine content along hair shafts as an indicator of changes in smoking behaviour: evaluation in a smoking cessation programme with or without the aid of nicotine chewing gum. Br. J. Clin. Paharmacol. **39:** 665–669.
25. NILSEN, T., K. ZAHLSEN & O.G. NILSEN. 1994. Uptake of nicotine in hair during controlled environmental air exposure to nicotine vapour: evidence for a major contribution of environmental nicotine to the overall nicotine found in hair from smokers and non-smokers. Pharmacol. & Toxicol. **75:** 136–142.
26. ZAHLSEN, K. & O.G. NILSEN. 1994. Nicotine in hair of smokers and nonsmokers: sampling procedure and gas chromatographic/mass spectrometric analysis. Pharmacol. & Toxicol. **75:** 143–149.
27. NAFSTAD, P., G. BOTTEN, J.A. HAGEN, K. ZAHLSEN et al. 1995. Comparison of three methods for estimating environmental tobacco smoke exposure among children aged between 12 and 36 months. Int. J. Epidemiol. **24:** 88–94.
28. NAFSTAD, P., J.J. JAAKKOLA, J.A. HAGEN, K. ZAHLSEN & P. MAGNUS. 1997. Hair nicotine concentrations in mothers and children in relation to parental smoking. J. Exposure Analysis & Environ. Epidemiol. **7:** 235–239.
29. MIZUNO, A., T UEMATSU, A. OSHIMA, M. NAKAMURA & M. NAKASHIMA. 1993. Analysis of nicotine content of hair for assessing individual cigarette smoking behaviour. Therap. Drug Monitor. **15:** 99–104.
30. COULTAS, D.B., J.M. SAMET, J.F. MCCARTHY & J.D. SPENGLER. 1990. A personal monitoring study to assess workplace exposure to environmental tobacco smoke. Am. J. Public Health **80:** 988–990.
31. PATRICK, D.L., A. CHEADLE, D.C. THOMPSON, P DIEHR, T. KOEPSELL & S. KINNE. 1994. The validity of self-reported smoking: a review and meta-analysis. Am. J. Public Health **84:** 1086–1093.
32. WOODWARD, A. 1988. Passive smoking and acute respiratory illness in childhood. Ph.D. Thesis. University of Adelaide, Adelaide.

33. COULTAS, D.B., G.T. PEAKE & J.M. SAMET. 1989. Questionnaire assessment of lifetime and recent exposure to environmental tobacco smoke. Am. J. Epidemiol. **8130:** 338–347.
34. PRON, G.E., J.D. BURCH, G.R. HOWE et al. 1988. The reliability of passive smoking histories reported in a case-control study of lung cancer. Am. J. Epidemiol. **127:** 267–273.
35. COULTAS, D.B., J.M. SAMET & J.F. MCCARTHY et al. 1990. Variability of measures of exposure to environmental tobacco smoke in the home. Am. Rev. Respir. Dis. **142:** 602–606.
36. HENDERSON, F.W., H.F. REID, R. MORRIS, O. WANG, P.C. HU et al. Home air nicotine levels and urinary cotinine excretion in preschool children. Am. Rev. Respir. Dis. **140:** 197–201.
37. DE WAARD, F., J.M. KEMMEREN, L.A. VAN GINKEL & A.A. STOLKER. 1995. Urinary cotinine and lung cancer risk in a female cohort. British J. Cancer. **72:** 784–787.
38. WANG, X., I.B. TAGER, H. VAN VUNAKIS, F.E. SPEIZER & J.P. HANRAHAN. 1997. Maternal smoking during pregnancy, urine cotinine concentrations, and birth outcomes. A prospective cohort study. Int. J. Epidemiol. **26:** 978–988.
39. CASALE, R., D. COLANTONIO, M. CIALENTE, V. COLORIZIO, R. BARNABEI & P. PASQUALETTI. 1991. Impaired pulmonary function in schoolchildren exposed to passive smoking. Detection by questionnaire and urinary cotinine levels. Respiration **58**(3–4): 198–203.
40. COOK, D.G., P.H. WHINCUP, O. PAPACOSTA, D.P. STRACHAN et al. 1993. Relation of passive smoking as assessed by salivary cotinine concentration and questionnaire to spirometric indices in children. Thorax **48:** 14–20.
41. MORGAN, G.M. & M. HENRION. 1990. Uncertainty—A Guide to Dealing with Uncertainty in Quantitative Risk and Policy Analysis. Cambridge University Press, New York.
42. DOULL, J., K.K. ROZMAN & M.C. LOWE. 1996. Hazard evaluation in risk assessment: whatever happened to sound scientific judgement and weight of evidence? Drug Metab. Reviews **28:** 285–299.
43. OGDEN, M.W. 1996. Estimating exposure to environmental tobacco smoke (Letter). J.A.M.A. **276:** 603–604.
44. GORI, G.B. 1994. Science, policy and ethics: the case of environmental tobacco smoke. J. Clin. Epidemiol. **47:** 325–334.
45. NILSSON, R. 1996. Environmental tobacco smoke and lung cancer: a reappraisal. Ecotoxicol. Env. Safety **334:** 2–17.
46. HOWARD, G., G.L. BURKE, M. SZKLO, G.S. TELL, J. ECKFELDT, G. EVANS et al. 1994. Active and passive smoking are associated with increased carotid wall thickness. Arch. Int. Med. **154:** 1277–1282.
47. BARNES, D.E. & L.A. BERO. 1998. Why review articles on the health effects of passive smoking reach different conclusions. J.A.M.A. **279:** 1566–1570.
48. BRUNK, C.G., L. HAWORTH & B. LEE. 1991. Value Assumptions in Risk Assessment. A Case Study of the Alachlor Controversy. Wilfrid Laurier University Press, Waterloo.
49. VAN ASSELT, M.B.A. & J. ROTMANS. 1996. Uncertainty in perspective. Global Environ. Change **6:** 121–157.
50. EHRLICH, R., M. KATTAN, J. GODBOLD, D.S. SALTZBERG, K.T. GRIMM, P.J. LANDRIGAN et al. 1992. Childhood asthma and passive smoking. Urinary cotinine as a biomarker of exposure. Am. Rev. Respir. Dis. **145**(3): 594–599.
51. CHILMONCZYK, B.A., L.M. SALMUN, K.N. MEGATHLIN, L.M. NEVEUX et al. 1993. Association between exposure to environmental tobacco smoke and exacerbations of asthma in children. N. Engl. J. Med. **328:** 1665–1669.
52. REBAGLIATO, M., F. BOLUMAR & C. DU V. FLOREY. 1995. Assessment of exposure to environmental tobacco smoke in nonsmoking pregnant women in different environments of daily living. Am. J. Epidemiol. **142:** 525–530.
53. RYLANDER, E., G. PERSHAGEN, M. ERIKSSON & G. BERMANN. 1995. Parental smoking, urinary cotinine and wheezing bronchitis in children. Epidemiol. **6:** 289–293.

54. TUNSTALL-PEDOE, H., C.A. BROWN, M. WOODWARD & R. TAVENDALE. 1995. Passive smoking by self report and serum cotinine and the prevalence of respiratory and coronary heart disease in the Scottish heart health study. J. Epidemiol. Community Health **49:** 139–143.
55. HADDOW, J.E., G.J. KNIGHT, G.E. PALOMAKI, E.M. KLOZA & N.J. WALD. 1987. Cigarette consumption and serum cotinine in relation to birthweight. Br. J. Obstet. Gynaecol. **94:** 678–681.
56. WOODWARD, A., R.M. DOUGLAS, N.M.H. GRAHAM & H. MILES. 1990. Acute respiratory illness in Adelaide children: breast feeding modifies the effect of passive smoking. J. Epidemiol. Comm. Health **44:** 224–230.
57. PEREZ-STABLE, E.J., N.L. BENOWITZ & G. MARIN. 1995. Is serum cotinine a better measure of cigarette smoking than self-report? Prev. Med. **24:** 171–179.

The Contribution of Environmental Monitoring in the Epidemiological Assessment of Exogenous Risk

The Experience of ARPA in the Emilia-Romagna Region of Italy

A. ZAVATTI[a] AND P. LAURIOLA

Regional Agency for Prevention and Environment (ARPA), Emilia-Romagna Region, via Po 5, 40139 Bologna, Italy

ABSTRACT: The aim of the Emilia Romagna-Region Agency for Prevention and Environment (ARPA) is to define and improve interactions among the various prevention departments of the Emilia-Romagna Local Health Authorities in order to attain better knowledge about the health status of the population by using epidemiology and etiology studies, as well as predictive models. This is the basis for the environmental health risk assessment strategy of ARPA. The priority activity areas for ARPA are: urban areas, environmental and health effects of traffic (atmospheric pollution and noise pollution); industrial areas (Ravenna chemical plants, Modena/Reggio-Emilia ceramic factories and Ferrara chemical plants); high-speed trains; pesticides; asbestos; and pollution of the Adriatic Sea.

INTRODUCTION

In the past 20 years there has been growing interest in the environment and quality of life in Italy. One effect has been the creation and development of public environmental health preventive services. As a result of a referendum held in 1993, in 1994 the national and regional Environmental Protection Agencies network was established, engaging personnel from environmental and health laboratories, and from National Health Services. This rearrangement offered an opportunity to reconsider environmental and health prevention services in the Emilia-Romagna region where these services had been established in the 1970s and 1980s. At present, 15 out of 21 Italian regions have legislated environmental agencies, although not all of these have as yet been constituted, see FIGURE 1.

FEATURES OF ARPA EMILIA-ROMAGNA

ARPA Emilia-Romagna has adopted the following *mission*: "To conduct environmental controls oriented towards general prevention and safeguarding of natural resources and health so as to guarantee ongoing social and economic development in

---

[a]Address for correspondence: 39-051-6223811 (voice); 39-051-6223861 (fax).
e-mail: a.zavatti@sc.arpa.emr.it

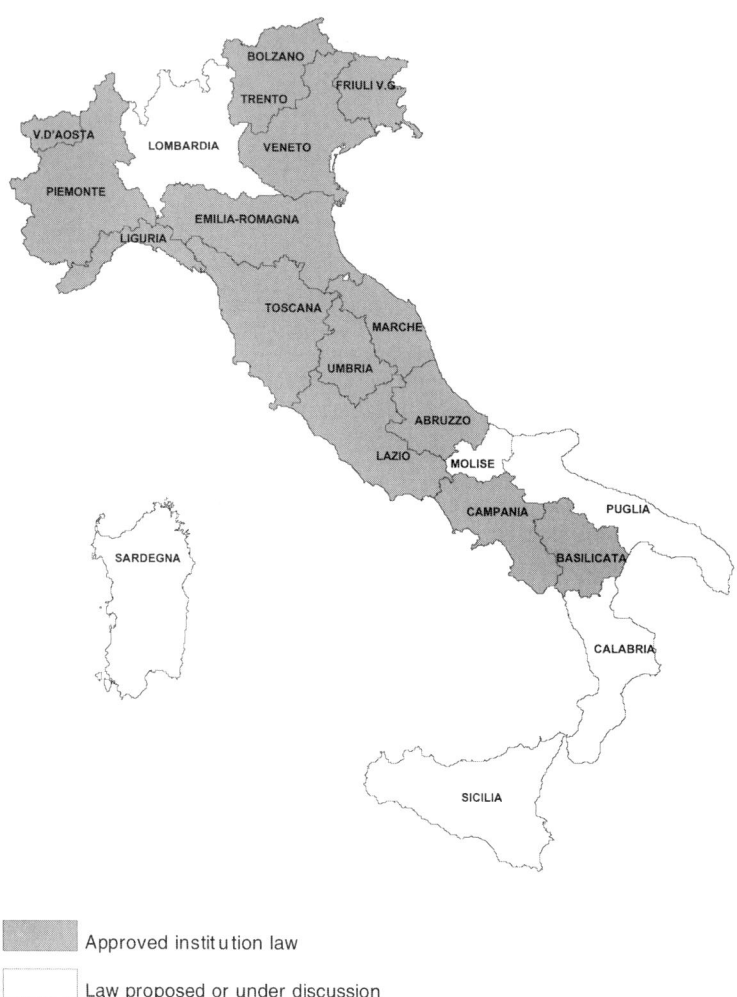

FIGURE 1. Institution of regional agencies for the environment (in accordance with Law 61/94).

ecological-environmental terms." This sees ARPA as developing and disseminating, in collaboration with private and public sectors, information about monitoring and preventive procedures, with the aim of improving the quality of environment and health protection; and to do so by means of the harmonization of a services network that is capable of producing and exchanging knowledge and innovation.

Among the main tasks for ARPA are:
1. control and surveillance of the application of environmental norms;
2. investigation and research for the approval of environmental projects;
3. technical support for environmental planning;
4. operational/technical support for the Health Service;
5. management of the environmental information system;
6. laboratory analyses to assess health and environmental status.

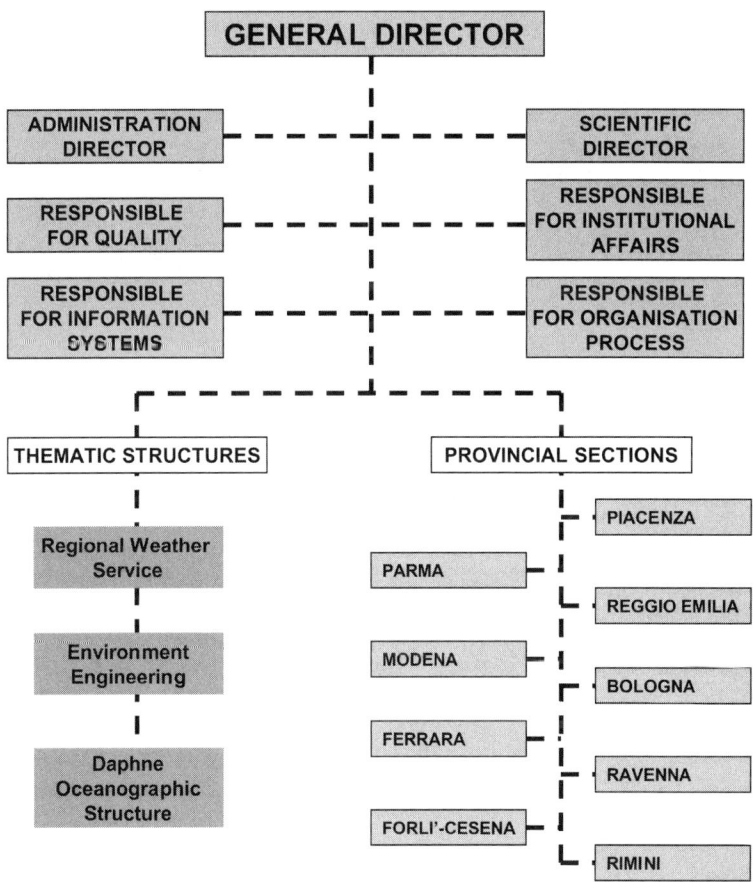

FIGURE 2. ARPA management structure.

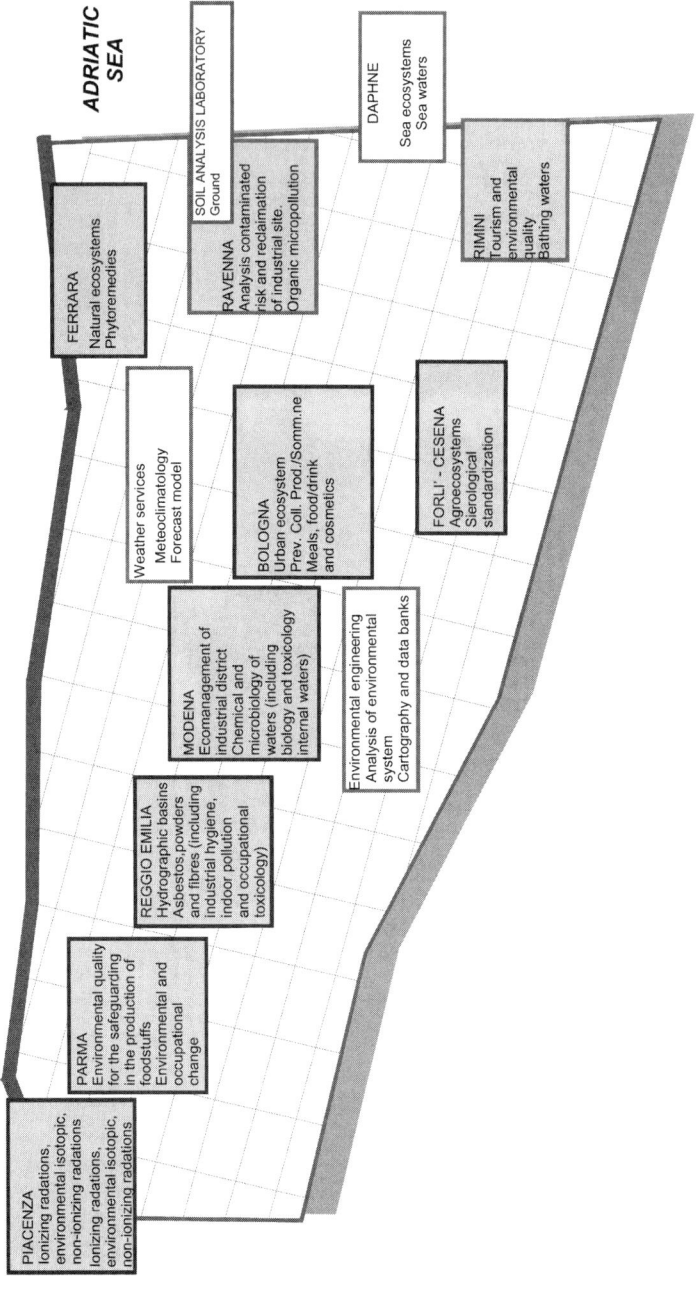

FIGURE 3. ARPA excellence and specialization network.

Its management structure is shown in FIGURE 2. The professional network that exploits excellence and specialization is shown in FIGURE 3.

INFORMATION MANAGEMENT AND USE

Acquisition of knowledge is the primary condition for a continuous process of adjustment of programming and planning. The ARPA management should be the result of a synthetic-detailed dissemination of information among the various sites of activity integration: European Environmental Agency, regional/national environmental protection agencies, Ministries, other national scientific and administrative bodies, Regions, Provinces, and Local Health Authorities.

In particular, this information involves the various ARPA environmental monitoring networks that deal with:

- Surface waters, monitored by means of 250 measuring stations surveyed monthly with 23 analytical parameters (see FIGURE 4).
- A network for qualitative and quantitative measurement of ground waters (500 wells in the Po Plain aquifer (see FIGURE 5).
- Atmospheric survey by means of 90 measuring stations with 500 analyzers (see FIGURE 6).
- The Adriatic Sea, by means of an oceanographic ship (Daphne) that monitors eutrophication emergencies (see FIGURE 7).
- Soil, a pedologic regional map in 1:25,000 scale from which a survey of contaminated sites has been developed.
- Environmental radioactivity monitoring, performed by taking 2,000 samples per year from various environmental matrices on the whole regional territory.
- Noise pollution, surveyed by drawing a noise map in each provincial capital town.
- Other significant sample cases surveyed including work environment, asbestos, foodstuffs, acid rain, land subsidence, and pollen.

An essential feature is the integration of all these networks to adequately underpin decisions orientated toward sustainable development, by the incorporation of Agenda 21 guidelines in an ecosystemic approach to environmental problems. In particular, use of environmental information will be aimed toward:

- favouring the passage from forms of environmental management of the *command and control* type to preventive safeguards;
- supporting the decisions of planning and implementation;
- informing citizens on the conditions of environmental quality, satisfying their *right to know*;
- supporting environmental analysis or projects;
- directing monitoring and control actions.

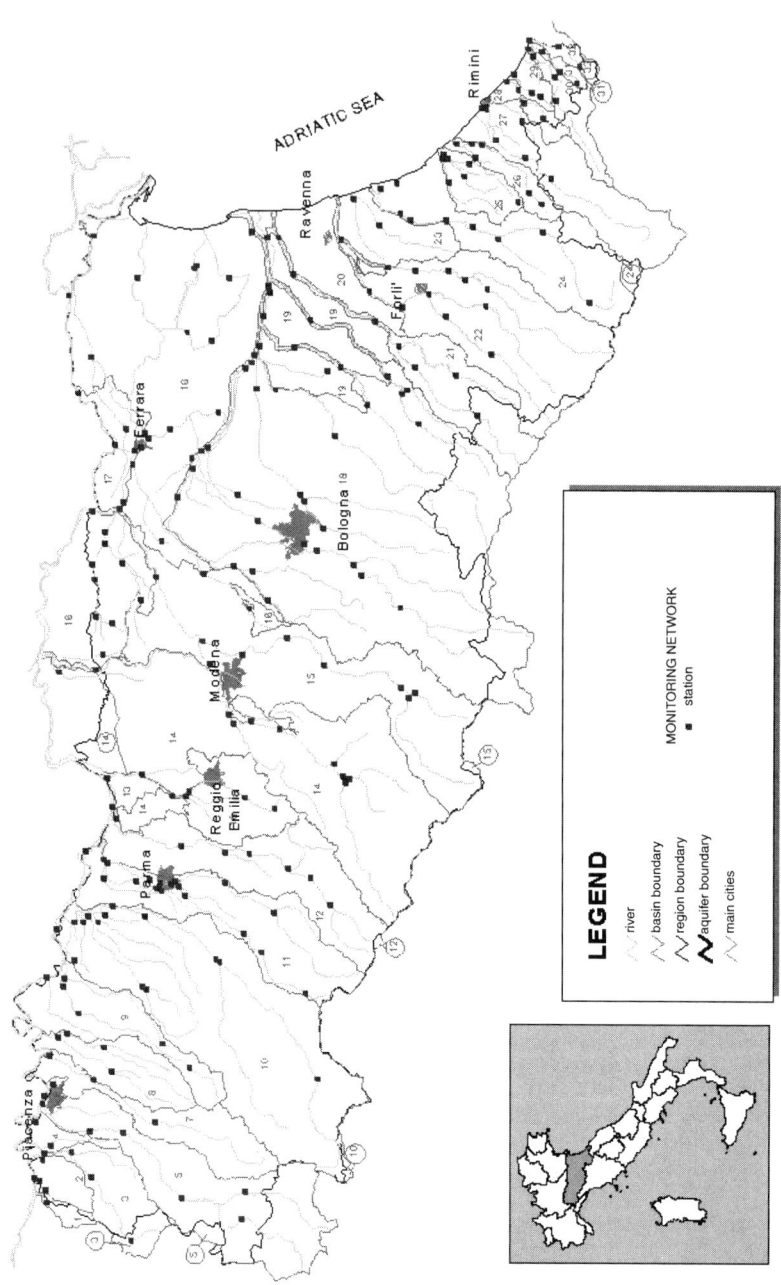

FIGURE 4. Surface water monitoring network.

ZAVATTI & LAURIOLA: ENVIRONMENTAL MONITORING 179

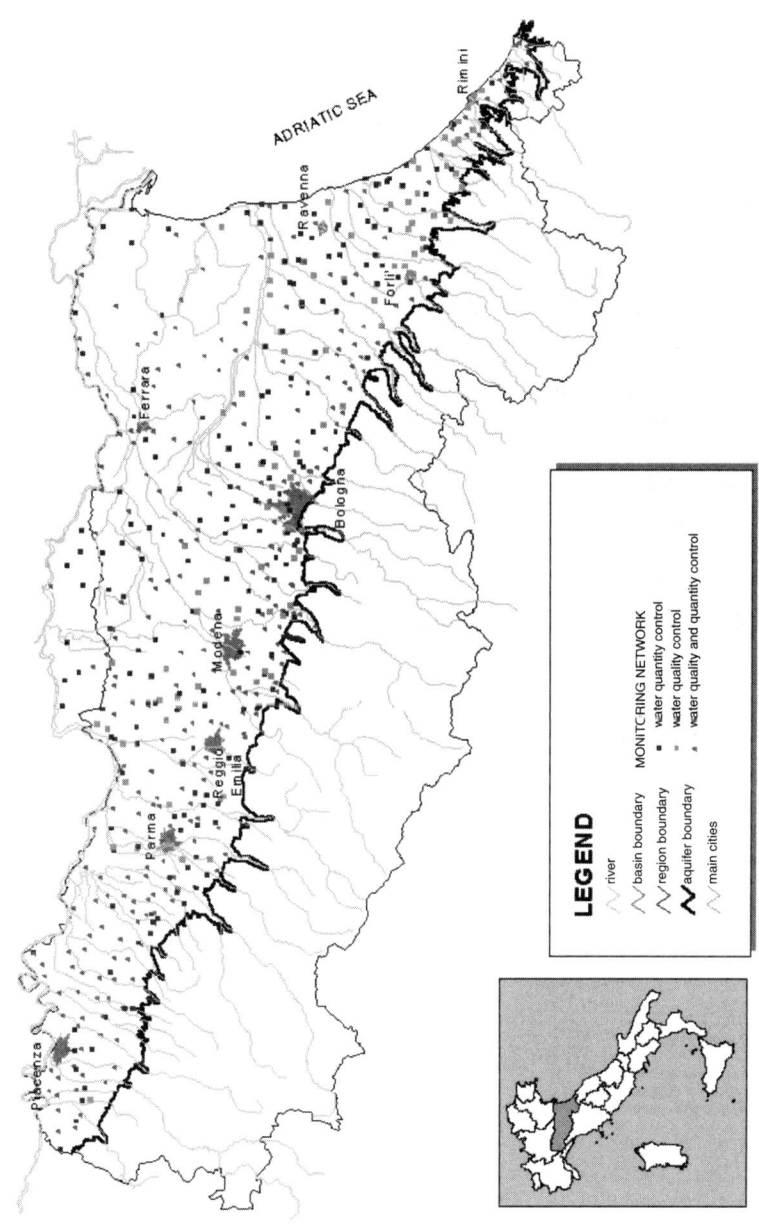

FIGURE 5. Ground water monitoring network.

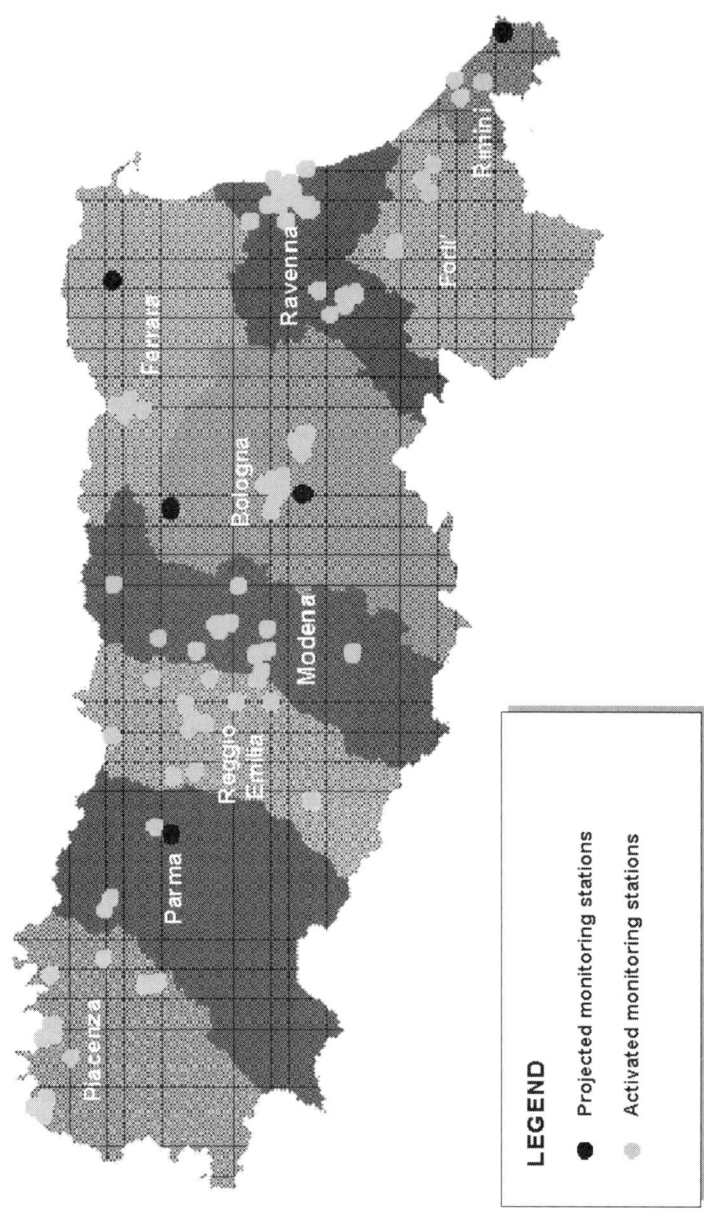

FIGURE 6. Air quality monitoring network.

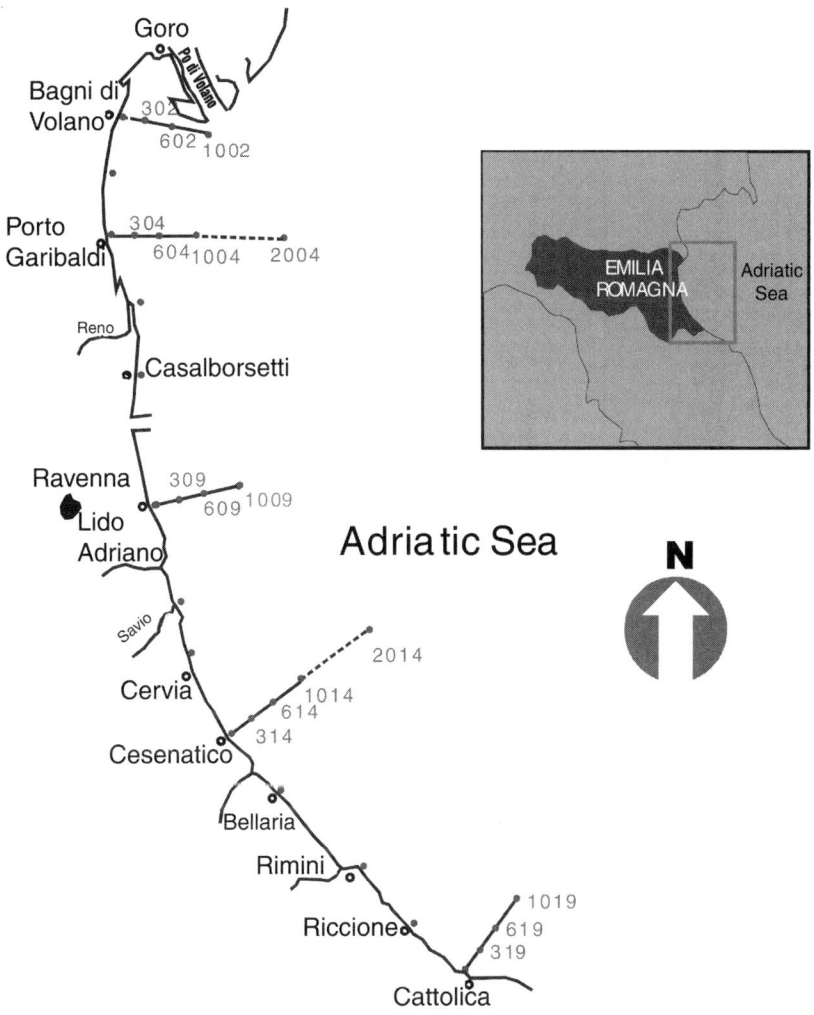

FIGURE 7. Sea eutrophication monitoring service.

All of these objectives are summarized in the so-called *virtuous circle for environmental data* (see FIGURE 8) that applies in both public and private contexts. In this respect, a preliminary condition for public/private integration is the effective organization of environmental monitoring, intended for the production of information relating to the carrying capacity, vulnerability, and critical conditions of the state of the environment (see FIGURE 9).

This means that the information is available to citizens, with due respect for the rights of companies and individuals according to the following principle: "ARPA

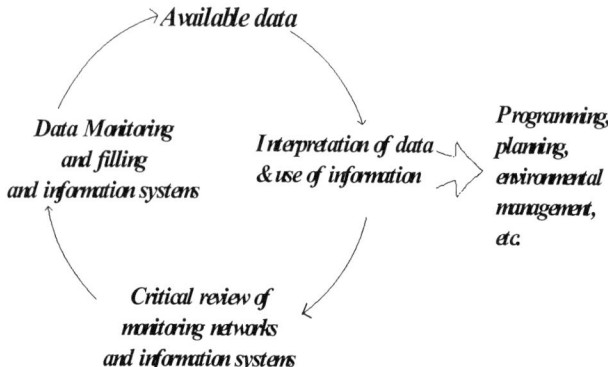

FIGURE 8. Virtuous circle for environmental data.

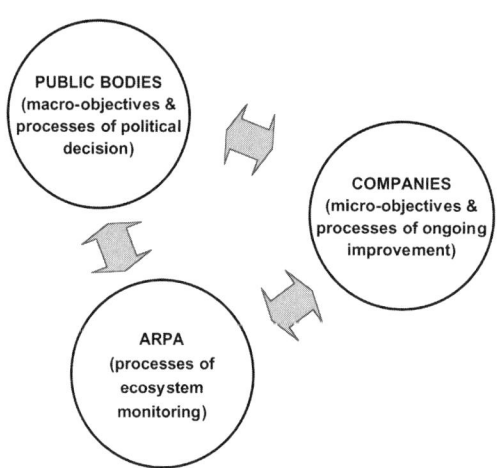

FIGURE 9. The role of ARPA in a context of public/private integration.

makes all data gathered through monitoring and control systems available to administrations, firms, and citizens by the most suitable means available—annual reports, web sites, etc.—by transferring and adapting the analysis of environmental components (in the air, water, ground, noise, radiation, etc.) to ecosystems (aquatic, urban, natural and agro ecosystems, etc.)."

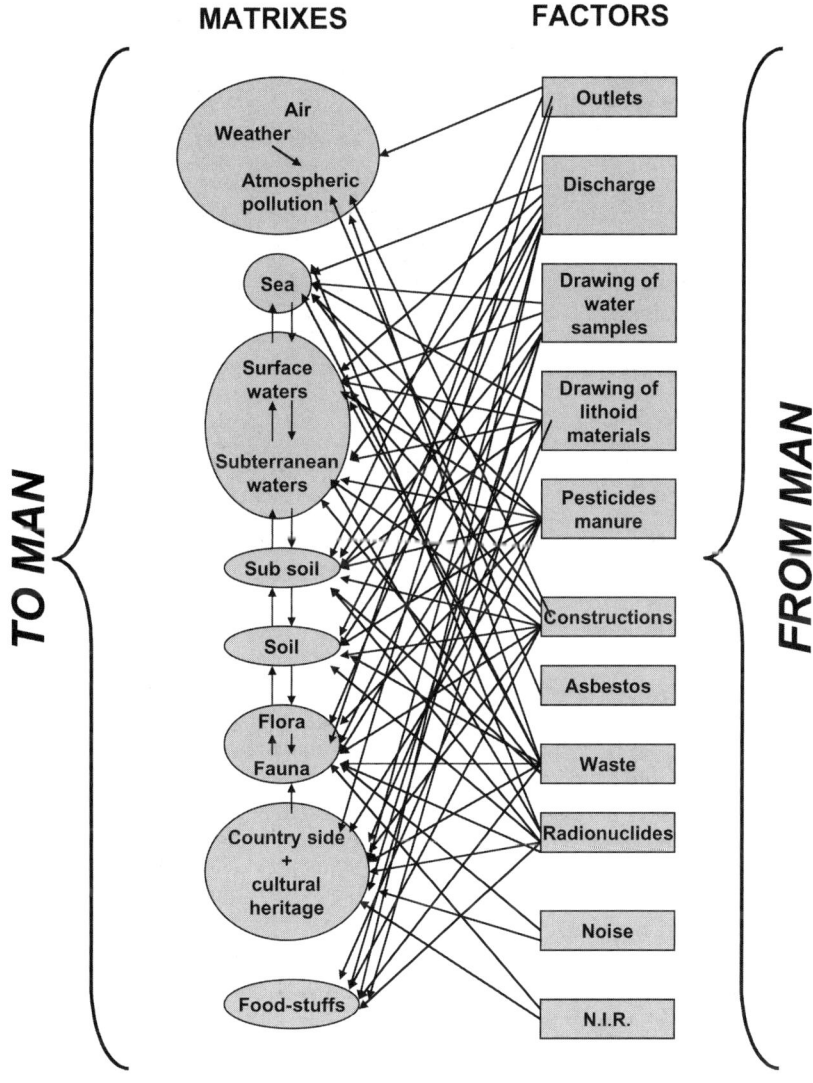

FIGURE 10. Role of human activity in environmental pollution.

ENVIRONMENTAL MONITORING AND HEALTH RISK ASSESSMENT

The investigation of the nature, causes and effects of environmental pollution involves evaluating the role of human activity in environmental pollution, as well as how people are affected (see FIGURE 10). To explain these relations implies an assessment of the relationship between environment and health that crucially underpins *sustainable development*. In other words, the relationship between humankind and nature must be understood as an interactive process, in which certain favorable conditions are offered for use (potentialities) but where constraints, or even prohibitions on certain uses, are also present. Consequently, thresholds are established that make use of the environmental indicators and indexes needed to implement agreed comparison statements defined quantitatively:

- anthropic pressures;
- conditions of the state of the environment and the capacity of ecosystems for endurance;
- the responses from the social system to attain the preformulated aims in the matter of *sustainable development*.

It is, therefore, useful to define a framework of environmental indicators and indices:

- descriptive picture of national reference;
- a common group of indicators/indexes to be monitored that are shared by environmental management bodies (core set);
- an integration of the *core set* in each individual territorial region with many other particular groups of indices and indicators.

As a corollary, the need for an interdisciplinary approach is evident in the study of each individual environmental matrix or polluting factor. This is even more evident if the complexity of the interdisciplinary and *interfactorial* relations are considered.

All of these considerations could be basically taken as the premise of the following statement: "The ecosystemic approach is the foundation of preventive health policies." Even starting from a different point of view, the same statement is supported by the authoritative epidemiologist, Professor Rose, who proved by using a quantitative epidemiology approach that *population-oriented prevention* is more effective than *risk group prevention*,[1] especially if the ethical issues are also taken into account—weaker people, such as the elderly and the unemployed, are more highly protected. The same has been concluded by the World Health Organisation (WHO) in stating[2] the *health and environment cause-effect framework* (se FIGURE 11), derived from the OECD *sustainable development indicators*.[3] It also states that reducing the effect of driving forces or the environmental pressures that produce the hazards, is the most effective long-term intervention.

On the basis of this option, ARPA Emilia-Romagna is developing epidemiology projects in collaboration with Local Health Authorities. This objective is also supported by the notion that the relation between risk factors (chemical, physical, or bi-

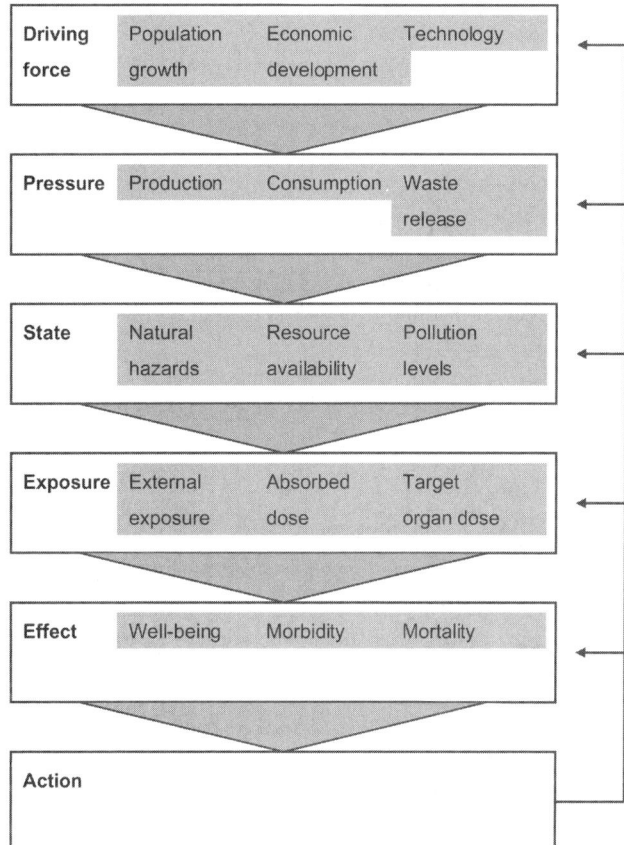

FIGURE 11. Health and environment cause-effect framework.

ological) cannot be summarized in a simple exposure-damage relation. In some cases, exposure to a risk factor causes no damage, in other cases it may change the susceptibility or defences of the host and/or cause functional or prepathologic changes. Even human behavior can be influenced by environmental factors, for instance physical factors such as light, noise and heat.[4]

For these reasons ARPA decided to use health data in order to quantify and assess the sustainability of development. In this context it is useful to remember what the UN declared at the Rio Conference in *Principle 1*: "Human beings are at the centre of concerns for sustainable development. They are entitled to a healthy and productive life in harmony [with] nature."[5]

ENVIRONMENTAL EPIDEMIOLOGY ACTIVITY IN ARPA EMILIA-ROMAGNA

A definition of environmental epidemiology, given by an anonymous health worker, was reported by B. Terracini in 1992: "it studies at different levels, but mainly on a local basis, connections between supposed factors of chemical-physical-biological and social risks present in the everyday environment and pathological or pre-pathological manifestations or health-related events."[6] Based on this definition the general objective of ARPA is to stimulate, support, and, where appropriate, to accredit local knowledge emphasizing a positive approach. In particular, the attempt is to insert an environmental-health preventive context into the administrative and legal norms.

In more detail, ARPA Environmental Epidemiology:

1. Promotes, coordinates, and activates programmes and initiatives for probing knowledge about the effects on human health of environmental risks situation.
2. Promotes, coordinates, and activates collaboration and close relations with organizations, bodies, and institutions aiming to,
   • launch initiatives of training and education in tune with epidemiologic evaluation of environmental risks,
   • carry out evaluations of environmental impact concerning the health component,
   • probe health problems consequent on environmental risk situations.
3. Contributes in finding priorities in control and prevention with the aim of safeguarding health, through the definition of levels of risk arising from analysis carried out by evaluation of data, indicators and technical-scientific indexes.

Some of the epidemiological studies in which ARPA is involved are as follows.

- Molecular epidemiology: validation study of the Ames test for mutagenicity of airborne particulate in association with levels of aromatic DNA adducts and other markers of biological and genetic damage in persons occupationally and nonoccupationally exposed to polcycyclic aromatic hydrocarbons.

- Epidemiologic surveillance of acute pesticide intoxication.

- Vehicle accident investigation: statistical investigation on determinants, implementation of mathematical simulation models to predict and evaluate preventive interventions, social and health costs, and emergency care evaluation.

- Cross-sectional studies on acute effects of air pollution on children and adults in rural, industrial, and urban areas.

- Studies on carcinogenic effects of environmental pollution due to vehicle traffic and agriculture by collaborating with experimental studies.

- Studies on pollen allergy.

In general terms it is expected that the results of these studies will not only produce the information that is required to assess the damage caused by environmental determinants, but especially to estimate and, whenever possible forecast, the risk by fully integrating all information collected by environmental monitoring, social and health observations, biochemical, microbiological, and genetic investigations. All this information will be used to prevent health hazard and risk.

ARPA collaborates with the following research centres:

- International Programme on Chemical Safety (IPCS-WHO)
- European Centre for Environmental Health (ECEH-WHO)
- International centre for pesticide safety (ICPS-WHO)
- European Ramazzini Foundation
- Istituto Nazionale di Statistica (ISTAT)
- Istituto Superiore di Sanità (ISS)
- Consiglio Nazionale delle Ricerche (CNR-FISBAT)
- Istituto Oncologico Romagnolo
- Local Health Authority—Preventive Departments.

ACKNOWLEDGMENTS

The authors are particularly grateful to Allison Eames for her thorough revision of the text and helpful suggestions.

REFERENCES

1. ROSE, G. 1992. The Strategy of Preventive Medicine. Oxford University Press, Oxford.
2. WHO. 1997. Health and Environment in Sustainable Development, Five Years After the Earth Summit. WHO, Geneva.
3. OECD. 1993. OECD core set of indicators for environmental performance reviews. Environmental Monograph N. 83. O.E.C.D., Paris.
4. IPCS. 1983. IPCS-WHO Guidelines On Studies In Environmental Epidemiology Environmental Health Criteria 27. WHO, Geneva.
5. UN 1990. Agenda 21: the United Nations programme of action from Rio. UN, New York.

Combining Uncertainty Factors in Deriving Human Exposure Levels of Noncarcinogenic Toxicants

RALPH L. KODELL[a] AND DAVID W. GAYLOR[b]

[a]*Division of Biometry and Risk Assessment, National Center for Toxicological Research, U.S. Food and Drug Administration,[c] 3900 NCTR Road, Jefferson, Arkansas 72079, U.S.A*

[b]*Office of Risk Assessment Policy and Research,
National Center for Toxicological Research,
U.S. Food and Drug Administration,[c] 3900 NCTR Road, Jefferson, Arkansas 72079, U.S.A*

ABSTRACT: **Acceptable levels of human exposure to noncarcinogenic toxicants in environmental and occupational settings generally are derived by reducing experimental no-observed-adverse-effect levels (NOAELs) or benchmark doses (BDs) by a product of uncertainty factors (Barnes and Dourson, Ref. 1). These factors are presumed to ensure safety by accounting for uncertainty in dose extrapolation, uncertainty in duration extrapolation, differential sensitivity between humans and animals, and differential sensitivity among humans. The common default value for each uncertainty factor is 10. This paper shows how estimates of means and standard deviations of the approximately log-normal distributions of individual uncertainty factors can be used to estimate percentiles of the distribution of the product of uncertainty factors. An appropriately selected upper percentile, for example, 95th or 99th, of the distribution of the product can be used as a combined uncertainty factor to replace the conventional product of default factors.**

INTRODUCTION

Human exposure levels of toxic substances, whether environmental or occupational, are established through the process of risk assessment. Such exposure levels are predicted to pose acceptable (usually zero or negligible) risks of adverse health effects to humans under specified exposure conditions. Often, the objective of a risk assessment is to establish a daily exposure level that is considered safe for a lifetime, or working lifetime, of exposure. Almost always, risk assessment involves extrapolation from the conditions under which the data are observed to an unobserved or unobservable exposure situation. Whenever possible, the process of risk assessment uses human data from epidemiology studies, but it generally focuses on absolute risk rather than relative risk. Because of the usual lack of suitable human data, risk assessment is most often based on data observed in experiments with animals.

---

[a]Address for correspondence: 870-543-7008 (voice); 870-543-7662 (fax).
e-mail: rkodell@nctr.fda.gov
[c]The opinions expressed in this paper are those of the authors and not necessarily those of the U.S. Food and Drug Administration.

Meaningful extrapolation of experimental data to the applicable human situation presents significant challenges. Various exposure conversions must be made in order to account for differences between the observed conditions of exposure and the conditions of exposure for which acceptable levels are desired. Often this involves route-to-route, duration-to-duration and species-to-species conversions. Furthermore, conversion of external exposures to target-tissue doses is required. Unfortunately, in most practical applications of risk assessment, insufficient data are available to make precise, scientific conversions for all the exposure extrapolations that need to be made. Hence, it is common practice to employ a set of uncertainty factors (also called safety factors) to reduce observed exposure levels to levels that are believed to be safe for humans.[2]

For toxic effects other than cancer, no-observed-adverse-effect levels (NOAELs) obtained from animal experiments are the observed exposure levels that commonly serve as starting points for deriving safe doses. A NOAEL is loosely defined as the highest experimental dose level for which no difference in the occurrence of adverse effects is observed in test animals, relative to the control group. In experiments where a NOAEL is not established, only a lowest-observed-adverse-effect-level (LOAEL) will be available for risk assessment. A LOAEL generally corresponds to a response in the range of 1% to 10%. Recently, there has been a movement to use benchmark doses (BDs) instead of NOAELs and LOAELs, as starting points for establishing safe exposure levels.[3-10] A BD_p is defined in the same way as the traditional ED_p; it is the effective dose of a substance that yields a response of level p. BD_p values in the range $0.01 \leq p \leq 0.10$ are considered to be the most appropriate starting values. In particular, BD_{01} has been recommended as a replacement for the NOAEL and BD_{10} has been recommended as a replacement for the LOAEL.[11] In practice, statistical lower confidence limits (e.g., 95% lower limits) on BD_p values are used more commonly as starting points, than are central estimates.

Like the NOAEL and the LOAEL that they approximate, BD_{01} and BD_{10} are merely starting points for establishing safe exposure levels, but they have more precise definition and determination than the NOAEL and LOAEL. Like the NOAEL and LOAEL, they can be interpreted to correspond to negligible or very low risk levels, rather than to precise numerical values. The exposure levels that result from reducing NOAELs and LOAELs (or BD_{01}s and BD_{10}s) by uncertainty factors, need not have specific risk connotations attached to them, but may simply be expected to provide adequate safety.

The most common uncertainty factors employed in risk assessment are U_H, a factor to account for uncertainty with respect to differential sensitivities among humans; U_A, a factor to account for uncertainty concerning the relative sensitivities of animals and humans; U_S a factor to capture uncertainty in extrapolating from subchronic-exposure data to the chronic-exposure situation; and U_L, a factor to account for uncertainty in extrapolating from a low-risk level (LOAEL or BD_{10}) to a zero-risk or negligible-risk level (NOAEL or BD_{01}). Frequently, the default value for each uncertainty factor is 10, which is the maximum value in the 1–10-range that is considered in practice.

Each uncertainty factor is designed to account for one specific source of uncertainty, for which either the direction of the difference or the magnitude of the difference between an estimated value and the true value is unknown. Each factor is presumed to account for extreme differences that might exist between estimated values and true values. Because not all true differences are expected to be at their extremes simultaneously, reducing an observed exposure value by a product of default uncertainty factors may lead to undue conservatism, in the sense that the resulting acceptable exposure level is lower than is necessary to provide the desired health protection. Various authors have written recently about the appropriate accounting of uncertainty from a product of uncertainty factors.[12–17] This paper proposes using an estimate of an upper percentile of the distribution of the product of uncertainty factors as a statistically valid way of combining uncertainty factors to provide the desired high degree of assurance of health protection without inducing undue conservatism.

METHODS

Implicit in the use of uncertainty (safety) factors is the assumption that true conversion factors for the various types of extrapolation are random variables. Furthermore, it is explicitly assumed that the value of each individual factor that is used (e.g., 10) is large enough to capture a high percentage of the range over which that factor varies. Recent work by various authors has shown that several of these uncertainty factors do indeed behave as random variables and that their probability distributions may be approximated by the log-normal distribution.[18,19]

To extrapolate from a LOAEL to a NOAEL, Abdel-Rahman and Kadry[20] observed that the median ratio of LOAEL to NOAEL for 24 chemicals used to establish RfDs was 3.5, with 96% (i.e., 23/24) of the ratios falling below 10. Swartout[21] observed that the median ratio of doses that produced equivalent NOAELs and LOAELs in approximately 100 subchronic and chronic rat studies was 2, and that the 95th percentile of the distribution was 17. (The default value of 10 fell at the 90th percentile.) Results of Calabrese and Baldwin[22] from the analysis of marine-life LC_{50} data on more than 500 agents can be used to infer that the median ratio for extrapolation between animals and humans is 1, with an estimated upper 97.5th percentile of 26. (Calabrese and Baldwin reported an upper 95% confidence limit of 64.8 on this percentile.) For human-to-human extrapolation, the median sensitivity ratio is unity by definition, and Dourson and Stara[2] deduced that 92% of 490 chemicals evaluated in acute lethality studies had interspecies adjustment factors of at most 10.

The data just cited provide representative means (medians) and standard deviations for the distributions of natural logarithmic uncertainty factors, $\ln(U_L)$, $\ln(U_S)$, $\ln(U_A)$, and $\ln(U_H)$. Representative mean (median) estimates are obtained as $m_{\ln(U_I)} = \ln(U_{I,0.5})$, where $U_{I,0.5}$ is the observed median of the distribution of uncertainty factor U_I ($I = L, S, A$, or H). Representative standard deviation estimates can be found by solving for $s_{\ln(U_I)}$ in the relationship

$$m_{\ln(U_I)} + z_\alpha s_{\ln(U_I)} = \ln(U_{I, 1-\alpha}),$$

where z_α is the $100(1-\alpha)$th percentile of the standard normal distribution and $U_{I, 1-\alpha}$ is the observed $100(1-\alpha)$th percentile of the distribution of uncertainty factor U_I.

From the data of Abdel-Rahman and Kadry,[20] the estimated mean (median) of $\ln(U_L)$ is $m_{\ln(U_L)} = \ln(3.5) = 1.25$. Given that 96% of their observed LOAEL-to-NOAEL ratios were less than 10, an estimate of the standard deviation, $s_{\ln(U_L)}$ can be obtained by solving

$$1.25 + z_{0.04} s_{\ln(U_L)} = \ln(10),$$

where $z_{0.04}$ is the 96th percentile of the standard normal distribution. This gives an estimate of 0.60 for $s_{\ln(U_L)}$. Similarly, from the results of Swartout,[21] the estimated mean (median) of $\ln(U_S)$ is $m_{\ln(U_S)} = \ln(2) = 0.69$ and the estimated standard deviation, $s_{\ln(U_S)}$, is found to be 1.30 by solving

$$0.69 + z_{0.05} s_{\ln(U_S)} = \ln(17),$$

where 17 was the observed 95th percentile of the distribution of subchronic-to-chronic dose ratios. For both $\ln(U_A)$ and $\ln(U_H)$, the estimated mean (median) is $\ln(1) = 0$. Results of Calabrese and Baldwin[22] provide an estimate of 1.66 for $s_{\ln(U_A)}$ from the equation

$$0 + z_{0.025} s_{\ln(U_A)} = \ln(26),$$

where 26 as an estimate for the upper 97.5th percentile of the distribution of animal-to-human dose ratios. This value agrees closely with an interspecies ln-standard deviation of 1.74 reported by Kodell and Gaylor[23] for carcinogenic potencies. The data of Dourson and Stara[2] give an estimated value of 1.64 for $s_{\ln(U_H)}$ as the solution to

$$0 + z_{0.08} s_{\ln(U_H)} = \ln(10),$$

based on the observation that 92% of interspecies adjustment factors had values of 10 or less.

Each individual factor can be thought of as a point estimate of the $100(1 - \alpha)$th percentile of its distribution of uncertainty, where z_α is the $100(1 - \alpha)$th percentile of the standard normal distribution. Each of these factors can be standardized to estimates of upper 95th percentiles, $U(95)$, by calculating

$$U(95) = \exp\{m_{\ln(U)} + z_{0.05} s_{\ln(u)}\}.$$

The value of $U_S(95)$ is already given as 17. The upper 95th percentile estimates for the other factors are $U_L(95) \doteq 9$, $U_A(95) \doteq 15$, and $U_H(95) \doteq 15$ (see TABLE 1).

The objective, then, is to provide a way to obtain an estimate of an upper percentile, say 95th, of the distribution of the product, $U_H \times U_A \times U_S \times U_L$, that will be sufficiently protective but not overly conservative. Standard statistical techniques for estimating upper tolerance limits of distributions of sums of independent random variables (in this case, log-normal) can be used to accomplish this. Specifically, a point estimate for the upper 95th percentile of the combined range of uncertainty can be obtained from

$$U_{HASL}(95) = \exp\{m_{\ln(U_H)} + m_{\ln(U_A)} + m_{\ln(U_S)} + m_{\ln(U_L)} \\ + 1.645[s_{\ln(U_H)}^2 + s_{\ln(U_A)}^2 + s_{\ln(U_S)}^2 + s_{\ln(U_L)}^2]^{1/2}\}.$$

The remaining sections are devoted to discussing and illustrating the use of this *combined factor*, as well as to comparing it with the conventional default method and with other new methods.

TABLE 1. Estimated upper percentiles of distributions of uncertainty factors

Uncertainty factor	95th Percentile		97.5th Percentile point estimate	99th Percentile point estimate	Product of default factors
	Point Est.	95% UCL			
U_L	9	13 (24)[a]	11	14	10
U_S	17	23 (100)	25	41	10
U_A	15	18 (500)	26	48	10
U_H	15	17 (490)	25	45	10
U_{HA}	46		97	228	100
U_{HS}	62		124	260	100
U_{HL}	62		107	203	100
U_{AS}	64		124	269	100
U_{AL}	64		111	212	100
U_{SL}	73		115	195	100
U_{HAS}	161		374	998	1000
U_{HAL}	184		392	950	1000
U_{HSL}	250		496	1103	1000
U_{ASL}	256		511	1143	1000
U_{HASL}	629		1489	4067	3000[b]

[a]Sample size, that is, number of chemicals, in parentheses.
[b]Maximum conventional value for four uncertainty factors (EPA, Ref. 25).

COMPARISON TO ALTERNATIVE METHODS

The above formula for U_{HASL} gives a statistically sound, combined uncertainty factor that is less conservative than the conventional approach of simply multiplying together a set of uncertainty factors. For example, the conventional product of two $U(95)$ uncertainty factors, say $U_H(95)$ and $U_A(95)$, can be expressed as

$$U_H(95) \times U_A(95) = 15 \times 15$$
$$= \exp\{m_{\ln(U_H)} + m_{\ln(U_A)} + 1.645[s_{\ln(U_H)} + s_{\ln(U_A)}]\},$$

because each represents an estimate of the 95th percentile of its respective distribution of uncertainty. As can be seen by comparing this expression with the correct statistical formula of the previous section, the conservatism of the simple product arises from implicit use of $[s_{\ln(U_H)} + s_{\ln(U_A)}]$ to estimate the standard deviation of the sum of random variables instead of the correct quantity $[s^2_{\ln(U_H)} + s^2_{\ln(U_A)}]^{1/2}$. The degree of conservatism, which for these two factors can be expressed by

$$\exp\{z_\alpha[s_{\ln(U_H)} + s_{\ln(U_A)} - (s^2_{\ln U_H} + s^2_{\ln U_A})^{1/2}]\},$$

increases as the number of uncertainty factors increases. For $U_H(95)$ and $U_A(95)$,

$$\exp\{1.645[1.64 + 1.66 - (1.64^2 + 1.66^2)^{1/2}]\} \doteq 5,$$

which implies that the product of factors ($15 \times 15 = 225$) is five times larger than the overall uncertainty factor needs to be (46, using the statistically correct formula), for 95% assurance (TABLE 1). When all four factors are considered, the correct combined uncertainty factor for 95% assurance is calculated to be 629 (TABLE 1), which is 50-fold less than the factor of 34,425 obtained from the simple product of the four $U(95)$ values.

The statistically correct uncertainty factor proposed in the previous section represents a point estimate for the upper $100(1 - \alpha)$th percentile of the overall distribution of uncertainty, just as the individual factors represent point estimates for their respective distributions. This use of point estimates is consistent with Monte Carlo approaches to estimating composite distributions of uncertainty.[15,17] Some risk assessors have discussed using statistical upper confidence limits on $100(1 - \alpha)$th percentiles of individual uncertainty factors, instead of merely using point estimates.[19,22] This does represent a more conservative approach. However, for combinations of uncertainty factors, because the combined distribution is really not sampled in practice, it can be difficult to determine the appropriate tolerance factor to use, since it depends on the sample size (see, e.g., Beyer[24]). If more conservatism is warranted, it may be appropriate to use a larger percentile than the 95th percentile, but to still use a point estimate.

TABLE 1 contains point estimates for the 95th, 97.5th, and 99th percentiles for each individual uncertainty factor, and for combinations of two, three, and four factors, along with the conventional default factors. In addition, for the individual factors, upper 95% confidence limits on 95th percentiles are given for each factor. Except for LOAEL-to-NOAEL uncertainty, the conventional default factor of 10 used for an individual source of uncertainty falls below the estimated 95th percentiles of the individual uncertainty-factor distributions (i.e., a factor of 10 does not appear to provide 95% assurance of protection). The product of two default factors, $10 \times 10 = 100$, is near the estimated 97.5th percentile for two uncertainty factors, while the product of three default factors, $10 \times 10 \times 10 = 1000$ approximates the esti-

TABLE 2. Comparison with other approaches for estimating upper percentiles of distributions of uncertainty factors

Uncertainty factor	95th Percentile point estimate			99th Percentile point estimate		
	P[a]	S	B	P	S	B
U_{HA}	46	51	50	228	104	220
U_{HAS}	161	234	126	998	544	586
U_{HAL}	184	234	192	950	544	825
U_{HASL}	629	1040	484	4067	2700	2261

[a]P, Present method; S, method of Swartout *et al.* (Ref. 17); B, method of Baird *et al.* (Ref. 15).
NOTE: The values under S represent *generic* values for any sets of two, three, or four uncertainty factors.

mated 99th percentile. The default factor of 3,000 recommended by EPA[25] for four factors also approaches the estimated 99th percentile.

TABLE 2 compares selected values from TABLE 1 with values obtained from Monte Carlo analysis by Baird et al.[15] and by Swartout et al.[17] The present calculated values appear to coincide more closely with the values of Baird et al.[15] than with those of Swartout et al.[17] The present values and the Baird values are uniformly lower (by as much as a factor of two) than the Swartout values for the 95th percentile, but they are generally higher (by as much as a factor of two) for the 99th percentile. However, the values of Swartout et al., are not specific to the particular sources of uncertainty indicated. Rather, they represent *generic* values for any sets of two, three, or four uncertainty factors. Considering the different assumptions and different numerical values on which the various analyses were based, the agreement in TABLE 2 appears quite good.

DISCUSSION

The particular values used to characterize the distributions of uncertainty obviously have a major impact on the results. The values presented here are thought to be representative. As more information on the individual distributions of uncertainty becomes available, parameter values can be updated to reflect the most current knowledge. As pointed out by Baird et al.,[15] uncertainty factors could be tailored to specific classes of chemicals if sufficiently refined data were to become available.

The combined uncertainty factor proposed in this paper represents a viable alternative to the use of a product of default factors to establish acceptable human exposure levels of toxic substances. The combined factor provides assurance of health protection with a known level of confidence, without unnecessarily compounding the conservatism built into each individual factor. Although the proposed combined factor gives similar results to other recently proposed probabilistic approaches (Baird et al.[15] and Swartout et al.[17]), it is simpler to implement, and it does not require extensive Monte Carlo simulations.

REFERENCES

1. BARNES, D.G. & M. DOURSON. 1988. Reference dose (RfD): description and use in health risk assessment. Regul. Toxicol. Pharmacol. **8:** 471–486.
2. DOURSON, M.L. & J.F. STARA. 1983. Regulatory history and experimental support of uncertainty (safety) factors. Regul. Toxicol. Pharmacol. **3:** 224–238.
3. CRUMP, K.S. 1984. A new method for determining allowable daily intakes. Fundam. Appl. Toxicol. **4:** 854–871.
4. KODELL, R.L. & R.W. WEST. 1993. Upper confidence limits on excess risk for quantitative responses. Risk Analysis **13:** 177–182.
5. ALLEN, B.C., R.J. KAVLOCK, C.A. KIMMEL & E.M. FAUSTMAN. 1994. Dose-response assessment for developmental toxicity. II. comparison of generic benchmark dose estimates with no observed adverse effect levels. Fundam. Appl. Toxicol. **23:** 487–495.
6. KREWSKI, D. & Y. ZHU. 1995. A simple data transformation for estimating benchmark doses in developmental toxicity experiments. Risk Analysis **15:** 29–39.
7. CRUMP, K.S. 1995. Calculation of benchmark doses from continuous data. Risk Analysis **15:** 79–89.

8. BOSCH, R.J., D. WYPIJ & L.M. RYAN. 1996. A semiparametric approach to risk assessment for quantitative outcomes. Risk Analysis **16:** 657–665.
9. BAILER, A.J. & J.T. ORIS. 1997. Estimating inhibition concentrations for different response scales using generalized linear models. Environ. Toxicol. Chem. **16:** 1554–1559.
10. MURRELL, J.A., C.J. PORTIER & R.W. MORRIS. 1998. Characterizing dose-response I: critical assessment of the benchmark dose concept. Risk Analysis **18:** 13–26.
11. GAYLOR, D.W., R.L. KODELL, J.J. CHEN & D. KREWSKI. 1999. A unified approach to risk assessment for cancer and noncancer endpoints based on benchmark doses and uncertainty/safety factors. Regulatory Toxicology and Pharmacology. **29:** 151–157.
12. BOGEN, K.T. 1994. A note on compounded conservatism. Risk Analysis **14:** 379–381.
13. SLOB, W. 1994. Uncertainty analysis in multiplicative models. Risk Analysis **14:** 571–576.
14. GAYLOR, D.W. & J.J. CHEN. 1996. A simple upper limit for the sum of risks of the components in a mixture. Risk Analysis **16:** 395–398.
15. BAIRD, S.J.S, J.T. COHEN, J.D. GRAHAM, A.I. SHLYAKHTER & J.S. EVANS. 1996. Noncancer risk assessment: a probabilistic alternative to current practice. Human Ecol. Risk Assess. **2:** 79–102.
16. RAI, S.N. & D. KREWSKI. 1998. Uncertainty and variability analysis in multiplicative risk models. Risk Analysis **18:** 37–45.
17. SWARTOUT, J.C., P.S. PRICE, M.L. DOURSON, H. CARLSON-LYNCH & R.E. KEENAN. 1998. A probabilistic framework for the reference dose (probabilistic RfD). Risk Analysis **18:** 271–282.
18. DOURSON, M.L., S.P. FELTER & D. ROBINSON. 1996. Evolution of science-based uncertainty factors in noncancer risk assessment. Regul. Toxicol. Pharmacol. **24:** 108–120.
19. HATTIS, D. 1998. Strategies for assessing human variability in susceptibility, and using variability to infer human risks. *In* Human Variability in Response to Chemical Exposures: Measures, Modeling, and Risk Assessment. D. Neumann & C. Kimmel, Eds.: 27–57. ILSI Press, Washington, DC.
20. ABDEL-RAHMAN, M.S. & A.M. KADRY. 1995. Studies on the use of uncertainty factors in deriving RfDs. Human Ecol. Risk Assess, **1:** 614–624.
21. SWARTOUT, J. 1996. Subchronic-to-chronic uncertainty factor for the reference dose (Abstract F2.03). Society for Risk Analysis Annual Meeting. New Orleans.
22. CALABRESE, E.J. & L.A. BALDWIN. 1995. A toxicological basis to derive generic interspecies uncertainty factors for application in human and ecological risk assessment. Human Ecol. Risk Assess. **1:** 555–564.
23. KODELL, R.L. & D.W. GAYLOR. 1997. Uncertainty of estimates of cancer risks derived by extrapolation from high to low doses and from animals to humans. Intl. J. Toxicol. **16:** 449–460.
24. BEYER, W.H. 1968. Handbook of Tables for Probability and Statistics, 2nd. ed. 135–139. The Chemical Rubber Company. Cleveland.
25. U.S. ENVIRONMENTAL PROTECTION AGENCY (EPA). 1991. General Quantitative Risk Assessment Guidelines for Noncancer Health Effects. ECAD-CIN-538. Environ. Criteria Office, Off. Health and Environ. Assessment, Cincinnati.

Statistical Methods for Developmental Toxicity Analysis of Clustered Multivariate Binary Data

LOUISE RYAN[a] AND GEERT MOLENBERGHS[b]

[a]*Harvard School of Public Health and Dana-Farber Cancer Institute,
44 Binney Street, Boston, MA 02115, USA*

[b]*Biostatistics, Center for Statistics, Limburgs Universitair Centrum,
Universitaire Campus, B-3590 Diepenbeek, Belgium*

> ABSTRACT: This paper discusses some of the statistical issues that arise from developmental toxicity studies, wherein pregnant mice are exposed to chemicals in order to assess possible adverse effects on developing fetuses. We begin with a review of some current approaches to risk assessment, based on NOAELs, and provide justification for the use of methods based on dose-response models. Due to the hierarchical nature of the data, such models are more complicated in the present context than, say, in cancer studies. For example, multivariate binary outcomes arise when each fetus in a litter is assessed for the presence of malformations and/or low birth weight. We describe a multivariate exponential family model that works well for these data and that is flexible in terms of allowing response rates to depend on cluster size. Maximum likelihood estimation of model parameters and the construction of score tests for dose effect are briefly discussed. Results are illustrated with data from several NTP studies.

INTRODUCTION

Society is becoming increasingly concerned about environmental impacts on fertility and pregnancy, birth defects, and developmental abnormalities. Consequently, regulatory agencies such as the U.S. Environmental Protection Agency (EPA) and Food and Drug Administration (FDA) have placed an increased priority on researching and identifying causes of these problems to protect the public from environmental exposures that may contribute to these risks. Although standard study designs and statistical methods for quantitative risk assessment have emerged for evaluating cancer risks, the area of quantitative risk assessment for developmental and reproductive toxicity remains a relatively new field of study. In general, risk assessment for reproductive and developmental toxicity must rely heavily on data from controlled chemical experiments, since epidemiologic data tend to be limited in this area. Because such laboratory studies involve considerable time and expense, as well as large numbers of animals, it is essential that appropriate, efficient statistical models are used to assess these types of non-cancer risks.

[a]Address for correspondence: 617-632-3602 (voice); 617-632-2444 (fax).
e-mail: ryan@jimmy.harvard.edu

Regulatory approaches for developmental toxicity currently employed by both the EPA and the FDA are based on calculation of no-observed-adverse-effect levels (NOAELs). One of the underlying assumptions that has motivated use of NOAELs is that there is a threshold of exposure for each environmental agent below which developmental effects will not occur. The NOAEL is defined as the experimental dose level immediately below the lowest dose that produces a statistically or biologically significant increase in adverse effects as compared to the control group. An *acceptably safe* daily dose level for humans is then calculated by dividing the NOAEL by a safety factor, usually 100 or 1000, to account for sensitive subgroups of the population and extrapolation from animal data to human risk. The EPA refers to this safe daily concentration as the *reference dose* (RfD), whereas the FDA uses the term *allowable daily intake* (ADI). In the event that the lowest experimental dose shows significant changes from control, it is termed a LOAEL (lowest observed adverse effect level) and the safety factor used to determine the RfD or ADI is increased tenfold.

The use of the NOAEL-safety factor approach to determine reference doses has been widely acknowledged as being subject to a number of serious statistical drawbacks (see Refs. 1 and 2). Estimation of the NOAEL is highly sensitive to the experimental design, in terms of the number and spacing of dose groups and the total sample size. As the sample size increases, NOAEL estimation becomes anticonservative. That is, large studies have higher power to detect small changes and, therefore, produce lower NOAELs than smaller studies. Another disadvantage of this approach is that it does not provide measures of the statistical variability in estimating the NOAEL. Thus, no estimates of the upper bound on the risk corresponding to the NOAEL or RfD are available. The actual risk levels of an adverse effect at the NOAEL or RfD may vary considerably from one developmental toxicity study to the next, making it difficult to compare environmental agents and prioritize risk management. Yet another problem with the NOAEL approach is that it typically relies on analysis of individual outcomes, rather than forming part of a risk assessment procedure that considers the entire process of fetal development. In other words, a separate NOAEL is computed for each adverse effect of interest (for example, death, malformation, and low birth weight), and the minimum NOAEL is selected for regulatory purposes. This strategy may appear to be conservative, but can actually be anticonservative in situations where there are subtle but consistent changes in a number of outcomes.

Because of the limitations in using the NOAEL safety factor approach, interest in developing techniques for dose-response modeling of developmental toxicity data has increased, and new regulatory guidelines[3] emphasize the use of quantitative methods for risk assessment similar to those developed for cancer risk assessment. An alternative approach to using NOAELs that has recently gained enthusiasm from both toxicologists and statisticians is estimation of *benchmark doses* (BD).[1] An appropriate dose-response model is first fitted to the animal data to estimate the reference dose, or dose corresponding to a moderate increase (e.g., 1% or 10%) in risk over the background rate. The BD is then defined as the lower 95% or 99% confidence limit on the reference dose.[1] Although it is acknowledged that estimation of risk levels at very low doses can be very sensitive to the choice of a dose-response model, the BD generally occurs within the range of experimental data so that its estimation is fairly robust to model choice. Fitting dose-response models to data from developmental toxicity studies is somewhat more complicated than determining a NOAEL, but it offers a number of important advantages. First, estimated benchmark doses provide a measure of the degree of variability in risk estimation. Second, dose-response models are much more flexible in describing the fetal development process and can account for special features of developmental toxicity data, such as litter effects and multiple outcomes. Finally, the use of dose-response models allows for the incorporation of other covariates of interest that may affect the risk of adverse effects, such as the litter size or the duration and timing of exposure.

Several experimental protocols are used in reproductive and developmental studies. Three test designs (Segments I, II, and III) were established by the U.S. FDA in 1966 to assess specific types of effects.[4] The Segment I design, or fertility and reproduction study, is designed to assess male and female fertility and general reproductive ability. Such studies are typically conducted in one species (usually the rat) and involve exposing males for 60 days and females for 14 days prior to mating. Females continue to be exposed after they have been mated, usually until mid-pregnancy.[5] The Segment III design, or peri- and postnatal study, focuses on effects later in gestation and involves exposing pregnant animals from day 15 of gestation through lactation.[5]

We focus on data collected from a Segment II design, which is suitable when interest lies in the effects of exposure during the period of major organogenesis and structural development. These experiments have been often referred to as "teratology" studies, since historically, the primary goal was to study malformations. Rats, mice, and occasionally rabbits, are usually chosen as the animal model for these experiments. Administration of the exposure is generally by the clinical or environmental route(s) most closely mimicking human exposure (for example, via food or water, or by inhalation). Timed-pregnant animals (dams) are exposed during the critical period of major organogenesis (days 6–15 for mice and rats, 6–19 for rabbits) and sacrificed just prior to normal delivery, at which time the uterus is removed and the contents are thoroughly examined.

Dose levels for the Segment II design consist of a control group and three or four different dose groups exposed to the test substance. The standard recommendation is to choose the lowest dose to produce no observable maternal toxicity, and increase dose levels gradually to a maximum dose designed to produce some toxicity, but no more than ten percent maternal deaths.[3] Typically, doses are chosen at equally-spaced intervals on a linear or log-spaced scale. Ordinarily between 20 and 30 pregnant dams are randomized to each dose group and control, and typical litter sizes (number of live-born offspring) for control animals range from about eight in the rabbit to about 12–14 in mice and rats, respectively.

To motivate the methods to be presented later, we consider five developmental toxicity studies conducted by the Research Triangle Institute under contract to the National Toxicology Program (NTP). The studies investigated the effects in mice of five different chemicals: di(2-ethyhexyl)-phthalate (DEHP),[6] ethylene glycol (EG),[7] triethylene glycol dimethyl ether (TGDM),[8] diethylene glycol dimethyl ether (DYME),[9] and theophylline (THEO).[10] Each study involved a control group and three or four dosed groups, each including 20 to 30 dams with between 2 and 17 offspring per litter. For these experiments, malformations were classified as being external, visceral, and skeletal. Several animals were found to have more than one malformation type. TABLE 1 summarizes the data for each of the studies. The fetuses in a given dose group are cross-classified according to presence or absence of the three malformation indexes, thereby collapsing over litters. For example, the column labeled (1, 1, 1)′ denotes the number of fetuses with all three malformations. Similarly, the column labeled (1, 0, 0)′ denotes those with only external malformation.

Although the analysis might be simplified by collapsing to litter-specific summaries, it is natural here to consider statistical models that account for the multivariate nature of the response, as well as the litter effect induced by the clustering of off-

TABLE 1. Developmental toxicity studies

Study	Dose	Dams	Live fetuses	1 1 1	1 1 0	1 0 1	1 0 0	0 1 1	0 1 0	0 0 1	0 0 0
DEHP	0.000	30	330	0	0	0	0	0	5	4	321
	0.025	26	288	0	0	0	3	0	1	1	283
	0.050	26	277	0	5	2	8	2	13	8	239
	0.100	24	137	3	0	5	16	6	12	11	84
	0.150	25	50	8	7	8	4	1	9	7	6
EG	0	25	297	0	0	0	0	0	0	1	296
	750	24	276	0	0	1	2	0	0	23	250
	1500	23	229	0	0	1	3	0	2	83	140
	3000	23	226	1	0	12	3	8	0	105	97
TGDM	0	27	319	0	0	0	1	0	0	0	318
	250	26	275	0	0	0	0	0	0	0	275
	500	26	262	0	0	0	1	0	0	1	260
	1000	28	286	0	0	1	11	0	1	20	253
DYME	0.00	21	282	0	0	0	0	0	1	0	281
	62.50	20	225	0	0	0	0	0	0	0	225
	125.00	24	290	0	0	0	3	0	1	3	283
	250.00	23	261	0	0	2	5	0	2	50	202
	500.00	23	141	16	1	58	18	10	1	28	9
THEO	0.000	26	296	0	0	0	1	0	0	0	295
	0.075	26	278	0	0	0	2	0	0	0	276
	0.150	33	300	0	0	0	5	0	1	1	293
	0.200	23	197	0	0	0	4	0	1	0	192

NOTE: Cross-classification of all individual fetuses by study and dose group, with respect to external, visceral, and skeletal malformations, respectively. 1 denotes presence and 0 denotes absence.

spring within dams. Furthermore, since the number of viable fetuses can sometimes be related to the response probability, a model should be flexible enough to allow cluster size to affect response probabilities.

As a result of the research activity over the past 10 to 15 years, there are presently several different schools of thought concerning the best approach to the analysis of correlated binary data. Unlike in the normal setting, marginal, conditional, and random-effects approaches tend to give dissimilar results, as do likelihood, quasi-likelihood and *generalized estimating equations* (GEE) based inferential methods (for excellent reviews, see Refs. 11–14).

Several likelihood based methods have been proposed. Fitzmaurice and Laird[15] incorporate marginal parameters for the main effects in this model and quantify the degree of association by means of conditional odds ratios. Fully marginal models are available that use marginal correlations,[16,17] or a dichotomized version of a multivariate normal[18] to analyze multivariate binary data. Alternatively, marginal odds ratios can be used.[19–21] Cox[17] also describes a model whose parameters have interpretations in terms of conditional probabilities. Similar models were proposed by Rosner[22] and by Liang and Zeger.[23] Random-effects approaches have been studied by Stiratelli, Laird, and Ware,[24] Zeger, Liang, and Albert,[25] Breslow and Clayton,[26] and by Wolfinger and O'Connell.[27] Generalized estimating equations were developed by Liang and Zeger.[28]

The debate about the relative merits of the different approaches continues. For several years it seemed that marginal models, particularly GEEs, were the most popular, perhaps due to their relative computational ease and the availability of good software. It is noteworthy that the recent renewed interest in random-effects models is partly provoked by the availability of the NLMIXED procedure in SAS. There are merits and disadvantages to all three model families and generally no simple transformations between the three families exist. Arguably, model choice has to depend not only on the application of interest but also on the specific analysis goals.

Because of the need to account for litter effects, all these issues of modeling strategy arise with developmental toxicity data. Several additional issues complicate the analysis. For example, cluster sizes vary and can affect response rates, perhaps due to competition between littermates or underlying health of the mother.[29] Also, it is often important to account for the multivariate nature of the outcomes measured on each littermate. Random-effects models (beta-binomial[30]) were among the first proposed for developmental toxicity data.[31] However, they do not extend naturally to multivariate outcomes. Lefkopoulou, Moore, and Ryan[32] apply generalized estimating equations ideas to model multiple binary outcomes measured on clusters of individuals. Although their approach is simple to apply and it leads to easily interpreted tests, a disadvantage is lack of a likelihood basis. Furthermore, there are some regions of the parameter space in which the method can be quite inefficient.[33] The approach does not lend itself well to quantitative risk assessment.

Due to the popularity of marginal (especially GEE) and random effects models for correlated binary data, conditional models have received relatively little attention, especially in the context of multivariate clustered data. A notable exception is Liang and Zeger,[23] although this approach was criticized (see page 147 in Ref.11) because the interpretation of the dose effect on the risk of one outcome is conditional on the responses of other outcomes for the same individual, outcomes of other individuals, and the litter size. As Molenberghs and Ryan[34] discuss, however, there are some advantages to conditional models and with appropriate care the disadvantages can be overcome. This paper aims to discuss conditional models and their relative merits. Molenberghs, Declerck, and Aerts[20] and Aerts, Declerck, and Molenberghs[35] have compared marginal, conditional, and random-effects models for univariate clustered data when the focus is on either testing for dose effect or on benchmark dose estimation. Their results are encouraging for the conditional model. They combine a likelihood basis with numerical stability and reasonable computing time. In addition to inferential agreement between the models, especially when the likelihood ratio statistic is chosen, an unrestricted parameter space and computational convenience are among the main advantages. The model proposed here exhibits a high flexibility in capturing different patterns of nonlinear dependencies of the marginal probabilities on the cluster size.

In the next section we present the conditional probability model of Molenberghs and Ryan,[34] which allows for clustering, as well as for multiple outcomes. In the absence of clustering, the model reduces to the conditional model of Cox.[17] the third section describes likelihood based inferential techniques, including a score test. The fourth section applies the model to the NTP data introduced earlier, and compares the results with those obtained by applying other available techniques for multiple outcomes.

MODEL FORMULATION

Consider an experiment involving N clusters, the ith of which contains n_i individuals, each of whom are examined for the presence or absence of M different responses. In the NTP data, we have $M = 2$, referring to malformation and weight. Suppose that $y_{ijk} = 1$ when the kth individual in cluster i exhibits the jth response, and -1 otherwise. We use this coding rather than 1 and 0 since it provides a parametrization that more naturally leads to desirable properties when the roles of success and failure are reversed.[36] Let Y_i represent the vector of outcomes for the ith individual, and x_i an associated vector of cluster level covariates. To develop our approach, we first consider a model for unclustered outcomes, then extend it to clustered outcomes in the univariate and multivariate settings. The joint densities are presented in this section and the log-likelihood is constructed in the next section.

No Clustering

First, suppose there is no clustering ($n_i = 1$; $i = 1,...,N$). Because $k \equiv 1$ in this setting, we drop this index temporarily from our notation. The observable outcome is thus $Y_i = (y_{i1},...,y_{iM})^T$. We assume the following probability mass function:

$$f_Y(y_i; \Theta_i, n_i) = \exp\left\{\sum_{j=1}^{M} \theta_{ij} y_{ij} + \sum_{j<j'} \omega_{ijj'} y_{ij} y_{ij'} - A(\Theta_i)\right\}, \quad (1)$$

where Θ_i represents the vector of all unknown natural parameters and $A(\Theta_i)$ is a normalizing constant, resulting from summing (1) over all possible outcomes. Covariate models for Θ_i will be discussed in the next section.

Expression (1) follows from the model proposed by Cox,[17] by setting the higher order interactions to zero. This model was also used by Zhao and Prentice[37] and by Fitzmaurice, Laird, and Rotnitzky,[12] who transformed to marginal parameters. Thélot[38] studied the case where $M = 2$. If $M = 1$, the model reduces to ordinary logistic regression.

Clustered Outcomes

Now consider a single clustered outcome. Because the index j always equals 1, we drop it temporarily from our notation. However, we re-introduce the subscript k to indicate an individual within a cluster. Using logic similar to that of the previous subsection, a natural candidate for the joint distribution of Y is:

$$f_Y(y_i; \tilde{\Theta}_i, n_i) = \exp\left\{\sum_{k=1}^{n_i} \tilde{\theta}_i y_{ik} + \sum_{k<k'} \tilde{\delta}_i y_{ik} y_{ik'} - A(\tilde{\Theta}_i)\right\}, \quad (2)$$

with $\tilde{\delta}_i$ describing the association between pairs of individuals within the ith cluster. If we define the number of individuals from cluster i with positive response to be z_i then (2) becomes

$$f_Y(y_i; \tilde{\Theta}_i, n_i) = \exp\left\{\tilde{\theta}_i(2z_i - n_i) + \tilde{\delta}_i\left[\binom{n_i}{2} - 2z_i n_i + 2z_i^2\right] - A(\tilde{\Theta}_i)\right\}.$$

On absorbing constant terms into the normalizing constant and a trivial reparametrization $\theta_i = 2\tilde{\theta}_i$ and $\delta_i = 2\tilde{\delta}_i$ we obtain

$$f_Y(y_i; \tilde{\Theta}_i, n_i) = \exp\{\theta_i z_i^{(1)} + \delta_i z_i^{(2)} - A(\tilde{\Theta}_i)\}, \quad (3)$$

with $z_i^{(1)} = z_i$ and $z_i^{(2)} = -z_i(n_i - z_i)$. Independence corresponds to $\delta_i = 0$. Positive and negative values of δ_i correspond to over- and underdispersion, respectively. It is worth noting that even for underdispersion no restrictions are required on the parameter space. This feature is in contrast to other models for clustered data, for example the Bahadur[16] model and the beta-binomial model.[39]

Model (3) has several desirable properties. First, it is clearly invariant to interchanging the codes of successes and failures; hence the tests, derived in the next section, will be invariant to this change as well. Second, consider the conditional probability of observing a positive response in a cluster of size n_i, given that the remaining littermates yield $z_i - 1$ successes:

$$P(y_{ik} = 1 | z_i - 1, n_i) = \frac{\exp[\theta_i + \delta_i(2z_i - n_i - 1)]}{1 + \exp[\theta_i + \delta_i(2z_i - n_i - 1)]}, \quad (4)$$

which decreases to zero when n_i increases and z_i is bounded, and approaches unity for increasing n_i and bounded $n_i - z_i^{(1)}$, whenever there is a positive association between outcomes. From (4) it is clear that the conditional logit of an additional success, given $z_i - 1$ successes, equals $\theta_i + \delta_i(2z_i - n_i - 1)$. Thus, on noting that the second term vanishes if $z_i - 1 = (n_i - 1)/2$, θ_i is seen to be the conditional logit for an additional success when about half of the littermates exhibit a success already. Similarly, the log odds ratio for the responses between two littermates is equal to $2\delta_i$, confirming the association parameter interpretation of the δ-parameter.

Finally, because our model is conditional in nature, the marginal expectation of $z_i^{(1)}/n_i$ is clearly a (non-linear) function of n_i. This expectation can be easily calculated and plotted to explore the relationship between cluster size and response probability. Alternatively, methods similar to those of Cox and Wermuth[36] could be applied to develop approximate expressions for the marginal means and odds ratios. In any case, both (4) and the mean function can be investigated graphically to assess the plausibility of the fitted model.

Consider now an extension of the proposed model to multiple outcomes, with the additional subscript j returning as in (1) to indicate outcome type. The joint distribution of the outcome vector Y is:

$$f_Y(y_i; \tilde{\Theta}_i, n_i) = \exp\left\{\sum_{j=1}^{M}\sum_{k=1}^{n_i} \tilde{\theta}_{ij} y_{ijk} + \sum_{j=1}^{M}\sum_{k<k'} \tilde{\delta}_{ij} y_{ijk} y_{ijk'} \right. \tag{5}$$

$$\left. + \sum_{j<j'}\sum_{k=1}^{n_i} \tilde{\omega}_{ijj'} y_{ijk} y_{ij'k} + \sum_{j<j'}\sum_{k \neq k'} \tilde{\gamma}_{ijj'} y_{ijk} y_{ij'k'} - A(\tilde{\Theta}_i)\right\},$$

where $A(\tilde{\Theta}_i)$ is again a normalizing constant, resulting from summing (5) over all 2^{Mn_i} possible outcomes. All model parameters depend on the subscript i, indicating that their values may vary from cluster to cluster through the covariate vector x_i for each cluster. The parameters θ_{ij} (main effect associated with the presence of outcome j for an individual in cluster i), δ_{ij} (association between two different individuals for the same cluster) and $\omega_{ijj'}$ (association between outcomes j and j' for a single individual within cluster i) have been discussed previously, in (1) and (3). Model (5) incorporates one further association parameter ($\gamma_{ijj'}$) to characterize the relationship between outcomes j and j' for two different individuals in the same cluster. The absence of individual-specific subscripts reflects the implicit exchangeability assumption between any two individuals within the same cluster.

After reparametrization and absorption of constant terms into the normalizing constant, model (5) can be rewritten parsimoniously as:

$$f_Y(y_i; \tilde{\Theta}_i, n_i) = \exp\left\{\sum_{j=1}^{M} \theta_{ij} z_{ij}^{(1)} + \sum_{j=1}^{M} \delta_{ij} z_{ij}^{(2)} \right. \tag{6}$$

$$\left. + \sum_{j<j'} \omega_{ijj'} z_{ijj'}^{(3)} + \sum_{j<j'} \gamma_{ijj'} z_{ijj'}^{(4)} - A(\tilde{\Theta}_i)\right\},$$

where the summary statistics $z_{ij}^{(1)}$ to $z_{ijj'}^{(4)}$ are defined as follows. Let z_{ij} be the number of individuals from cluster i positive on outcome j and let $z_{ijj'}$ be the number of individuals in cluster i with both outcomes j and j'. Then the summary statistics are

$$z_{ij}^{(1)} = z_{ij},$$
$$z_{ij}^{(2)} = -z_{ij}(n_i - z_{ij}),$$
$$z_{ijj'}^{(3)} = 2z_{ijj'} - z_{ij} - z_{ij'}, \tag{7}$$
$$z_{ijj'}^{(4)} = -z_{ij}(n_i - z_{ij'}) - z_{ij'}(n_i - z_{ij}) - z_{ijj'}^{(3)}.$$

For the ith cluster, these can be thought of as arising from the set of two-by-two tables obtained by cross-classifying every pair of outcomes as in TABLE 2.

TABLE 2. Cross-classification of littermates with respect to outcome variable pairs

	Outcome j	
Outcome j'	Absent	Present
Absent		
Present	$z_{ijj'}$	$z_{ij'}$
	z_{ij}	n_i

In the most general case, it is useful to think in terms of the three different types of associations captured in the model. They are depicted in FIGURE 1.

As discussed already in the single variable clustered case, model (6) is conditional in nature. Indeed, the model implies conditional odds and odds-ratios that are log-linear in the natural parameters. Furthermore, the conditional logit associated with the presence and absence of outcome j for an individual k in cluster i, depends on cluster size, as discussed above in the single outcome case. It also depends on the observed pattern of the remaining outcomes. Similar to (4), let us construct the logit of a success, conditional on all other outcomes in the same cluster. Let $\kappa_{ijk} = 1$ if the kth individual exhibits a success on the jth variable and 0 otherwise. Then

$$\log \frac{\text{pr}(Y_{ijk} = 1 | y_{ij'k'}, j' \neq j \text{ or } k' \neq k)}{\text{pr}(Y_{ijk} = -1 | y_{ij'k'}, j' \neq j \text{ or } k' \neq k)} = \theta_{ij} + \delta_{ij}(2z_{ij} - n_i - 1)$$
$$+ \sum_{j' \neq j} \omega_{ijj'}(2\kappa_{ij'k} - 1) + \sum_{j' \neq j} \gamma_{ijj'}(2z_{ij'} - n_i - 2\kappa_{ij'k} + 1).$$

This function clearly depends on the cluster size. The conditional log odds ratios, associated with any two components of the vector Y_i, reduce to:

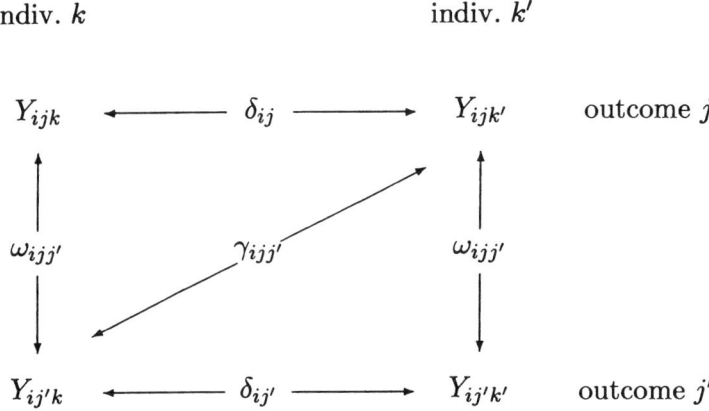

FIGURE 1. Association structure: outcomes j and j' individuals k and k', cluster i.

$$\log \text{OR}(Y_{ijk}, Y_{ijk'}|i) = 2\delta_{ij},$$
$$\log \text{OR}(Y_{ijk}, Y_{ij'k}|i) = 2\omega_{ijj'},$$
$$\log \text{OR}(Y_{ijk}, Y_{ij'k'}|i) = 2\delta_{ijj'}.$$

($j \neq j'$, $k \neq k'$), where $|i$ symbolizes the conditioning on all other outcomes in litter i.

Model (6) includes only pairwise interactions between outcomes. Clearly, in the spirit of log-linear modeling, it could be extended with three-way and higher-order interactions. Furthermore, subscripting the parameters in (5) with the index k allows the inclusion of fetus-specific covariates, such as sex or individual-specific dosing. However, Geys, Molenberghs, and Williams[40] have shown that the marginal success probability of one fetus then depends on the covariates of the other fetuses. This would restrict such an extension to a very limited number of applications.

Liang and Zeger[23] developed a similar model in which the number of outcomes per individual is variable as well, but neither cluster-level nor individual-level covariates are included. Since they do not code the responses as $-1/1$, their model is not invariant to reversing the coding.

MODEL FITTING AND INFERENCE

Consider now the issue of modelling covariate effects. A natural example occurs in the case of multigroup comparisons or dose-response modelling where the covariate x_i represents the treatment group or dose level for the ith cluster. In this section, we outline procedures for likelihood based parameter estimation and testing in this setting.

The first step is to group the summary statistics from (7) into a new vector z_i, ordered according to the set of natural parameters in the $q \times 1$ vector Θ_i. Let $\mu_i = E(z_i)$. Applying a linear link function, we assume $\Theta_i = X_i\beta$, with X_i a $q \times p$ design matrix, constructed from the cluster-specific covariates x_i, and β is a $p \times 1$ vector of unknown regression coefficients. Assuming a Poisson or multinomial sampling scheme, the kernel of the log-likelihood is proportional to

$$l = \sum_{i=1}^{N} \{z_i^T X_i \beta - A(X_i\beta)\},$$

whence the score function becomes

$$U(\beta) = \sum_{i=1}^{N} X_i^T (z_i - \mu_i).$$

The maximum likelihood estimator for β is defined as the solution to $U(\beta) = 0$.

Molenberghs and Ryan[34] derived a score test for the null hypothesis of no dose effect. Using logic similar to Rotnitzky and Jewell,[41] the use of empirically adjusted variances ensures the score test will remain valid under certain model misspecifications, in the sense of White.[42] In general, inference can be based on standard likelihood procedures, such as Wald and likelihood ratio statistics. General forms are implemented as GAUSS procedures.

ANALYSIS OF NTP DATA

TABLE 3 summarizes the results of the model fitting for the DEPH data, a detailed tabulation of which can be found in Lefkopoulou and Ryan.[33] The model includes main effects for each of the three outcomes: $\theta_{ij} = \sigma_{j1} + \sigma_{j2n_i} + \tau d_i$, including cluster size as a covariate and a common dose effect (τ), as well as association between animals on the same outcome ($\delta_{ij} = \delta_j$), within animal association parameters ($\omega_{ijj'} = \omega_{jj'}$), and association between animals on different outcomes ($\gamma_{ijj'} = \gamma_{jj'}$).

There is a strong dose effect. The association structure differs with the outcomes: there is a strong cluster effect for skeletal malformation, and the association between a pair of outcomes is higher if skeletal malformation is involved.

TABLE 4 shows the results of several different procedures for testing the null hypothesis of no dose effect ($\tau = 0$) in the DEHP data. Included are the results of likelihood ratio, Wald, and score tests, the latter two with either model based or empirically adjusted variances. All tests give a similar qualitative impression of a strong dose effect, the model based tests tend to have more extreme χ^2 values than their corresponding empirically adjusted counterparts.

TABLE 3. Parameter estimates for CEHP study

Parameter	Value	Naive		Robust	
		s.e.	pr > |Z|	s.e.	pr > |Z|
σ_{11}	−4.3484	0.2473	0.0000	0.2822	0.0000
σ_{12}	−0.6883	0.1776	0.0001	0.1983	0.0005
σ_{21}	−4.0325	0.2230	0.0000	0.2659	0.0000
σ_{22}	−0.5355	0.1607	0.0009	0.1812	0.0031
σ_{31}	−4.3913	0.2363	0.0000	0.2996	0.0000
σ_{32}	−0.2637	0.1612	0.1018	0.1663	0.1128
δ_1	0.1934	0.1517	0.2021	0.1562	0.2154
δ_2	0.2548	0.1275	0.0456	0.0890	0.0042
δ_3	0.4461	0.0608	0.0000	0.0649	0.0000
ω_{12}	0.0750	0.4043	0.8529	0.5023	0.8813
ω_{13}	1.1088	0.4060	0.0063	0.4215	0.0085
ω_{23}	0.6524	0.4174	0.1180	0.5353	0.2230
γ_{12}	0.1195	0.1161	0.3034	0.1373	0.3843
γ_{13}	−0.0651	0.0904	0.4712	0.1123	0.5621
γ_{23}	−0.2285	0.0977	0.0193	0.1249	0.0673
τ	18.4194	2.9029	0.0000	4.0660	0.0000

Log-likelihood: −530.47

TABLE 4. DEHP study. Tests for $H_0: \tau = 0$

Likelihood ratio	86.97
Wald model based	40.26
Wald empirical	20.52
Score model based	46.85
Score empirical	20.62

TABLE 5 compares different χ_1^2 score test procedures for a common dose parameter in all three outcomes for three of the five studies described in TABLE 1. The TGDM and THEO studies were omitted from this comparison after inspection of TABLE 1 revealed several marginal zeros. For instance, in the THEO study, there are no animals recorded with more than one malformation. This leads to estimates on the boundary of the parameter space. Due to this sparseness, exact inference would be more appropriate, a topic that is currently under investigation. For the three studies included in TABLE 5, using empirically corrected versions of the tests lead to similar results, whether applied to the Lefkopoulou and Ryan[33] model, or to that proposed in this paper. Again, model based tests yield substantially higher χ^2 values.

The observed discrepancy between model based and empirical tests suggests substantial lack of fit. One likely explanation is that the model assumes that association parameters are constant across clusters. In reality, the degree of association often depends on dose level.[43] This point is clearly illustrated with an example using the *external* and *visceral* outcomes from the DEHP study. Starting from a model with linear and quadratic dose effects on all parameters, a backward elimination proce-

TABLE 5. χ_1^2 Parameter estimates for CEHP study

Study	Univariate				Multivariate
	extern	visc	skel	any	
	Lefkopoulou-Ryan				
EG	7.16	7.42	29.21	30.34	26.21
DYME	22.97	11.32	29.18	32.56	29.05
DEHP	16.36	16.47	13.36	22.92	19.77
	MR, Empirically corrected				
EG	5.32	6.12	25.78	26.28	22.82
DYME	14.58	10.38	21.99	23.71	21.96
DEHP	15.25	22.78	12.68	25.74	20.62
	MR, model based				
EG	10.64	11.47	46.59	45.60	46.06
DYME	40.87	8.12	48.55	65.45	52.96
DEHP	31.14	26.95	33.16	53.29	46.85

dure, forced to include all intercepts, yields the following model (d_i represents dose level):

$$\theta_1(d_i) = -30.7 - 0.43n_i + 0.30d_i,$$
$$\theta_2(d_i) = -3.77 - 0.43n_i + 0.60d_i,$$
$$\delta_1 = 0.47,$$
$$\delta_2 = 0.36,$$
$$\omega(d_i) = -0.04 + 3.06d_i - 0.92d_i^2,$$
$$\gamma(d_i) = 0.12 - 0.25d_i + 0.07d_i^2.$$

Comparing this model to that with constant associations and linear-dose main effects gives a likelihood ratio statistic of 30.08 on four degrees of freedom, confirming that the constant association model is too simple for these data. Given this more complex model, we can construct a new test for the null hypothesis that $\theta_1(d_i)$ and $\theta_2(d_i)$ are dose independent. The model based and empirically corrected score test statistics for a dose main effect are 30.07 and 17.90 on two degrees of freedom, respectively. If we compare these statistics to the underspecified model with no dependence on cluster size, these statistics are 164.64 and 22.60. Of course, these latter quantities are not well defined, because the corresponding models are not invariant to recoding of the outcome. The discrepancy that is still observed between the model based and the robust version of the statistic could be due to over-simplification of the higher order association.

DISCUSSION

We have discussed the analysis of multivariate clustered binary data of the kind that arises in developmental toxicity studies. We described the likelihood based framework for clustered multivariate binary outcomes that has been proposed by Molenberghs and Ryan.[34] Particular emphasis was given to the construction of a score test for assessing dose response. Model based and empirically adjusted tests were considered. The model based test is a natural extension of the Cochran-Armitage test for trend, and corresponds exactly to that test in the absence of clustering and for a single outcome. When all cluster sizes are equal, the empirically adjusted score test is identical to the GEE-based score test derived by Lefkopoulou and Ryan.[33] For the variable cluster sizes (ranging between 2 and 12) encountered in the NTP data, the model based score test with empirical variance adjustment were numerically similar to the test derived by Lefkopoulou and Ryan.[33]

The likelihood basis of the proposed model has both advantages and disadvantages. An important advantage of our approach is that it lends itself well to formulation of exact inferential procedures, a topic that we are presently investigating. Another advantage is that when the model is correctly specified, then efficiency can be gained over other procedures such as GEE methods. This was seen with our example. A disadvantage is that in the absence of correct model specification, a model based variance will not always guarantee valid inference. The fact that our score test reduces, in special cases, to the GEE based test, however, suggests that there may be classes of models within which our methods may be relatively robust. Furthermore, this correspondence suggests that our derived score test will enjoy the same properties (including good power and an accurate type I error) as the GEE-based test.[13] These observations highlight the importance of careful modelling, and suggest the development of model assessment tools as a useful avenue for further research.

ACKNOWLEDGMENTS

We gratefully acknowledge support from National Institutes of Health Grant CA48061, the U.S. Environmental Protection Agency, and NATO Collaborative Research Grant 950648.

REFERENCES

1. CRUMP, K. 1984. A new method for determining allowable daily intakes. Fund. Appl. Toxicol. **4:** 854–871.
2. LEISENRING, W. & L.M. RYAN. 1992. Statistical properties of the NOAEL. Regulatory Toxicology and Pharmacology **15:** 161–171.
3. U.S. ENVIRONMENTAL PROTECTION AGENCY. 1991. Guidelines for developmental toxicity risk assessment. Federal Register. **56:** 63798–63826.
4. FOOD AND DRUG ADMINISTRATION. 1966. Guidelines for reproduction and studies for safety evaluation of drugs for human use. Bureau of Drugs. Rockville, MD.
5. KIMMEL, C.A. & C.J. PRICE. 1990. Developmental toxicity studies. *In* Handbook of in Vivo Toxicity Testing. 271–300. Academic Press.
6. TYL, R.W., M.C. PRICE, M.C. MARR & C.A. KIMMEL. 1988. Developmental toxicity evaluation of dietary di(2-ethylhexyl)phthalate in Fisher 344 rats and CD-1 mice. Fund. Appl. Toxicol. **10:** 395–412.
7. PRICE, C.J., C.A. KIMMEL, J.D. GEORGE & M.C. MARR. 1987. The developmental toxicity of diethylene glycol dimethyl ether in mice. Fund. Appl. Toxicol. **8:** 115–126.
8. GEORGE, J.D., C.J. PRICE, C.A. KIMMEL, & M.C. MARR. 1987. The developmental toxicity of triethylene glycol dimethyl ether in mice. Fund. Appl. Toxicol. **9:** 173–181.
9. PRICE, C.J., C.A. KIMMEL, R.W. TYL & M.C. MARR. 1985. The developmental toxicity of ethylene glycol in rats and mice. Toxico. Appl. Pharmacol. **81:** 113–127.
10. LINDSTROM, P., R.E. MORRISSEY, J.D. GEORGE, C.J. PRICE, M.C. MARR, C.A. KIMMEL & B.A. SCHWETZ. 1990. The developmental toxicity of orally administered theophylline in rats and mice. Fund. Appl. Toxicol. **14:** 167–178.
11. DIGGLE, P.J., K.-Y. LIANG & S.L. ZEGER. 1994. Analysis of Longitudinal Data. Clarendon Press, Oxford.
12. FITZMAURICE, G.M., N.M. LAIRD & A. ROTNITZKY. 1993. Regression models for discrete longitudinal responses. Stat. Sci. **8:** 284–309.
13. LEGLER, J.M., M. LEFKOPOULOU, & L.M. RYAN. 1995. Efficiency and power of tests for multiple binary outcomes. J. Am. Stat. Assoc. **90:** 680–693.
14. PENDERGAST, J.F., S.J. GANGE, M.A. NEWTON, M.J. LINDSTROM, M. PALTA & M.R. FISHER. 1996. A survey of methods for analyzing clustered binary response data. Int. Stat. Rev. **64:** 89–118.
15. FITZMAURICE, G.M. & N.M. LAIRD. 1993. A likelihood-based method for analysing longitudinal binary responses. Biometrika **80:** 141–151.

16. BAHADUR, R.R. 1961. A representation of the joint distribution of responses to n dichotomous items. *In* Studies in Item Analysis and Prediction. H. Solomon, Ed.: Stanford Mathematical Studies in the Social Sciences VI. Stanford University Press, Stanford.
17. COX, D.R. 1972. The analysis of multivariate binary data. Appl. Stat. **21:** 113–120.
18. ASHFORD, J.R. & R.R. SOWDEN. 1970. Multivariate probit analysis. Biometrics **26:** 535–546.
19. DALE, J.R. 1986. Global cross-ratio models for bivariate, discrete, ordered responses. Biometrics. **42:** 909–917.
20. MOLENBERGHS, G., L. DECLERCK. & M. AERTS. 1997. Misspecifying the likelihood for clustered binary data. Computational Statistics and Data Analysis **26:** 327–349.
21. MOLENBERGHS, G. & E. LESAFFRE. 1994. Marginal modelling of correlated ordinal data using a multivariate Plackett distribution. J. Am. Stat. Assoc. **89:** 633–644.
22. ROSNER, B. 1984. Multivariate methods in ophtalmology with applications to other paired-data situations. Biometrics **40:** 1025–1035.
23. LIANG, K.-Y. & S.L. ZEGER. 1989. A class of logistic regression models for multivariate binary time series. J. Am. Stat. Assoc. **84:** 447–451.
24. STIRATELLI, R., N.M. LAIRD & J.H. WARE. 1984. Random-effects models for serial observations with binary response. Biometrics **40:** 961–971.
25. ZEGER, S.L., K.-Y. LIANG & P.S. ALBERT. 1988. Models for longitudinal data: a generalized estimating equation approach. Biometrics **44:** 1049–1060.
26. BRESLOW, N.E. & D.G. CLAYTON. 1993. Approximate inference in generalized linear mixed models. J. Am. Stat. Assoc. **88:** 9–25.
27. WOLFINGER, R. & M. O'CONNELL. 1993. Generalized linear mixed models: a pseudolikelihood approach. J. Stat. Comp. Simul. **48:** 233–243.
28. LIANG, K.-Y. & S.L. ZEGER. 1986. Longitudinal data analysis using generalized linear models. Biometrika **73:** 13–22.
29. RAI, K. & J. VAN RYZIN. 1985. A dose-response model for teratological experiments involving quantal responses. Biometrics **47:** 825–839.
30. WILLIAMS, D.A. 1975. The analysis of binary responses from toxicological experiments involving reproduction and teratogenicity. Biometrics **31:** 949–952.
31. CHEN, J.J. & R.L. KODELL. 1989. Quantitative risk assessment for teratological effects. J. Am. Stat. Assoc. **84:** 966–971.
32. LEFKOPOULOU, M., D. MOORE & L.M. RYAN. 1989. The analysis of multiple correlated binary outcomes: application to rodent teratology experiments. J. Am. Stat. Assoc. **84:** 810–815.
33. Lefkopoulou, M. & L.M. Ryan. 1993. Global tests for multiple binary outcomes. Biometrics **49:** 975–988.
34. MOLENBERGHS, G. & L.M. RYAN. 1998. Likelihood inference for clustered multivariate binary data. Environmetrics **10:** 279–300.
35. AERTS, M., L. DECLERCK & G. MOLENBERGHS. 1997. Likelihood misspecification and safe dose determination for clustered binary data. Environmetrics **8:** 613–627.
36. COX, D.R. & N. WERMUTH. 1994. A note on the quadratic exponential binary distribution. Biometrika **81:** 403–408.
37. ZHAO, L.P. & R.L. PRENTICE. 1990. Correlated binary regression using a quadratic exponential model. Biometrika **77:** 642–648.
38. THÉLOT, C. 1985. Lois logistiques à deux dimensions. Annales de l'Insée. **58:** 123–149.
39. KLEINMAN, J.C. 1973. Proportions with extraneous variance: single and independent samples. J. Am. Stat. Assoc. **68:** 46–54.

40. GEYS, H., G. MOLENBERGHS & P. WILLIAMS. 1997. Analysis of clustered binary data with covariates specific to each observation. *In* Good Statistical Practice, Proc. 12th International Workshop on Statistical Modelling, Band 5. C.E. Minder and H. Friedl, Eds. Schriftenreihe der Österreichischen Statistischen Gesellschaft, Wien.
41. ROTNITZKY, A. & N.P. JEWELL. 1990. Hypothesis testing of regression parameters in semiparametric generalized linear models for cluster correlated data. Biometrika **77:** 485–497.
42. WHITE, H. 1982. Maximum likelihood estimation of misspecified models. Econometrica. **50:** 1–25.
43. KUPPER, L.L., C. PORTIER, M.D. HOGAN & E. YAMAMOTO. 1986. The impact of litter effects on dose-response modeling in teratology. Biometrics **42:** 85–98.

Sources of Uncertainty in Dose-Response Modeling of Epidemiological Data for Cancer Risk Assessment

LESLIE STAYNER,[a] A. JOHN BAILER, RANDALL SMITH, STEPHEN GILBERT, FAYE RICE, AND EILEEN KUEMPEL

Education and Information Division, Department of Health and Human Services, Centers for Disease Control and Prevention, National Institute for Occupational Safety and Health, Robert A. Taft Laboratories, 4676 Columbia Parkway, MSC-15, Cincinnati, Ohio 45226, USA

ABSTRACT: Epidemiologic data is increasingly being used for dose-response analysis in risk assessment. The Environmental Protection Agency (EPA) and other U.S. agencies have expressed a preference for using epidemiologic data rather than toxicologic data when possible. However, there are a number of important sources of uncertainty in using epidemiologic data for this purpose that need to be clearly recognized and, when possible, quantified. This paper presents a critical review of the major sources of uncertainty in the use of epidemiologic data for cancer risk assessment. These may include: (1) study design issues such as potential confounding and other biases, inadequate sample size, and followup, (2) the choice of the data set, (3) specification of the dose-response model, (4) estimation of exposure and dose, and (5) unrecognized variability in susceptibility. Examples from risk assessments for cadmium, asbestos, and diesel exhaust are used to illustrate the potential magnitude of some of these sources of uncertainty. It is shown that the overall uncertainty from these various sources combined may often result in highly uncertain risk estimates from dose-response modeling of epidemiologic data. For this reason, we believe it is best to present a range of possible risk estimates, which, to the extent possible, reflects the variability and uncertainty inherent in the dose-response evaluation of epidemiologic data.

INTRODUCTION

Most regulatory agencies in the United States have expressed a clear preference for using human data, when available, instead of toxicologic data from animal studies, to quantify the risks associated with environmental and occupational carcinogenic hazards. However, most quantitative risk assessments that have been performed to date have been based on dose-response modeling of animal bioassay data. This situation appears to be changing as data from epidemiologic studies become an increasingly important source of information for dose-response modeling

---

[a]Address for correspondence: 513-533-8365 (voice); 513-533-8224 (fax).
e-mail: lts2@cdc.gov

in the quantitative assessment of human health risks. This change is probably related to the increasing criticism of animal models for predicting human risks;[1] and to improvements in the quality of the available epidemiologic database.

There are several major potential sources of uncertainty that may arise in using epidemiologic data for dose-response assessments. These sources of uncertainty need to be considered, and when possible quantified, in any risk assessment that uses dose-response data from epidemiologic studies. This paper presents a review of the major sources of uncertainty, with examples from risk analyses that have been conducted by the authors.

STUDY DESIGN

The lack of adequate exposure information is probably the most frequently cited limitation of epidemiologic data for risk assessment purposes. Although this certainly is an important factor, which we discuss below, there are several other major limitations on epidemiologic study design that may be as important. Epidemiologic studies, by definition, are observational in nature and, consequently, it is generally impossible to randomize the assignment of exposures. Thus, serious questions often arise about the potential for confounding, selection bias, and other sources of bias. The frequent use of general population rates as the referent group for occupational cohorts often introduces a form of selection bias due to the well known *healthy worker effect*.[2] The impact of this potential bias may be mitigated in many occupational studies, simply by restricting the dose-response analysis to the exposed and non-exposed (if available) subjects within the cohort. However, workers must generally remain healthy to stay employed, a phenomenon that has been termed the healthy worker survivor effect (HWSE),[3] a fact that may exert a strong influence on the dose-response relationship. Steenland *et al.*[4] have shown that a negative bias in exposure-response relationships, attributable to the HWSE, may often be observed in occupational cohort studies.

In addition to potential biases, one has to consider other potential problems arising from limitations in the design of the study. An important question is whether or not the period of observation (follow-up) of the cohort was adequate? Many occupational and environmental cancers have an average latency period of approximately 15 to 20 years, and thus the cohort should be followed for at least this long in order to observe an excess from these health outcomes. One also needs to consider whether the methods for case ascertainment are adequately sensitive. For example, studies based on mortality data may be inadequately sensitive for cancers that are treatable and have long survival times, such as leukemia.

Finally, the size of the study is an extremely important consideration. Sample size estimates for different levels of excess risk are presented in TABLE 1 for a hypothetical study of lung cancer in an occupational cohort. It should be noted that similar results would be obtained for case-control studies nested within a cohort. These sample size estimates are based on a 5% false-positive rate (alpha) and 80% sensitivity (power) for detecting different levels of excess risk. Most cohort mortality studies have at least 1,000 workers and very few have more than 100,000 workers. As this table illustrates, these studies would generally be incapable of detecting an excess

TABLE 1. Sample size estimates for detecting varying levels of excess lung cancer risk in a hypothetical retrospective cohort mortality study

Excess risk	Relative risk (SMR)[a]	Expected deaths[b]	Person years[c]	Number of workers[d]
10^{-2}	1.20	170	217,161	4,343
10^{-3}	1.02	15,605	2.0×10^7	399,605
10^{-4}	1.002	1.5×10^6	2.0×10^9	39.6×10^6
10^{-5}	1.0002	1.5×10^8	2.0×10^{11}	39.6×10^{10}

[a]Relative risks calculated using a background risk (cumulative probability) of 0.06 for developing lung cancer for males over age 15, based upon the proportion of deaths from lung cancer among U.S. males over age 15 in 1982.
[b]Expected number of deaths calculated assuming 80% power $(1 - \beta)$, α level of 0.05 (single tail) and the calculated relative risk.
[c]Person years calculated by dividing the expected number of deaths by the lung cancer rate (7.8×10^{-4}) among males between the ages of 45–54 based upon U.S. mortality rates from 1982 (NCHS 1986) which is approximately the average of the hypothetical population.
[d]Number of workers calculated by assuming each worker contributed 50 person-years to the study.

risk of less than 1 per 1,000 workers. It should also be noted that an excess risk of 1 per 1,000 corresponds to relative risk of 1.02, which most epidemiologists would be highly reluctant to consider meaningful even if it were statistically significant. The U.S. Occupational Safety and Health Administration (OSHA) generally considers a risk of greater than 1 per 1,000 to be significant, and the Environmental Protection Agency (EPA) generally considers a risk of 1 per 1,000,000 to be significant.[5] Thus epidemiologic studies generally have low power for detecting the levels of risk that are of regulatory concern in the United States. Conversely, epidemiologic studies that demonstrate a statistically significant excess are likely to identify risks that are of regulatory concern.

IS THERE A CAUSAL RELATIONSHIP?

Because of the design issues discussed above, it is often difficult, if not impossible, to draw firm conclusions about whether or not a causal association exists between an exposure and disease based on a single or even several epidemiologic studies. Hertz-Picciotto[6] has suggested that epidemiologic data should only be used for extrapolation in risk assessments (that is, for dose-response modeling) if: (1) a moderate to strong positive association exists, (2) strong biases can be ruled out, (3) confounding is well-controlled or limited, and (4) exposures have been well-characterized quantitatively. However, we believe that these criteria, particularly the first, are too restrictive. It may be informative to conduct dose-response analyses using epidemiologic data even if the study is negative or shows only a weak association (i.e., Criterion 1). This type of analysis may at least inform decision makers on what an upper bound estimate or best estimate of risk might be. Similarly a risk analysis based on epidemiologic data may also be informative, even if confounding or other biases cannot be completely ruled out. For example, such analyses could be used to assess the credibility of other analyses based on animal data or other epidemiologic studies.

CHOICE OF DATA

There is frequently more than one epidemiologic data set that may be used for a dose-response analysis. Not surprisingly, given the issues of study design discussed above, there may be a great deal of heterogeneity in the results from dose-response analyses from different epidemiologic studies. For example, in FIGURE 1 the results from an exposure-response analysis that we performed for chrysotile asbestos and lung cancer, based on a study of textile workers,[7] are contrasted with estimates of risk based on another study of chrysotile miners from Quebec.[8] The slopes from these two studies differ by more than one order of magnitude. It is very difficult for risk assessors and risk managers to deal with this kind of difference, since it is frequently impossible to identify a single study as providing the "best" data for the risk analysis. An example of an approach that has been used is the OSHA final rule for asbestos, where they chose to use the geometric mean of slopes from several studies.[9] An attractive alternative to this problem would be to conduct a meta-analysis or to pool the results from all of the studies available and conduct dose-response anal-

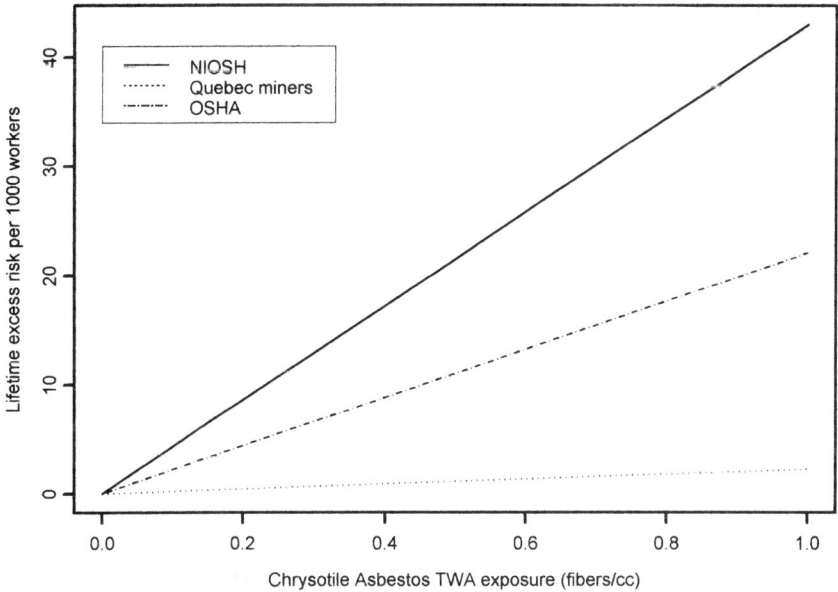

FIGURE 1. Comparison of lung cancer excess risk estimates and chrysotile asbestos exposure based on NIOSH Stayner *et al.* (1997) study of textile workers, McDonald *et al.* (1980) study of Quebec miners and millers, and the OSHA asbestos risk assessment.

yses based on the combined data set. We are currently attempting to perform such a pooled analysis for silica and lung cancer risk in collaboration with scientists at the International Agency for Research on Cancer (IARC).

CHOICE OF THE DOSE-RESPONSE MODEL FORM

Choosing an appropriate dose-response model is a critical step and another major source of uncertainty. In the past, many risk assessments simply assumed a linear relationship between relative risk and cumulative exposure.[10] In part, the justification for this assumption seems to have been based on the multistage theory of carcinogenesis,[11] which suggests that the carcinogenic effects of chemicals would be low-dose linear. However, this model is not truly consistent with an Armitage-Doll model, except when the model has two stages. These models essentially assume the following relationship:

$$RR = 1 + \beta(X)$$

where RR is the relative risk, β is the slope, and X is the cumulative exposure. However, restricting attention to such simple models no longer seems justifiable when modern methods and computing easily permit examination of alternative models with different functional forms.[12] In addition, current theories of carcinogenesis suggest chemicals may act on cell growth and differentiation as well as mutational

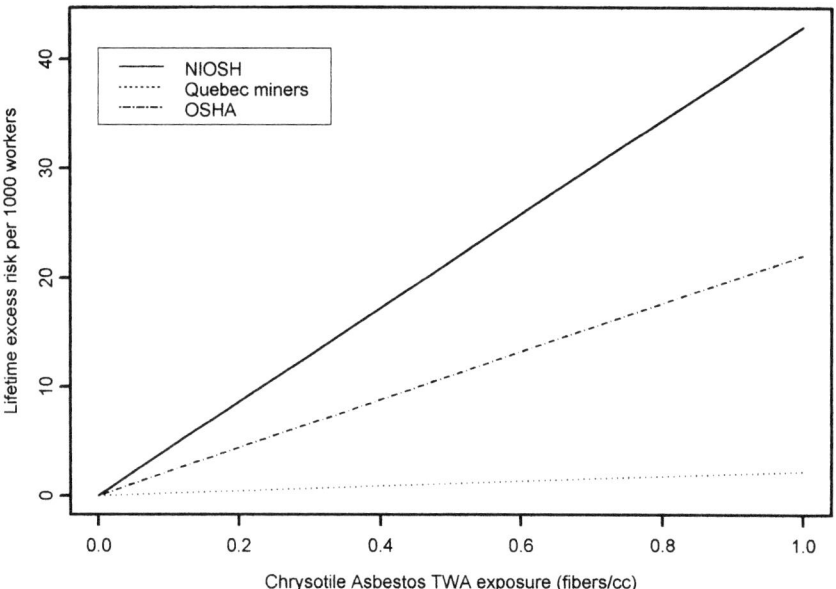

FIGURE 2. Comparison between excess risk estimates derived from various models fitted to lung cancer data from the NIOSH study of cadmium exposed workers. (Adapted from Stayner *et al.* Ref. 12.)

events.[13] Hence a chemical may exert an effect on any number of several available pathways, and the resulting exposure-response relationship may not always be low-dose linear.

The choice of a dose-response model may have a dramatic effect on the resulting estimates of risk, particularly at exposure levels that are well below the levels experienced by subjects of the epidemiologic study. Poisson regression or Cox proportionate hazard models using alternative parametric forms (i.e., log-linear, additive relative risk, and power), as well as biologic models (i.e., multistage or two-stage clonal expansion) may be fitted to the data. In FIGURE 2, estimates of risk are presented for several alternative dose-response models from an analysis performed by Stayner et al.[12] of occupational cadmium exposure and lung cancer risk. It can be seen from this figure that the estimates of risk vary by nearly an order of magnitude depending on the dose-response model used.

Splines[14] and other data smoothers offer an attractive new and flexible method for evaluating the shape of the dose-response by making few, if any, parametric assumptions. This method is illustrated in FIGURE 3 from an analysis of chrysotile asbestos and lung cancer risk that we performed.[7] The restricted cubic spline model yielded a very similar fit to the data as that obtained from the additive relative rate model. This result added confidence to our choice of the additive relative rate model as the best parametric form for our risk analysis. Alternatively, one could use the spline model itself for the risk analysis, which in this example would have yielded essen-

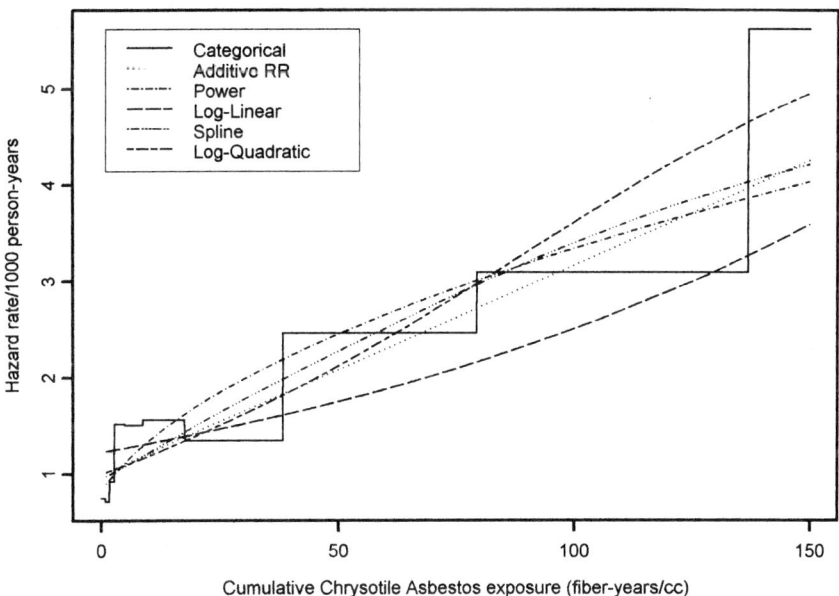

FIGURE 3. Lung cancer mortality rates as a function of cumulative chrysotile asbestos exposure predicted by alternative models for white males, age 50 in 1940–1969. (Adapted from: Stayner et al. Ref. 7.)

tially the same result. However, there could be instances where a spline or other smoothers might yield dose-response models with questionable fitted values, since they can be so flexible that they are sensitive to local random variations leading to over fitting the data.

Finally, a critical concern in a risk analysis is whether or not there is a threshold below which the exposure has no effect on the disease risk. The assumption that there is no threshold for carcinogens is increasingly being questioned. Some epidemiologists have argued that there is a threshold at cut points in their data where they no longer see a significant excess risk. This is clearly inappropriate, since there will generally be a level of exposure in an epidemiologic study where one no longer sees an excess risk simply due to a lack of sufficient sample size and associated study power limitations. Furthermore, if exposures are categorized, it may be easily shown that the choice of cut-points (which is generally arbitrary in epidemiologic studies) can influence the determination of the no-adverse-effect level.[15]

Ulm[16] has suggested a formal statistical method for estimating a threshold parameter from epidemiologic data that has continuous exposure information. This is a useful method, although what it yields should probably not be called a "threshold", but rather a point in the data below which there is no evidence of an excess risk. This is because the parameter estimate is influenced by the study design (for example, sample sizes and exposure data) and should not thus be viewed as a true biologic threshold. We applied this method in our analysis of lung cancer risk and exposure to chrysotile asbestos,[7] and we found that the maximum likelihood estimate for this parameter was zero. This may often be the case with epidemiologic data, or the confidence intervals on this parameter may be extremely broad. Even if a true threshold exists, the reality is that epidemiologic studies will seldom be able to detect it. Thus, unless there is other biologic evidence for a threshold, it would be ill-advised to use a threshold model for human health risk assessments. Furthermore, even if there were evidence of a threshold, a single number would not apply to all individuals, and it is more plausible to think in terms of a distribution of thresholds among the population.

ERRORS IN EXPOSURE ESTIMATES

The fact that epidemiologic studies of cancer require information on exposures from 20 or more years prior to the end of the study makes the reconstruction of exposures an extremely difficult exercise, one that is generally fraught with potential errors. Despite this well-recognized fact, most epidemiologic studies and risk assessments based on these studies, treat the exposures as if they were known and without error. It is also commonly assumed in epidemiology that errors in exposure estimates that are non-differential with respect to disease will lead to an underestimate of the true dose-response slope. However, this is not always the case, and errors in exposure may in fact either inflate or deflate the slope of the dose-response relationship depending on the structure of the error.[17]

We are currently working on an analysis of the effects of errors in exposure estimates on the dose-response relationships in a study of railroad workers exposed to diesel exhaust particles.[18] This study has several potential sources of error that may

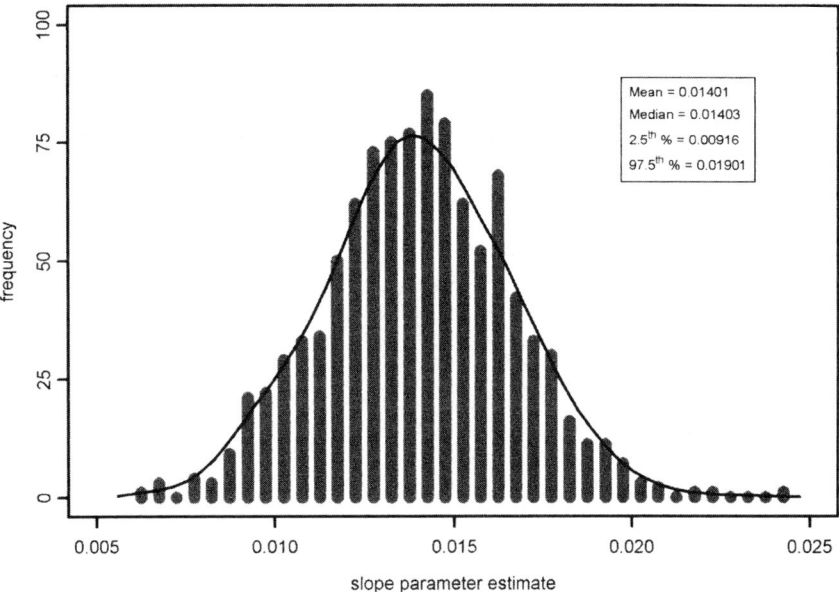

FIGURE 4. Histogram of parameter estimates from 1,000 Monte Carlo simulations of duration of diesel exposure using a linear relative risk model based on data from Garshick *et al.* (1986).

have contributed to a distortion of the dose-response relationship, including errors that effect estimation of both the duration and intensity of exposure. We are exploring the use of Monte Carlo methods to evaluate the potential uncertainty introduced by these exposure estimation errors on quantifying the dose-response relationship. Preliminary results from the Monte Carlo simulation of errors affecting the estimates of duration of exposure are illustrated in FIGURE 4. This figure shows that the slope of the linear relative rate regression model varied by a factor of approximately four (minimum versus maximum) with 95% of the results lying within a factor of two. This range reflects only a part of the overall uncertainty, which is likely to increase as we consider the other sources of uncertainty in the exposure estimates used in this analysis.

ERRORS IN USING EXPOSURE RATHER THAN DOSE

At best, epidemiologic studies of cancer risk rely on estimates of external exposure from personal breathing zone samples and work history information for estimating exposure. The delivered dose, or the actual dose that reaches the target tissue, is rarely available in epidemiologic studies of chronic diseases like cancer. If exposure is proportional to dose, then external exposure would be a reasonable surrogate for tissue dose, which would differ by some constant factor. However, if exposure is not proportional to dose (for example, when saturation occurs in capacity-limited processes such as uptake, metabolism, or clearance), then external exposure measures would not necessarily represent dose over the entire distribution of exposures. Similarly, if there are systematic differences among individuals in the exposure-dose relationship (for example, genetic polymorphisms resulting in metabolic differences, such as fast or slow acetylators; or pre-existing conditions such as bronchitis, which can alter deposition and clearance in the lungs), then exposure might not be a good representation of dose.

Dose information may be available from autopsy or clinical studies, particularly if the substance is biopersistent. For example, a strong association has been observed in most case-control studies of mesothelioma and dose (lung burdens) of amphibole asbestos, but not of chrysotile asbestos. This may be explained by the fact that chrysotile asbestos has a relatively short half-life in the lung; whereas, amphiboles have a long half-life.[19]

Dosimetric models have been developed for a relatively few occupational and environmental epidemiologic studies.[20] Kuempel[21] recently developed a human dosimetric lung model of the long-term retention of particulates, using autopsy data of U.S. coal miners, information on job-specific duration and intensity of exposure to respirable coal mine dust, and other human data on breathing rates, particle deposition in the lungs, and initial clearance rates. She found that measured lung dust burden was a stronger predictor of the probability for developing pulmonary fibrosis than was cumulative exposure, and that the model-predicted lung burdens also showed statistically significant dose-response, with similar coefficients to those for measured lung dust burdens. Furthermore, she found a different pattern of exposure-dose in humans than that observed in animal studies with chronic exposures to particles. This illustrates the potential usefulness of dosimetric models in risk assessment, which can represent biologic processes that affect dose.

Clearly our inability to use biologic markers for dose and our reliance on using measures of external exposure introduces uncertainty into the use of epidemiologic data in the risk assessment process. It is difficult at this time to judge the extent of this uncertainty, but it may be large in some cases, particularly when individual characteristics are known to modify the absorption, metabolism and delivery of the exposure to the target tissue.

HUMAN VARIABILITY IN SUSCEPTIBILITY

The effects of human variability in susceptibility to exposure on the results from risk analyses from epidemiologic studies have largely been neglected to date. We generally fit our models to epidemiologic data by assuming all of the individuals in the study are from the same population, and then extrapolate our findings to other populations who may have quite different characteristics that effect susceptibility. The reason we have done so is simply because of our near total ignorance of what these factors are, and how they are distributed in our study population. We are becoming increasingly aware of how bad this assumption is, and of the existence of subpopulations in our studies with genetic polymorphisms that influence their risk.

In fact, it may often be the case that the individuals at the greatest risk are those that have some combination of different genetic polymorphisms. For example, in a recent case-control study of lung cancer, Hirvonen[22] evaluated interactions between asbestos exposure, GSTM1 genotype, and N-acetyltransferase slow acetylator genotype (NAT-2). Being either $GSTM1^{null}$ or a slow acetylator (NAT-2^{*slow}) was associated with an approximately twofold increased risk of lung cancer. Having both *at-risk* genotypes ($GSTM1^{null}$ and NAT-2^{*slow}) was associated with an approximately fourfold increase in risk. Having both *at-risk* genotypes and being highly exposed to asbestos was associated with an approximately eightfold increase in risk. Hence the results from this study suggest a multiplicative relationship between *GSTM1, NAT-2* and high asbestos exposure. This example illustrates how large the differences in risk may be for subpopulations in our studies, and in the populations for which we are trying to estimate risk. Our failure to recognize these difference may lead to large errors in our risk estimates particularly for certain members of the population.

CONCLUSION

In this paper we have attempted to briefly discuss and illustrate some of the major sources of uncertainty in using epidemiologic data for dose-response analyses. Several of these sources have the potential to result in relatively large errors in the estimation of risk. Our cadmium example illustrates that just varying the statistical model may result in risk estimates that span an order of magnitude. Other sources of uncertainty reviewed in this paper may also easily result in errors in predicted risks that are as large. The overall uncertainty from these various sources combined may often result in risk estimates from dose-response modeling of epidemiologic data that are highly uncertain. For this reason, we believe that it is best to present a range of possible risk estimates, which, to the extent possible, reflects the variability and uncertainty inherent in the dose-response evaluation of epidemiologic data.

REFERENCES

1. AMES, B.N. & L.S. GOLD. 1990. Chemical carcinogenesis: too many rodent carcinogens. Proc. Natl. Acad. Sci. **87:** 7772–7776.
2. MCMICHAEL, A.J. 1976. Standardized mortality ratios and the "Healthy Worker Effect": scratching beneath the surface. J. Occupational Medicine **18**(3): 165–168.
3. ROBBINS, J. 1990. A graphical approach to the identification and estimation of causal parameters in mortality studies with sustained exposure periods. J. Chronic Dis. **40**(Suppl. 2): 1091–1098.
4. STEENLAND, K., J. DEDDENS, A. SALVAN & L. STAYNER. 1996. Negative bias in exposure-response trends in occupational studies: Modeling the healthy workers survivor effect. Am. J. Epi. **143**(2): 202–210.
5. RODERICKS, J.V., S.M. BRETT & G.C. WRENN. 1987. Significant risk decisions in federal regulatory agencies. Regulatory Toxicol. and Pharmacol. **7:** 307–320.
6. HERTZ-PICCIOTO, I.H. 1995. Epidemiology and quantitative risk assessment: a bridge from science to policy. Am. J. Public Health **85:** 484–491.
7. STAYNER, L.T., R. SMITH, J. BAILER, S. GILBERT, K. STEENLAND, J. DEMENT, D. BROWN & R. LEMEN. 1997. Exposure-response analysis of respiratory disease risk associated with occupational exposure to chrysotile asbestos. Occupational Environmental Medicine **54:** 646–652.

8. MCDONALD, J.C., F.D.K. LIDDELL, G.W. GIBBS, G.E. EYSSEN & A.D. MCDONALD. 1980. Dust exposure and mortality in chrysotile mining, 1910-75. Br. J. Ind. Med. **37:** 11–24.
9. OSHA. 1986. Occupational exposure to asbestos, tremolite, anthophylite and actinolite. Federal Register **51:** 22612–22747.
10. SMITH, A.H. 1988. Epidemiologic input to environmental risk assessment. Arch. Environ. Health **43:** 124–127.
11. ARMITAGE, P. & R. DOLL. 1954. The age distribution of cancer and a multistage theory of carcinogenesis. Br. J. Cancer. **VIII**(1): 1–12.
12. STAYNER, L.T., R. SMITH, A. J. BAILER, G. E. LUEBECK & S.H. MOOLGAVKAR. 1995. Modeling epidemiologic studies of occupational cohorts for the quantitative assessment of carcinogenic hazards. Am. J. Ind. Med. **27:** 155–170.
13. MOOLGAVKAR, S.H. & G.E. LUEBECK. 1990. Two-event model for carcinogenesis: Biological, mathematical, and statistical considerations. Risk Analysis **10:** 323–341.
14. HASTIE, T.J. & R.J. TIBSHIRANI. 1990. Generalized Additive Models. Chapman & Hall, London.
15. BAILER, A.J., L.T. STAYNER, R.J. SMITH, E.D. KUEMPEL & M.M. PRINCE. 1997. Estimating benchmark concentrations and other noncancer endpoints in epidemiology studies. Risk Analysis **17:** 771–780.
16. ULM, K.W. 1990. Threshold models in occupational epidemiology. Mathematical Computer Modeling **14:** 649–652.
17. Wacholder, S. 1995. When measurement errors correlate with truth: Surprising effects of nondifferential misclassification. Epidemiology **6**(2): 157–161.
18. GARSHICK, E., M.B. SCHENKER, A. MUNOZ, M. SEGAL, T.J. SMITH, S.R. WOSKIE, S.K. HAMMOND & F.E. SPEIZER. 1988. A retrospective cohort study of lung cancer and diesel exhaust exposure in railroad workers. Am. Rev. Resp. Dis. **137:** 820–825.
19. STAYNER, L., D.A. DANKOVIC & R.A. LEMEN. 1996. Occupational exposure to chrysotile asbestos and cancer risk. A review of the "amphibole hypothesis". Am. J. Public Health **86**(2): 179–186.
20. KREIBEL, D. 1994. The dosimetric model in occupational and environmental epidemiology. Occ. Hyg. **1:** 55–68.
21. KUEMPEL, E. 1997. Development of a biomathematical lung model to describe respirable particle retention and to investigate exposure, dose and disease in U.S. coal miners. Dissertation, University of Cincinnati, Cincinnati, Ohio.
22. HIRVONEN, A. 1997. Combinations of susceptible genotypes and individual responses to toxicants. Environmental Health Perspectives **105:** 755–758.

Nonparametric Analysis of Dose-Response Relationships

K. ULM[a]

Institut für Medizinische Statistik und Epidemiologie,
Technische Universität München, Munich, Germany

> ABSTRACT: A nonparametric method, isotonic regression, is proposed for analyzing a dose-response relationship and for assessing a threshold value. There are several advantages of this method compared to parametric models. No specific form of the relationship (type of model and use of the covariates) is required. The only assumption is monotonicity. Rejection of specific hypothesis can be based on the result of a permutation test. Several applications (para-aramid, crystalline silica, and PNOC) are presented. In these examples the dose-response relationships are analyzed. Where a relationship is present the existence of a threshold is investigated.

INTRODUCTION

The analysis of the dose-response relationship is an important criterion needed in establishing causality. Furthermore, if a relationship is present the question of consequences needs to be discussed. In occupational medicine the most important question is whether a threshold can be assessed. There are several statistical methods available for analysis of a given set of data. In the case of an ordinal response, several of these methods have been described in form of a tutorial.[1] In larger samples different methods tend to exhibit comparable results. In smaller samples, however, as well as for certain outcomes, the methods can lead to differing results.[2] In a binary response the logistic and the linear regression have been compared using the dose in the original form, and then transformed. The results are not always consistent. Assessment of a threshold value can also be based on a specific statistical model.[3] It is well-known that different models can lead to contradictory results.[4] Very recently it was shown that even if the same model is applied, the result may depend on the form in which the dose is used.[5]

In order to obtain a solution that is independent of the form in which the dose is used, a nonparametric method, isotonic regression,[6] is proposed. First, isotonic regression is described very briefly and subsequently several applications are presented.

---

[a]Address for correspondence: Prof. Dr. K. Ulm, Institute for Medical Statistics and Epidemiology, Technical University Munich, Ismaninger Straße 22, 81675 Munich, Germany. +49-89-4140-4321 (voice); +49-89-4140-4850 (fax).
 e-mail: kurt.ulm@imse.med.tu-muenchen.de

METHOD

Isotonic Regression

In many epidemiological studies, especially in occupational medicine, a monotonic dose-response relationship is assumed. Nearly all parametric models, for example, logistic regression, are based on this assumption. If only the dose is considered and p_i is the risk associated with dose level d_i, the assumption of monotonicity is fulfilled if the following relation holds:

$$p_1 \leq p_2 \leq \ldots \leq p_I. \qquad (1)$$

Using a model of the form

$$F(P(d)) = \alpha + \beta \cdot d,$$

where $F(\cdot)$ is a certain transformation of the response probability $P(d)$, relation (1) always holds. However, the estimates of $P(d)$ can depend on how d is used in the model—in the original or transformed form. Sometimes the dose is grouped into several categories and in this situation the same problems also occur. Therefore, a method independent of the form in which the dose is used has certain advantages. Isotonic regression provides a maximum likelihood estimate for the response probability $P(d)$ that satisfies relation (1) and is independent of the form of the dose. Any monotonic transformation of the dose leads to an identical result.

With only one variable the algorithm is simple. If the relation (1) fails to hold for the observed response rates within pair $(j, j+1)$, both groups are pooled using the size (n_j, n_{j+1}) as weights. This method is called the pooling adjacent violators algorithm.[6]

$$p_j^* = p_{j+1}^* = \frac{p_j \cdot n_j + p_{j+1} \cdot n_{j+1}}{n_j + n_{j+1}}$$

Proof of a dose-response relationship is based on likelihood ratio statistics R, by comparing the appropriate likelihood function under H_0 (all response rates are identical) and under H_1 (result of isotonic regression). The large sample distribution of the test-statistic is non standard and is a weighted sum of χ^2-distributions with different degrees of freedom.[6] For smaller samples the performance of a permutation test is recommended in order to calculate the appropriate p-value.[2]

The same procedure can also be used to take additional covariates into account. In the case of two covariates the algorithm provided by Dykstra and Robertson can be applied.[7] In this case the restriction of monotonicity means

$$p_{ij} \leq p_{i'j'}$$

with $i \leq i'$ and $j \leq j'$.

To test the influence of both covariates again the likelihood ratio statistic R can be used. However, if one is interested in the effect of a single covariate, dose for example, given the influence of the other covariate, for example, time since first exposure, no standard test procedure is available. The problem is related to the appropriate number of degrees of freedom. One solution to this problem is again the performance of a permutation test.

If more than one additional covariate is taken into account, no algorithm for estimating the response rates is available. In this case the model has to be specified, for example, an additive isotonic model.[8]

Permutation Test

Based on the observations, a large number of permutations (e.g., $m = 10.000$) can be analyzed. Each individual is characterized by a data pair, (d_i, δ_i), $i = 1, ..., n$, with d_i denoting the dose and δ_i the status ($\delta_i = 0$ without event and $\delta_i = 1$ with event). For the permutation test this pair is separated and the dose and the status are combined randomly. Within each permutation H_0 (equal risk in all dose-groups) is considered. Each permutation is analyzed by the test proposed and leads to a test statistics t_{perm}. If t_{obs} is the observed value of the test statistic of the original data, the p-value is merely the probability that the result of a permutation is equal to t_{obs} or exceeds it.

$$p = Pr(t_{perm} \geq t_{obs}) = \sum I_+(t_{perm} \geq t_{obs})/m.$$

Sometimes the numerator and the denominator are increased by unity, which has no impact if m is large. If the p-value is less than the predefined significance level α, H_0 is rejected and a dose-response relationship can be assumed.

This idea can be extended to analyze the influence of a certain covariate, d, given the effect of other covariates, $x = (x_1, x_2, ..., x_n)$. The data are then given in the form (d_i, x_i, δ_i), $i = 1, ..., n$. This vector is now separated into two parts (d_i) and (x_i, δ_i) that are randomly combined. The same procedure as that described for the univariate situation can be applied.

Estimation of a Threshold Value

The use of isotonic regression can be extended to estimate a threshold value following a proposal of Schell and Singh.[9] The idea is simply to amalgamate adjacent groups and to compare the corresponding likelihood functions. If the difference between the values of the likelihood functions is too small both groups can be pooled, otherwise a threshold can be assessed.

For example, assume $p_1 < p_2 < ... < p_I$ are the results of the isotonic regression with $\ln L$ the value of the corresponding likelihood function. In the first step, dose level 1 and 2 are pooled leading to a response rate of p_{12} with $\ln L_{12}$ the value of the corresponding likelihood function. The difference

$$D = 2 \cdot (\ln L - \ln L_{12})$$

is of interest. If D is small the difference between p_1 and p_2 can be ignored. The test statistic D should follow approximately a χ^2-distribution with one degree of freedom. If D is less than, for example, 2.71 ($= \chi^2_{1, 90\%}$), both groups can be amalgamated and the procedure continued. If D exceeds that critical level, dose d_1 can be assessed as threshold value.

RESULTS

Para-aramid

The classification of man-made mineral fibers as carcinogenic is still controversial. One type of fiber, para-aramid, is especially, under discussion. The main source for classifying this type of fiber is an animal experiment that has been evaluated many times. The latest update is given in TABLE 1.

TABLE 1. Data from para-aramid study (Ref. 10)

dose[$\cdot 10^6$ F/m^3]	0	2.5	25	100	400
number of tumors[a]	1	1	1	4	3
number of animals	137	133	132	137	92

[a]Adenoma, bronchido-alveolar without squamous-cell carcinoma.

One of the methods used to analyze this study is logistic regression. Three forms of the dose assignment (dose, log-dose, and index) are applied (see TABLE 2). The best fit is obtained in using the index ($p = 0.024$). However, if dose is used, the hypothesis of an association cannot be accepted ($p = 0.053$). The level is slightly less than significant. The log-dose assignment leads also to significant value ($p = 0.04$). A similar result was obtained by applying the usual test for trend from Cochran and Armitage.[2]

Our data were also analyzed by isotonic regression. The observed response rates already fulfill the criterion of monotonicity and are therefore the result of isotonic regression. The corresponding test statistic yields a value $R = 4.99$. The p-value obtained from the large sample approximation is slightly above 0.05 ($p = 0.058$). The hypothesis H_0 cannot be rejected. The exact p-value based on the permutation test ($m = 10,000$ permutations) also exceeds 0.05 ($p = 0.111$).

From this analysis one can conclude that there is no statistically significant correlation between dose and tumor rate. However, the results are only slightly below the significance level. IARC concluded[10] that an increased incidence of cystic keratinizing squamous-cell carcinomas was reported. The biological significance of these lesions is unclear. There is inadequate evidence from experimental animals for the carcinogenicity of para-aramid fibers.

Silica Dust

The question of whether silica dust itself is carcinogenic is still open. IARC has classified crystalline silica as category 1, which means that it is carcinogenic to humans.[10] One study that had great impact on this decision is that from Checkoway.[11] In order to investigate the dose-response relationship, cumulative exposure has been classified into five categories. The lowest category serves as a baseline. The data are presented in TABLE 3.

TABLE 2. Results of the analysis of the para-aramid data (see TABLE 1) with the logistic model and isotonic regression

Type of regression	Dose Assignment		
	dose	log(dose + 0.01)	index
logistic p-value	0.053	0.040	0.024
isotonic p-value (exact)	0.11		

TABLE 3. Result of isotonic regression analyzing the study by Checkoway (Ref. 11) of the association between crystalline silica and lung cancer

Cumulative exposure (mg/m³ years)	lung cancer					isotonic regression			reduced isotonic regression		
	obs	exp	SMR	RR	$\ln L(H_0)$	SMR	RR	$\ln L(H_1)$	SMR	RR	$\ln L(H_2)$
0–0.5	17	15.25	1.12	1.00	4.27	0.99	1.00	−0.18	1.07	1.00	1.09
0.5–1.1	14	11.73	1.19	1.07	3.52	0.99	1.00	−0.14	1.07	1.00	0.90
1.1–2.1	7	11.41	0.61	0.55	1.76	0.99	1.00	−0.07	1.07	1.00	0.45
2.1–5.0	15	11.30	1.33	1.19	3.77	1.33	1.34	4.24	1.07	1.00	0.96
5.0+	24	10.20	2.35	2.11	6.03	2.35	2.38	20.53	2.35	2.21	20.53
sum	77	59.90	1.29		19.34			24.38			23.94
							R	10.39			9.21

There is a significant trend toward using Poisson regression.[11] The main problem associated with this type of regression analysis is quantification of dose. In the situation where each category contains a range of exposures, several dose-assignment options are possible. The mean or median of that category, or just the index, are frequently used. These can lead to different results.

The expected values are not given in Reference 11. They are estimated according to the total number of expected values and the relative risks. In the observed estimates for the relative risk, the monotonicity constraint fails between the second ($RR = 1.07$) and third ($RR = 0.55$) category. Pooling both categories, an SMR of 0.91 is observed, which is smaller than the risk in the first category. Therefore, the three lowest categories need to be pooled leading to an SMR of 0.99. The fourth category has an SMR of 1.33. The highest category exhibits an SMR of 2.35 based on 24 cases (see TABLE 3). The likelihood ratio statistic for isotonic regression yields a statistically significant value $R = 10.09$ ($p = 2 \cdot (24.38 - 19.34)$; $p < 0.01$).

In order to assess a threshold value for the first step, the fourth category is amalgamated with the three lower categories already pooled by isotonic regression. The value of the corresponding likelihood function is reduced to $\ln L_{12} = 23.94$. The difference between the values of both likelihood functions leads to $D = 0.88$. This difference is too small to indicate an increase in the risk from the three lower categories to the fourth category. Therefore, only the fifth category leads to the significant increase in risk. The difference then shows a value $D = 9.20 = 2 \cdot (23.94 - 19.34)$, which is too large to indicate equal risks. Based on this analysis a threshold value of about $5 \cdot mg/m^3$ can be assumed.

PNOC

Recently the assessment of a threshold for particles not otherwise classified (PNOC) has been investigated. An analysis of one particular cohort is given below. The data of that cohort are described in TABLE 4 (for details see Ref. 5).

The data have been analyzed by various logistic models leading to different results.[5] The result is highly dependent on the form in which the dose is used (linear or log-transformed). Without any transformation, a nonsignificant threshold value of 2 mg/m^3 is obtained ($p = 0.07$). Using a log-transformation, a statistically significant threshold of 3.75 mg/m^3 is obtained ($p < 0.01$).

The same set of data has been analyzed by isotonic regression. To simplify the analysis the data are grouped into five-year time categories and dust intervals of

Table 4. Description of smokers in the cohort (PNOC-study)

	with CBR	without CBR	total
sample size	241 (26.2%)	679 (73.8%)	920
		median (min-max)	
total inhalable dust concentration (in mg/m^3)	4.6 (0.3–12.1)	1.1 (0.2–15)	1.4 (0.2–15)
time since first exposure (in years)	28 (6–9)	24 (3–5)	23 (3–51)

0.5 mg/m^3. Without any covariate the likelihood function has a value of $2 \cdot \ln L/H_0 = -1058.17$. Using time as a covariate, this value is reduced to $2 \cdot \ln L/H_0 = -1004.62$. The difference, $R = 54.55$, indicates a statistically significant influence of time since first exposure.

If time is used without grouping the fit is only slightly better. Taking into account the possible influence from dust, the value of the likelihood function further increases to $2 \cdot \ln L(\text{time, dust}) = -954.08$. The corresponding likelihood ratio statistic R yields a value of $R = 50.54$ indicating a statistically significant influence from dust based on the permutation test ($p < 0.01$). The result of the isotonic regression depicted in FIGURE 1.

In order to assess a threshold value, the dose groups are pooled starting with the two lowest groups. In the first step, the likelihood function is changed to -954.85 (see TABLE 5). The difference of $D = 0.77$, is too small to indicate a significant increase in risk. The change in risk over the time categories 10–15 and 15–20 years is either too small or the number of individuals in that subgroups is too low. Pooling the next dose group with the two lowest groups, the difference of $D = 0.86$ again is too small to indicate a threshold. In the next four dose groups up to 3 mg/m^3 there is no change in the risk. Therefore, the value of the likelihood function remains the same. Pooling the next three groups (up to 4.5 mg/m^3) the difference gives a value $D = 0.26$. If the next dose group (4.5–5 mg/m^3) is aggregated the difference attains a value $D = 7.68$. This difference is large enough to indicate a significant increase in risk from that dose and beyond. Therefore, based on isotonic regression, a threshold level of 4.5 mg/m^3 is obtained.

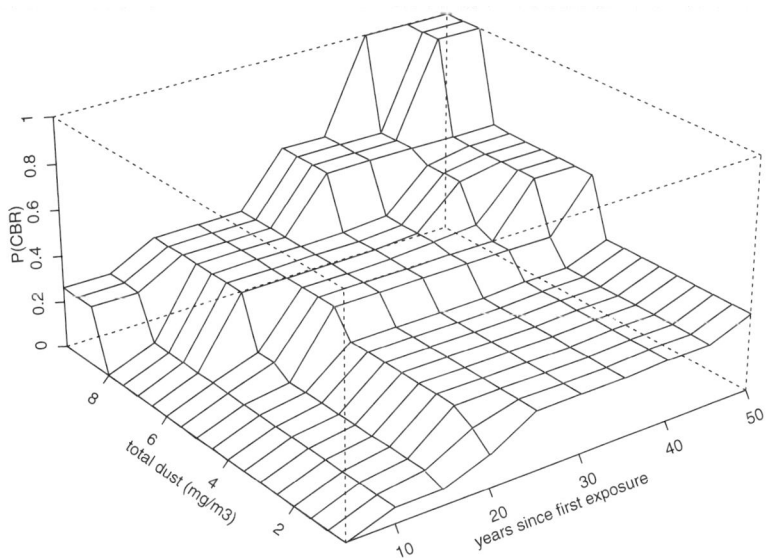

FIGURE 1. Isotonic regression analysis of the data presented in TABLE 4.

TABLE 5. Result of the isotonic regression on the data from TABLE 4.

	$-2\cdot\ln L$
no covariate	1058.17
time	1004.62
time + dust	954.08
aggregating dust—categories (mg/m^3)	
−1.0	954.85
−1.5	955.71
−2.0	955.71
−2.5	955.71
−3.0	955.71
−3.5	955.71
−4.0	955.97
−4.5	955.97
−5.0	963.65

DISCUSSION

The analysis of a dose-response relationship, as well as the existence and value of a threshold, are of great importance in occupational epidemiology. These results are essential to the safety of the workforce and to the economic aspects. Several statistical methods are available for these analyses. However, the various methods can lead to different results. Some of the models may indicate a significant dose-response relationship, whereas others may fail to do so. The outcome of the analysis can depend on several aspects (form of the relationship and transformation of covariates). The isotonic regression method is independent of these assumptions. The only requirement is monotonicity. However, this seems to be of no limitation, since all the parametric models imply this assumption.

There are at least two problems related to isotonic regression. The first concerns the appropriate test statistics. The likelihood ratio statistic, R, can be used. However the distribution of R under H_0 is known only for large samples and with an equal number of observations in each of the various subgroups. This problem can be solved by applying a permutation test. By performing a large number of permutations an adequate p-value is obtained. The other problem is related to the number of covariates used in the analysis. The program presently available can handle up to only two covariates. For more variables an additive model needs to be applied.

Isotonic regression can also be used to assess a threshold value. The main problem here is again related to the appropriate test statistics. In order to give a reasonable solution to that problem, the χ^2-distribution is proposed. However, the question concerns the number of degrees of freedom. In the examples presented, it was possible to assess a threshold value. More work remains to be done in order to use this method.

REFERENCES

1. CHUANG-STEIN, C. & A. AGRESTI. 1997. Tutorial in biostatistics: a review of tests for detecting a monotone dose-response relationship with ordinal response data. Statistics in Medicine **16**: 2599–2618.
2. ULM, K., F. DANNEGGER & U. BECKER. 1998. Test on trends in binary response. Discussion paper 115, SFB 386. University of Munich.
3. ULM, K. 1999. A statistical method for assessing a threshold in epidemiological studies. Statistics in Medicine **10**: 341–349.
4. ULM, K. 1991. On the estimation of threshold values (correspondence). Biometrics **45**: 1324–1326.
5. KÜCHENHOFF, H. & K. ULM. 1997. Comparison of statistical methods for assessing threshold limiting values in occupational epidemiology. Computational Statistics **12**: 249–264.
6. ROBERTSON, T., F.T. WRIGHT & R.L. DYKSTRA. 1988. Order Restricted Statistical Inference. J. Wiley, New York.
7. DYKSTRA, R.L. & T. ROBERTSON. 1982. An algorithm for isotonic regression tests on multinomial and Poisson parameters: the sharpened restriction. Ann. Statistics **10**: 1246–1252.
8. BACCHETTI, P. 1989. Additive isotonic models. J. Am. Stat. Assoc. **84**: 289–294.
9. SCHELL, M.J. & B. SINGH. 1997. The Reduced Monotonic Regression Method. J. Am. Stat. Assoc. **92**: 128–135.
10. IARC-MONOGRAPHS. Silica, Some silicates, coal dust and par-aramid fibrils. World Health Organization. International Agency for Research on Cancer.
11. CHECKOWAY, H., N.J. HEYER, N.S. SEIXAS et al. 1997 Dose-response associations of silica with nonmalignant respiratory disease and lung cancer mortality in the diatomaceous earth industry. Am. J. Epidemiol. **145**: 680–688.

Estimates of the Proportions of Carcinogens and Anticarcinogens in Bioassays Conducted by the U.S. National Toxicology Program

Application of a New Meta-analytic Approach

KENNY S. CRUMP,[a,b] DANIEL KREWSKI,[c] AND CYNTHIA VAN LANDINGHAM[b]

[b]*The KS Crump Group, 602 East Georgia, Ruston, Louisiana 71270, USA*

[c]*Department of Epidemiology and Community Medicine, University of Ottawa, Room 3229C, 451 Smyth Road, Ottawa, ON K1H8M5, Canada*

ABSTRACT: A meta-analysis was performed in order to estimate the proportion of liver carcinogens, the proportion of chemicals carcinogenic at any site, and the corresponding proportion of anticarcinogens among chemicals tested in 397 long-term cancer bioassays conducted by the U.S. National Toxicology Program (NTP). Although the estimator used was negatively biased, the study provided persuasive evidence for a larger proportion of liver carcinogens (0.43, 90% CI: 0.35, 0.51) than was identified by the NTP (0.28). A larger proportion of chemicals carcinogenic at any site was also estimated (0.59, 90% CI: 0.49, 0.69) than was identified by the NTP (0.51), although this excess was not statistically significant. A larger proportion of anticarcinogens (0.66) was estimated than carcinogens (0.59). Despite the negative bias, it was estimated that 85% of the chemicals were either carcinogenic or anticarcinogenic at some site in some sex-species group. This suggests that most chemicals tested at high enough doses will cause some sort of perturbation in tumor rates.

INTRODUCTION

The National Toxicology Program (NTP) has been testing chemicals for carcinogenic potential for about 30 years. Of the roughly 400 chemicals that have been tested to date, about 50% have been identified as carcinogens. About 25% of the tested chemicals have been found to be carcinogenic to the liver, which is the most frequent site of carcinogenesis in NTP bioassays.[1,2]

Carcinogenicity test results obtained by the NTP are used extensively by regulatory agencies charged with protection of public health and by the scientific community concerned with carcinogenic risk assessment. Consequently, these studies have important health and economic consequences. Chemicals identified as carcinogenic in animal bioassays are generally regulated much more stringently than chemicals not so identified.

To achieve a high degree of sensitivity with limited numbers of animals, animal bioassays generally employ high doses in an attempt to enhance tumor occurrence.

[a]Address for correspondence: 318-242-5019 (voice); 318-255-4960 (fax).
e-mail: kcrump@icfconsulting.com

The highest dose used in an NTP bioassay is the maximum tolerated dose (MTD), defined as the highest dose that can be administered in a long-term experiment without reducing survival (other than as a result of tumor occurrence) or appreciably altering body weight gain.[3] Even though use of the MTD enhances the sensitivity of a bioassay, it is possible that some carcinogens may have remained undetected by the NTP. The present paper evaluates the extent to which that may have occurred.

To accomplish this goal, data from 397 NTP bioassays are used to estimate the portion of the chemicals that are carcinogenic to the liver, and the proportion that are carcinogenic at any site, in any experimental animal group. Estimates are also developed for the proportion of the 397 chemicals that are anticarcinogenic, or either carcinogenic or anticarcinogenic. A chemical that caused a dose-related increase in tumor incidence at one site and a dose-related decrease at a different site would be considered both a carcinogen and an anticarcinogen. Other accounts of this work may be found elsewhere.[4–5]

These estimates are based on a substantially different methodology than was used by the NTP to identify carcinogens.[6–7] Unlike the NTP approach, the estimation procedure used here does not involve determination of whether an individual chemical is carcinogenic. Rather, it examines the distribution of p-values obtained from statistical tests applied to each of the NTP bioassays. If there were no carcinogens present, these p-values would theoretically be uniformly distributed. The proportion of carcinogens is estimated by means of the pattern of departure from a uniform distribution. The approach does not rely upon a single cutoff for p-values (e.g., $p = 0.05$) and accounts for the proportion of p-values in any range (e.g., an excess of p-values in the range 0.1 to 0.2, or a deficit in the range 0.8 to 1.0).

METHODS

Data from 397 long-term carcinogenicity bioassays were obtained from NTP data archives.[4,5] Most of these studies involved mice and rats, and our analysis was restricted to these two species. Generally, males and females of a species were tested in separate experiments that involved two or three dose groups of about 50 animals each, in addition to a control group of the same size (although control groups in a few of the earlier studies contained as few as 10 animals). Experiments that the NTP considered inadequate for a determination of carcinogenicity were removed from consideration.

The procedure used to estimate the number of carcinogens in the NTP data base was based on the empirical distribution of p-values obtained from a statistical test applied to the individual studies,[6,7] and this is now briefly described. If none of the chemicals had any effect upon tumor rates, the p-values would be uniformly distributed between zero and one, which means that the cumulative distribution of p-values would graph as a straight line from the point (0,0) to the point (1,1), as illustrated in FIGURE 1A. However, if, for example, 60% of the chemicals were carcinogenic—so highly carcinogenic that the corresponding p-values were essentially zero (FIG. 1B), the cumulative distribution would still plot as a straight line, and this line would intersect the y-axis at 0.6, the proportion of carcinogens. FIGURE 1C depicts a more realistic case in which the proportion of carcinogens is still 60% but the carcinogenic

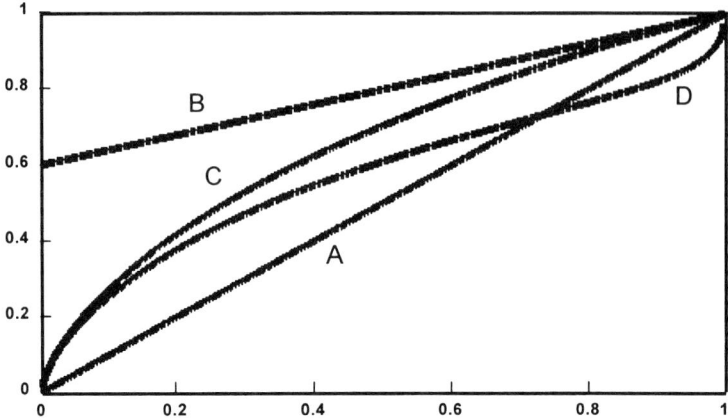

FIGURE 1. Theoretical distribution of p-values under various conditions. A, no carcinogens or anticarcinogens. B, 60% of chemicals are highly carcinogenic. C, 60% are carcinogenic, but not as extremely so as in B. D, 60% of chemicals are carcinogenic (as in C), and an additional 20% are anticarcinogenic.

responses are weaker, so that the p-values from the carcinogens are not all zero. In this case a tangent line drawn at any point on the theoretical cumulative distribution of p-values will intersect the y-axis at a point that is less than 0.6 (the proportion of carcinogens), but the intersection point will be nearer to 0.6 if the tangent line is drawn at a point closer to $p = 1$. Intuitively, this is because, for larger values of p, there are relatively fewer p-values present that correspond to carcinogens and influence the slope of $F(p)$. In fact, as illustrated by FIGURE 1C, under some general conditions, the tangent line at the point $p = 1$ intersects the y-axis exactly at the proportion of carcinogens.[6] FIGURE 1D is a modification of FIGURE 1C in which the proportion of carcinogens remains at 0.6, but, in addition, 20% of the chemicals are anticarcinogens. In this case, any tangent line will intersect the y-axis at a value that is less than 0.6. However, as suggested by FIGURE 1D, the point of intersection will be largest, and consequently nearer to the true proportion of carcinogens, when the tangent line is drawn through the inflection point of the curve.

This discussion suggests that the proportion of carcinogens should be estimated from the empirical distribution function, $\hat{F}(p)$ (defined as the proportion of studies with p-values not greater than p), by drawing a secant line through two points, a and b, of the graph of $\hat{F}(p)$, and using as an estimator the y-intercept of this secant line. This estimator is

$$\frac{b\hat{F}(a) - a\hat{F}(b)}{b - a},$$

and its variance is given by

$$\frac{b^2 F(a)[1 - F(a)] + a^2 F(b)[1 - F(b)] - 2ab F(a)[F(b) - F(a)]}{N(b - a)^2},$$

where F is the theoretical distribution of p-values (expected value of $\hat{F}$), and N is the number of p-values (studies). Under fairly general conditions, this estimator has the following properties,[7] all of which are suggested by the above discussion:
1. The estimator is biased low no matter how a and b are chosen.
2. This negative bias is smallest when a and b are selected near the inflection point of $F(p)$.
3. For a given value of b, the value of a that minimizes the bias is on the opposite side of the inflection point from b.
4. The variance of the estimator becomes large when a and b are close together.

These properties suggest selecting a and b near to, and on opposite sides of, the inflection point of the graph of $\hat{F}(p)$, but not so near to the inflection point that the variance becomes excessively large.

To use this procedure to estimate the proportion of NTP chemicals that were liver carcinogens, we first calculated p-values from the POLY3 test[8] applied to the liver tumor data from all dose groups of each sex-species-specific experiment, for each tested chemical. The POLY3 test is an age-adjusted test for trend, and it has recently been adopted by the NTP as the statistical test of choice for the NTP carcinogenesis bioassays.[9] The p-value for a test of the hypothesis that a chemical was carcinogenic to the liver in at least one sex-species group, was then defined as $1 - (1 - p_{min})^k$, where p_{min} is the minimum POLY3 p-value from all sex-species experiments and k is the number of such experiments for a chemical (for the majority of chemicals, $k = 4$, corresponding to the fact that separate experiments had been performed in males and females of mice and rats). This p-value can be theoretically shown to be uniformly distributed in the null case (when the exposure does not affect tumor rates in any sex-species group).

Calculation of the p-values needed to estimate the proportion of chemicals that were carcinogenic at any site in any sex and species group is somewhat more complicated. First the POLY3 test was applied to each of 93 tumor categories defined so that they were similar to the categories routinely analyzed by the NTP. The test statistic, T, for an effect in a sex-species experiment was the largest of these POLY3 test statistics, after application of a continuity correction, derived from any tumor category. In order to insure that the test based on T had the proper false positive rate, its p-value was determined using a randomization procedure.[10] In this procedure animals from a given sex-species experiment were randomly reassigned to treatment groups a total of 400 times and the POLY3 was reapplied to each set of randomized data. In order to control for potential treatment-related differences in life span among different treatment groups, animals were stratified into four groups according to elapsed time from beginning of study until death, and the total number of animals in each treatment-time category was kept fixed at its value in the original data. The p-value for the test statistic, T, was defined as the proportion of times (out of the total of 400) for which the largest POLY3 test statistic from a randomly created data set was equal to or exceeded T. The p-value for a test for an effect in any sex-species experiment was again defined as $1 - (1 - p_{min})^k$. The fact that p-values calculated in this manner exhibited a uniform distribution in the null case was verified by a simulation study in which ten sets of null data were fabricated from results of each NTP experiment by randomly reassigning animals in the manner described above.

RESULTS

TABLE 1 compares the results of the POLY3 test applied to liver tumor data from specific studies to the carcinogenicity determinations made by the NTP. The NTP classification for a specific sex-species group was considered positive if the evidence for liver carcinogenicity was coded as either P (positive), CE (clear evidence), or SE (some evidence). A study was considered positive for liver carcinogenesis if at least one of the sex-species groups was positive. The concordance was defined as the percent of studies for which the NTP classification was positive and the POLY3 p-value was less than or equal to the selected significance level plus the percent of studies in which the NTP classification was not positive, and the POLY3 p-value was greater than the selected significance level. Results are presented for two levels of significance (0.05 and 0.009). Using the level of 0.05, the correspondence between the NTP classification and the POLY3 test ranged from 91% to 93% for the different sex-species groups. However, correspondences were higher when a significance level of 0.009 was used—ranging from 94% for all sexes and species to 99% for female rats.

TABLE 1. Concordance between NTP classification and POLY3 test for liver carcinogenicity

	NTP classification			Concordance[a] using POLY3 p-value cutoff of	
	Total	Positive	Negative	$p = 0.05$	$p = 0.009$
Male mice	370	61	309	91%	95%
Female mice	370	81	289	91%	96%
Male rats	367	35	332	91%	97%
Female rats	367	30	337	93%	99%
All sexes and species	390	108	282	92%	94%

[a]Percent of experiments where POLY3 agreed with NTP classification.

TABLE 2. Concordance between NTP classification and POLY3 test for carcinogenicity at any site

	NTP classification			Concordance[a] ($p = 0.05$)
	Total	Positive	Negative	
Male mice	367	108	259	91%
Female mice	373	129	244	89%
Male rats	366	130	236	85%
Female rats	367	103	264	90%
All sexes and species	397	201	196	86%

[a]Percent of experiments where POLY3 agreed with NTP classification.

TABLE 2 provides a similar comparison for carcinogenicity at any site. This table was constructed in the same manner as TABLE 1, except that a chemical was considered to be carcinogenic by the NTP if it was positive at any site. Based on a significance level of 0.05, the correspondence between the POLY3 test results and the NTP classifications was lower than it was for liver carcinogenesis—ranging from 85% to 91%. Furthermore, the correspondence could not be substantially improved through use of a different level of significance.

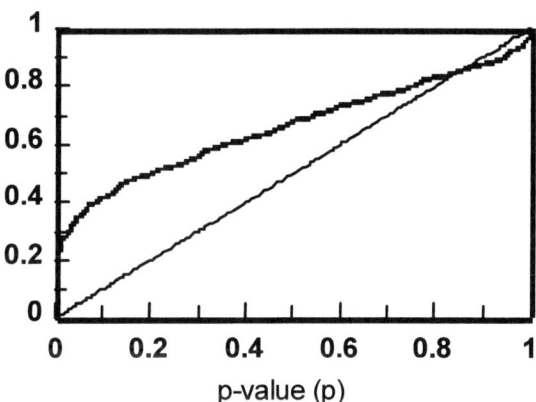

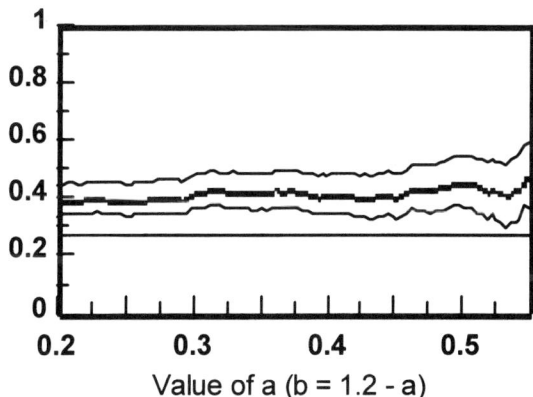

FIGURE 2. Results of analysis to estimate proportion of chemicals tested by NTP that were carcinogenic to the liver in any sex-species group. In the **lower part** of the figure: the *solid wavy line* is a point estimate; *narrower wavy lines* define 90% C.I. on point estimate; *horizontal line* indicates NTP estimate (0.28).

FIGURE 2 shows the results of the analysis used to estimate the number of liver carcinogens. The empirical distribution of POLY3 p-values is considerably above the line $y = x$ for small values of p, indicating the presence of liver carcinogens. This graph also shows some evidence of anticarcinogenesis since the graph lies slightly below the graph $y = x$ for p-values close to 1.0. This evidence for anticarcinogenesis was somewhat surprising, since this graph was based generally on p-values determined from a minimum of, generally, four p-values, and it might be expected that,

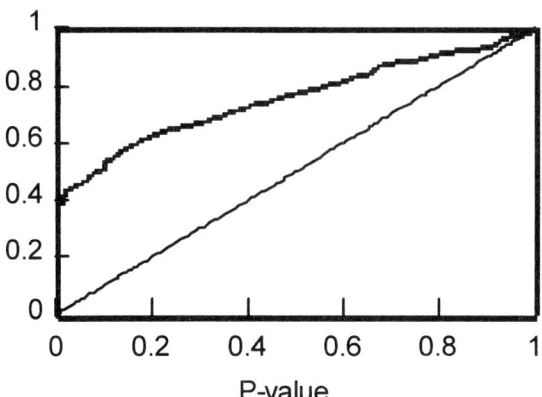

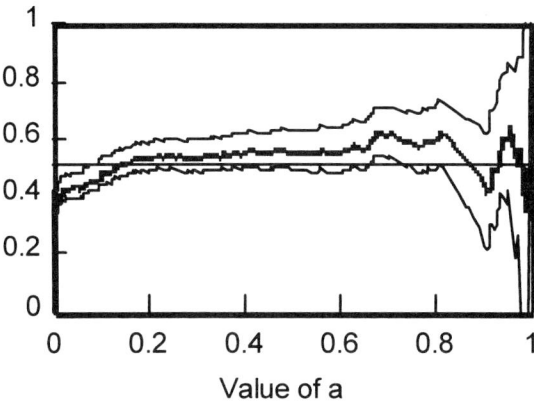

FIGURE 3. Results of analysis to estimate proportion of chemicals tested by NTP that were carcinogenic at any site in any sex-species group. In the **lower part** of the figure: the *solid wavy line* is a point estimate; *narrower wavy lines* define 90% C.I. on point estimate; *horizontal line* indicates NTP estimate (0.51).

for example, anticarcinogenicity in one sex-species group would have relatively little effect upon the minimum of four p-values. In fact, comparable graphs for specific sex-species groups showed much greater evidence of anticarcinogenesis.

FIGURE 2 also shows estimates of the number of liver carcinogens among the NTP-tested chemicals obtained for various values of the parameter a between 0.2 and 0.55, with b selected as $1.2 - a$. The solid wavy line is the point estimate and the lighter lines on either side depict the 90% confidence interval around the point esti-

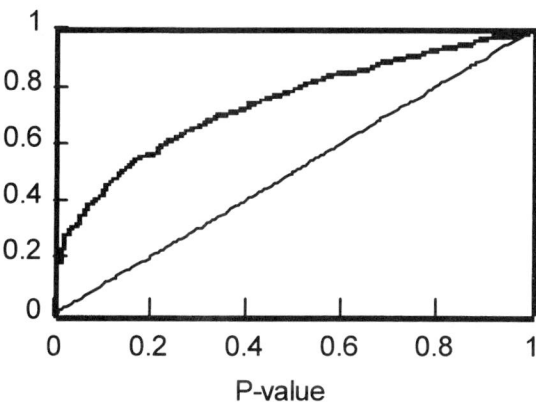

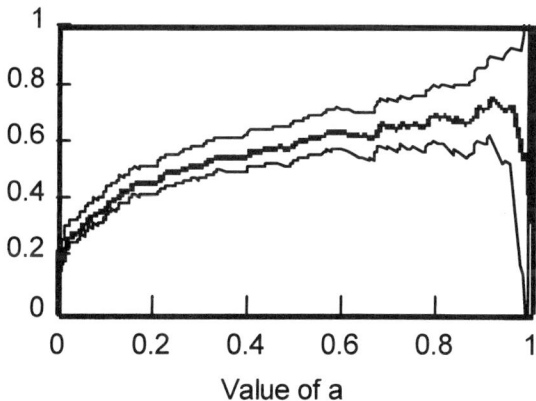

FIGURE 4. Results of analysis to estimate proportion of chemicals tested by NTP that were anticarcinogenic at any site in any sex-species group. In the **lower part** of the figure: the *solid wavy line* is a point estimate; *narrower wavy lines* define 90% C.I. on point estimate.

mate. The horizontal line shows the number of liver carcinogens (108) identified by the NTP. This graph provides evidence for more liver carcinogens than were identified by the NTP as both the point estimate and the 95% lower confidence bound is above the NTP estimate for all values of a.

FIGURE 3 presents results of the analysis to estimate the proportion of chemicals that were carcinogenic at any site in any sex-species group. The graph of the estimate of the proportion of carcinogens shows the estimate for all values of a between 0

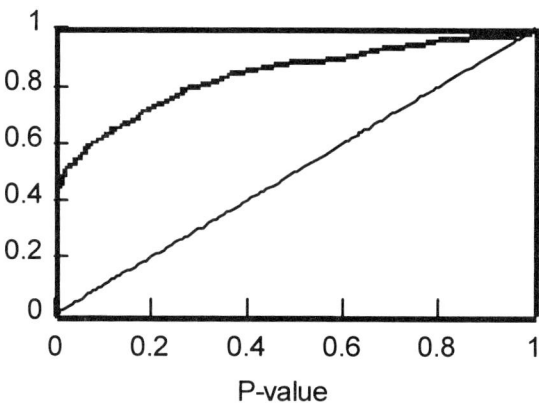

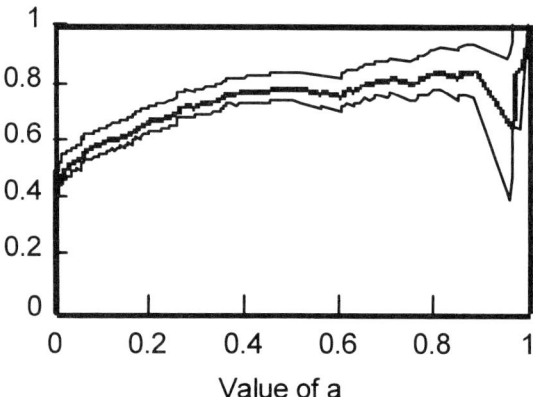

FIGURE 5. Results of analysis to estimate proportion of chemicals tested by NTP that were either carcinogenic or anticarcinogenic at any site in any sex-species group. In the **lower part** of the figure: the *solid wavy line* is point estimate; *narrower wavy lines* define 90% C.I. on point estimate.

TABLE 3. Representative estimates of the proportion of chemicals that were found to be carcinogenic or anticarcinogenic

	Estimated proportion	90% C.I.	NTP Estimate
Liver Carcinogenic[a]	0.43	(0.35, 0.51)	0.28
Carcinogenic overall[b,c]	0.59	(0.49, 0.69)	0.51
Anticarcinogenic overall[c,d]	0.66	(0.56, 0.75)	
Carcinogenic or anticarcinogenic overall[c,e]	0.85	(0.78, 0.91)	

[a]For any sex-species group. Obtained from FIGURE 2 using $a = 0.375$.
[b]At any site in any sex-species group.
[c]Obtained from FIGURE 3 using $a = 0.75$.
[d]Obtained from FIGURE 4 using $a = 0.75$.
[e]Obtained from FIGURE 5 using $a = 0.75$.

and 1, with b fixed at $b = 1$. Although the point estimate of the proportion of carcinogens is higher than the proportion identified by the NTP (0.51) for all values of a except the smallest (where the estimator has the greatest negative bias) and largest (where the variance of the estimator is greatest), the 95% lower bound on our estimate is close to or below the proportion of carcinogens obtained by the NTP for most values of a. Thus, evidence for an excess proportion of chemicals that were carcinogenic at any site over the proportion obtained by the NTP is weaker than the corresponding evidence for liver cancer.

FIGURES 4 and 5 contain results of the analyses used to obtain estimates of the proportion of chemicals that were anticarcinogenic, or either carcinogenic or anticarcinogenic, respectively, at any site in any sex or species. FIGURE 4 indicates the presence of a considerable anticarcinogenesis, and FIGURE 5 suggests that most chemicals were either carcinogenic or anticarcinogenic at some site in some sex-species group.

TABLE 3 contains representative estimates of the proportion of liver carcinogens (obtained by setting $a = 0.375$ in FIG. 2) and the proportion of chemicals that were carcinogenic, anticarcinogenic or either (obtained by setting $a = 0.75$ in FIGS. 3, 4, and 5, respectively). The estimated proportion of liver carcinogens was 0.43 (90% CI: 0.35, 0.51), which is significantly larger than the proportion identified by the NTP (0.28). Although the estimated proportion of chemicals carcinogenic at any site was 0.59 (90% CI: 0.49, 0.69), compared to the NTP estimate of 0.51 this excess was not statistically significant. The estimated proportion of anticarcinogens was 0.66, which was higher than the estimate of the proportion of carcinogens. The proportion of chemicals that were either carcinogenic or anticarcinogenic was estimated as 0.85 (90% CI: 0.78, 0.91).

DISCUSSION

Despite the fact that the NTP exposes animals to high doses, it is possible that some carcinogens may have remained undetected in NTP bioassays. To address this possibility, we made independent estimates of the proportion of liver carcinogens and the proportion of chemicals carcinogenic at any site among 397 chemicals tested by the NTP. We estimate that 43% of chemicals are carcinogenic to the liver, which is about 50% higher than the value of 28% obtained by the NTP. We further estimate that 59% of chemicals were carcinogenic at some site in some sex-species group compared to 51% classified as carcinogenic by the NTP, although this difference was not statistically significant. Thus, we obtained persuasive evidence of more liver carcinogens and some evidence of more carcinogens overall than were estimated by the NTP.

The difference in our findings with respect to liver carcinogenesis (persuasive evidence of more carcinogens than identified by the NTP) *vis-a-vis* carcinogenesis (only equivocal evidence of such an excess) may be due in part to the manner in which the NTP evaluated their results. The NTP tended to evaluate the data for each tumor site individually, and a chemical was labeled a carcinogen if it was deemed to be carcinogenic at any site. Since the NTP did not use a formal method for correcting for multiple comparisons, they may have been prone to accept weaker statistical evidence for an effect at any tumor site than for an effect at a particular site. In contrast, our analysis did adjust appropriately for multiple comparisons. Another factor that may have contributed to our finding a larger proportion of liver carcinogens than the NTP stems from the high frequency of dose-related increases among liver tumors, and the occurrence of some of these tumors through mechanisms that are of questionable relevance to humans. To compensate, the NTP may have used more stringent criteria for evaluating liver tumors than tumors at other sites. The fact that closer correspondence between the POLY3 test and the NTP classification for liver were obtained using a significance level of 0.009 instead of the conventional level of 0.05 also supports this notion.

The correspondence between the results of POLY3 test and the NTP classification of individual chemicals as liver tumors were high—ranging between 94% and 99% for the various sex-species groups, when a significance level of 0.009 was used. However, correspondences for carcinogenicity at any site were less strong—ranging between 85% and 91%. There are several potential reasons for these differences. Whereas we used a single statistical test for trend in our analysis (the POLY3 test), the NTP used a variety of statistical tests, including individual pairwise comparisons of a control group with each treatment group. The NTP pooled control groups from several studies in their statistical evaluations of some of the earlier studies. We did not have complete records for identifying these pooled controls and, consequently, we used matched controls in our analyses of some of these studies. The NTP sometimes took into account historical control data, but we did not. In some equivocal cases, the NTP generated additional data that were not recorded in our data base. Whereas we evaluated sex-species groups in isolation, the NTP sometimes labeled an insignificant trend in a particular sex as clear evidence of carcinogenicity if the evidence at the same site in the opposite sex was unequivocal. (However, this should not affect the overall determination of carcinogenicity in any sex-species group.) Male rats had a high background rate of testicular tumors, and dose-related trends in these tumors generally were not taken into account by the NTP (although removing chemicals from our analysis for which the strongest effect was seen in these tumors did not appreciably improve the concordance between our analysis that of the NTP). Finally, whereas our *p*-values were adjusted for multiple comparisons, the NTP had no formal procedure for doing this. We would not argue that our formal statistical analysis based on the POLY3 test provided a more (or less) accurate classification of the carcinogenicity of individual chemicals than the NTP procedure. However, we do maintain that our analysis was appropriate and valid for our primary purpose, which was not to classify individual chemicals, but to estimate the overall proportion of carcinogens. Whatever the reason for the differences between our analyses and those of the NTP for individual chemicals, they serve to remind us that the carcinogenicity classification of a chemical is sometimes uncertain.

Any carcinogens in the data base that were not detected by the NTP would tend to be those that caused, at most, marginal increases in tumor responses at the maximal tolerated dose (MTD). Do such undetected carcinogens present any appreciable risk to humans? This question is a difficult one to answer. If the dose response of such a carcinogen was linear, then the risk would be proportional to exposure. If humans were exposed to large amounts (relative to the MTD) of such a chemical, then the resulting risk could be higher than that from a carcinogen that caused unequivocal increases in a bioassay, but to which human exposures were much lower relative to the MTD. On the other hand, if the dose response of such a carcinogen was highly nonlinear, then the risk to humans would likely be minimal. This could be the case for chemicals whose tumorigenic effect is secondary to the toxic effect of testing at very high doses. Ames and Gold[11] have argued that many of the identified carcinogenic responses from animal studies are of this type, and if this is true, many of the undetected carcinogens are likely to be in this category also.

The present study estimated that there were more anticarcinogens (0.66) than carcinogens (0.59) among NTP chemicals. An analysis that used a conventional significance level of 0.05 to detect effects would not have discovered this, since the proportion of chemicals having a p-value less than 0.05 for anticarcinogenesis was smaller than the corresponding proportion for carcinogenesis. Estimating a larger proportion of anticarcinogens than carcinogens was unexpected because chemicals were selected for study by the NTP on the basis of suspected carcinogenicity, and also because anticarcinogenesis should be inherently more difficult to detect than carcinogenesis. More than 90% of the background incidences of the tumor categories used in our analysis were less than 0.05. It would be difficult to detect dose-related decreases in tumor responses in a tumor category having a background rate as small as 0.05 with a conventional bioassay design.

Haseman and Johnson[12] concluded that much of the anticarcinogenesis seen in NTP bioassays was indirectly caused by a dose-related reduction in weight gain. This mechanism may not be operative except at very high doses. However, this uncertainty is not limited to this mechanism or even to anticarcinogenesis since there is generally uncertainty about whether any effect seen in a high dose bioassay will occur at lower doses.

This study estimated that 85% of the chemicals studied by the NTP were either carcinogenic or anticarcinogenic at some site in some sex-species group of rodents. It should be kept in mind that the estimator used to obtain this estimate is inherently negatively biased. This suggests that most chemicals, when given at sufficiently high doses, may cause perturbations that affect tumor responses, causing increases at some sites and decreases at others.

ACKNOWLEDGMENT

The authors would like to thank Dr. Joe Haseman for his invaluable help with this project.

REFERENCES

1. HUFF J.E., J. CIRVELLO, J. HASEMAN & J. BUCHER. 1991. Chemicals associated with site-specific neoplasia in 1394 long-term carcinogenesis experiments in laboratory rodents. Environ. Health Perspect. **93:** 247–270.
2. FUNG, V.A., J.C. BARRETT & J.E. HUFF. 1995. The carcinogenic bioassay in perspective: application in identifying human cancer hazards. Environ. Health Perspect. **103:** 680–683.
3. NATIONAL RESEARCH COUNCIL. 1993. Issues in Risk Assessment. National Academy Press. Washington, DC.
4. CRUMP, K.S., D. KREWSKI & Y. WANG. 1998. Estimates of the number of liver carcinogens in bioassays conducted by the National Toxicology Program. Risk Anal. **18:** 299–308.
5. CRUMP, K.S., D. KREWSKI & C. VAN LANDINGHAM. 1998. Estimates of the proportion of chemicals that were carcinogenic, anticarcinogenic or either in bioassays conducted by the National Toxicology Program. Environ. Health Perspect. **107:** 83–88.
6. BICKIS, M., S. BLEUER & D. KREWSKI. 1996. Estimation of the proportion of positives in a sequence of screening experiments. Can. J. Stat. **24:** 1–16.
7. CRUMP, K.S. & D. KREWSKI. 1998. Estimation of the number of studies with positive trends when studies with negative trends are present. Can. J. Stat. **26:** 643–655.
8. BAILAR, A. & C. PORTIER. 1988. Effects of treatment-induced mortality and tumor-induced mortality on tests for cancer in small samples. Biometrics **44:** 417–431.
9. NATIONAL TOXICOLOGY PROGRAM. 1998. Toxicology and carcinogenesis studies of diethanolamine in F344/N rats and $B6C3F_1$ mice. National Toxicology Program Technical Report Series No. 478. U.S. Department of Health and Human Services, Public Health Service, National Institutes of Health.
10. FARRAR, D. & K.S. CRUMP. 1990. Exact statistical tests for any carcinogenic effect in animal bioassays. II. Age-adjusted tests. Fundam. Appl. Toxicol. **15:** 710–721.
11. AMES, B. & L. GOLD. 1990. Chemical carcinogenesis: too many rodent carcinogens. Proc. Natl. Acad. Sci. **87:** 7772–7776.
12. HASEMAN J. & F. JOHNSON. 1996. Analysis of National Toxicology Program rodent bioassay data for anticarcinogenic effects. Mutat. Res. **350:** 131–141.

Characterization of Uncertainty and Variability in Residential Radon Cancer Risks

D. KREWSKI,[a] S.N. RAI,[b] J.M. ZIELINSKI,[c] AND P.K. HOPKE[d]

[a]Faculty of Medicine, University of Ottawa,
451 Smyth Road, Ottawa, Ontario, Canada K1H 8M5

[b]Statistics Canada, Ottawa, Canada

[c]Health Canada, Ottawa, Canada

[d]Department of Chemistry, Clarkson University, New York, USA

ABSTRACT: Radon, a naturally occurring gas found at some level in most homes, is an established risk factor for human lung cancer. The U.S. National Research Council has recently completed a comprehensive evaluation of the health risks of residential exposure to radon and developed models for projecting radon lung cancer risks to the general population. This analysis suggests that radon may play a role in the etiology of 10–15% of all lung cancer cases in the United States, although these estimates are subject to considerable uncertainty. In this article, we present a detailed analysis of uncertainty and variability in estimates of lung cancer risk due to residential exposure to radon. We use a general framework for the analysis of uncertainty and variability that we developed previously. Specifically, we focus on estimates of the age-specific excess relative risk (*ERR*) and lifetime relative risk (*LRR*), both of which vary substantially among individuals. We also consider estimates of the population attributable risk (*PAR*), which reflects the proportion of the lung cancer burden attributable to radon. Variability in the *ERR* and *LRR* is largely determined by variability in residential exposure levels and in the dosimetric *K*-factor used to extrapolate from occupational to environmental settings. Uncertainty in the *ERR* and *LRR* is due to uncertainty in the model parameters, notably those reflecting the carcinogenic potency of radon and the modifying effect of attained age. Uncertainty in the *PAR* is determined by uncertainty about the values of the parameters in the risk models used to estimate the *PAR*. Uncertainty in radon levels in homes and the dosimetric *K*-factor contribute comparatively little to uncertainty in the *PAR*. These results suggest that reduction in uncertainty about the *PAR* for radon induced lung cancer can only be achieved if more reliable risk projection models can be developed.

INTRODUCTION

Radon, an inert gas naturally present in rocks and soils, is formed during the radioactive decay of uranium-238.[1] Radioactive decay products, or radon daughters, emit alpha particles, that can damage intracellular DNA to result in adverse health outcomes. In particular, underground miners, exposed to high levels of radon in the past, have been shown to be at excess risk of lung cancer,[2,3] raising concerns about potential lung cancer risks due to the presence of lower levels of radon in homes.[4–6] The U.S. Environmental Protection Agency[25] estimated that 7,000–30,000 cases of lung cancer in the United States might be attributable to residential radon exposures each year. They promoted voluntary testing of homes and exposure mitigation whenever the Agency guideline of 4 pCi/L was exceeded.

The U.S. National Academy of Sciences Committee on the Biological Effects of Ionizing Radiation (BEIR VI) recently affirmed residential radon as an important risk factor for lung cancer.[7] Using epidemiological data on underground miners exposed to radon, the Committee developed risk models for projecting risks to the general population, with the two preferred models leading to estimates of 15,000 and 22,000 of radon-induced lung cancer annually in the United States, respectively. These estimates are subject to considerable uncertainty, but this can be described by using current methods for uncertainty analysis.

There are many sources of uncertainty and variability in health risk assessment.[8] Many epidemiological investigations are based on occupational groups with higher levels of exposure than the general population, requiring extrapolation from occupational to environmental exposure conditions. For example, lung cancer risks experienced by underground miners exposed to high levels of radon gas in the past may be used to predict the potential risks associated with lower levels of radon present in homes.[9] Retrospective exposure profiles can be difficult to construct, particularly with chronic diseases, such as cancer, for which exposure data many years prior to the onset of disease are needed. Radon measurements in homes taken today may not reflect past exposures because of changes in address, recent building renovations, changes in lifestyle such as sleeping with the bedroom window open or closed, or inherent variability in radon measurements. Lack of accurate information on variables that effect radon risk, notably tobacco smoking which interacts synergistically with radon,[10] confer uncertainty on risk estimates.

It is important to clearly distinguish between uncertainty and variability in risk assessment.[11] Uncertainty represents the degree of ignorance about the precise value of a particular variable, such as the body weight of a given individual.[12–14] In this case, uncertainty may be due to systematic or random error associated with a simple scale or more sophisticated mass balance used to measure the body weight. On the other hand, variability represents inherent interindividual variation in the value of a particular parameter within the population of interest. In addition to being uncertain, body weight also varies among individuals. A variable, such as body weight, which can be determined with a high degree of accuracy and precision, may be subject to little uncertainty, but can be highly variable. Other parameters may be subject to little variability, but substantial uncertainty. Some may be both highly uncertain and highly variable.

Individual risks, such as the lifetime risk of developing lung cancer, vary within the population at risk depending on the conditions of exposure to radon, exposure to important risk modifying factors such as tobacco smoke, and possibly genetic susceptibility. For the purposes of population health risk assessment, it is important to describe this risk variation within the general population, and to identify high-risk subgroups. With population-based measures of risk such as the population attributable risk that indicate the proportion of the lung cancer burden attributable to radon, interindividual variation in risk is effectively averaged out since the excess lifetime relative risk is integrated across the population of interest. Thus, although subject-specific measures of risk can be both uncertain and variable, population average measures are subject only to uncertainty.

Currently, there is a trend in risk assessment toward a more complete characterization of risk using techniques for uncertainty analysis.[8,5,16] The results of these analyses can be summarized in the form of a distribution of possible risks within the exposed population, taking into account as many sources of uncertainty and variability as possible.

In this paper, we conduct a detailed analysis of uncertainty and variability in cancer risk due to residential radon exposures by using the general methods developed by Rai et al.[17] and by Rai and Krewski.[18] In the next section, we briefly describe our measures of uncertainty and variability in the special case of multiplicative risk models. The cancer risk models for residential radon exposure recently developed by the U.S. National Research Council[7] are described in the third section. Our analysis of uncertainty and variability in the age-specific excess relative risk (*ERR*) and the lifetime relative risk (*LRR*) are then presented in the fourth and fifth sections, respectively. Subsequently, we present our analysis of uncertainty in the population attributable risk (*PAR*). The implications of these results for radon risk management are discussed briefly in the concluding section.

UNCERTAINTY AND VARIABILITY ANALYSIS

Multiplicative Risk Models

Building on results developed by Krewski et al.[19] for pharmokinetic models and by Rai et al.[20] for time series with over-dispersion models, Rai et al.[17] developed a general framework for characterizing and analyzing uncertainty and variability for arbitrary risk models. In this section, we briefly outline the framework for the analysis of uncertainty and variability in the special case of multiplicative risk models described previously by Rai and Krewski.[18] Specifically, suppose that the risk R is defined as the product

$$R = X_1 \times X_2 \times \ldots \times X_p \tag{1}$$

of p risk factors $X_1, \ldots, X_p$. Each risk factor X_i may vary within the population of interest according to some distribution with probability density function $f_i(X_i|\theta_i)$, conditional upon the parameter θ_i. Uncertainty in X_i is characterized by a distribution $g_i(\theta_i|\theta_i^0)$ for θ_i, where θ_i^0 is a known constant. The total uncertainty/variability in X_i is then described by the density function $h_i(X_i|\theta_i^0) = \int f_i(X_i|\theta_i) g_i(\theta_i|\theta_i^0) d\theta_i$. If θ_i is a vector valued, then g_i is a multivariate distribution. Here, it is assumed that the forms of the distributions f, g, and h are known.

For any pair (i,j), let X_i and X_j have a joint distribution f_{ij}, conditional upon the parameter θ_{ij}, describing variability in X_i and X_j. The parameter vector θ_{ij} in turn has a (possibly multivariate) distribution g_{ij}, with known parameter θ_{ij}^0. As described below, the first two moments of these bivariate distributions can be used to describe uncertainty and variability in risk.

If θ_i is a known constant and the distribution f_i is not concentrated at a single point, X_i exhibits variability only. On the other hand, X_i is subject to both uncertainty and variability if both θ_i and f_i are stochastic. When f_i is concentrated at a single point θ_i, and θ_i is stochastic, X_i is subject to uncertainty but not variability. Consequently, the variables $X_1, \ldots, X_p$ can be partitioned into three groups: variables subject only to uncertainty, variables subject only to variability, and variables subject to both uncertainty and variability.

Relative Uncertainty/Variability

After logarithmic transformation, the multiplicative model (1) can be re-expressed as an additive model

$$R^* = \log(R) = \sum_{i=1}^{p} X_i^*, \qquad (2)$$

where $X_i^* = \log X_i$, ($i = 1, 2, \ldots, p$). The expected risk on a logarithmic scale is $E(R^*) = \sum_{i=1}^{p} E(X_i^*)$, with variance $Var(R^*) = Var(\sum_{i=1}^{p} X_i^*)$. Here, the expectation $E(\cdot)$ and variance $Var(\cdot)$ are taken with respect to the distribution of R^*, which can be derived from the joint distribution of the risk factors $X_1, \ldots, X_p$. Although the distribution of R^* is of interest (see *Risk Distributions* below), calculation of the first two moments of this distribution requires only the means $E(X_i^*)$ and covariances $Cov(X_i^*, X_j^*)$ of the risk factors ($i, j = 1, \ldots, p$).

Let $W(R^*) = Var(R^*)$ be the total uncertainty/variability in R^*. This variance can be decomposed into two components,

$$W(R^*) = Var(E(R^*|X_i)) + E(Var(R^*|X_i)).$$

We define $W_i(R^*) = Var(E(R^*|X_i))$ as the uncertainty in R^* due to the risk factor X_i. Note that when X_i is neither uncertain nor variable, $W_i(R^*)$ is zero. With this definition, $W_i(R^*)$ effectively represents the uncertainty/variability in $E(R^*|X_i)$, the conditional expectation of R^* given X_i.

For the transformed additive model (2),

$$W_i(R^*) = Var(X_i^*) + \sum_{j(\neq i)=1}^{p} \sum_{k(\neq i)=1}^{p} Cov(E(X_j^*|X_i), E(X_k^*|X_i)), \qquad (3)$$

with the total uncertainty/variability given by

$$W(R^*) = \sum_{i=1}^{p} Var(X_i^*) + \sum_{i=1}^{p} \sum_{j(\neq i)=1}^{p} Cov(X_i^*, X_j^*). \qquad (4)$$

If $X_1, \ldots, X_p$ are independent, the covariance terms in equations (3) and (4) vanish, so that $W_i(R^*) = Var(X_i^*)$ and $W(R^*) = \sum_{i=1}^{p} Var(X_i^*) = \sum_{i=1}^{p} W_i(R^*)$. We define relative uncertainty/variability in R^* due to the risk factor X_i as $W_i(R^*)/W(R^*)$.

Partitioning Uncertainty and Variability

We now introduce a measure $U(R^*)$ of uncertainty in R^* due to uncertainty in all of the risk factors combined. Similarly, we define a measure $V(R^*)$ of variability in R^* that encompasses variability in all the risk factors. Without loss of generality, we can assume that the variables $X_1, \ldots, X_{p_1}$ in (2) are subject only to uncertainty, that $X_{p_1+1}, \ldots, X_{p_2}$, exhibit only variability, and that the remaining $p - (p_1 + p_2)$ variables are subject to both variability and uncertainty. Thus,

$$R^* = \sum_{i=1}^{p_1} X_i^* + \sum_{i=p_1+1}^{p_2} X_i^* + \sum_{i=p_2+1}^{p} X_i^*. \tag{5}$$

Following Rai and Krewski,[18] we note that

$$U(R^*) = \sum_{i=1}^{p_1} Var(X_i^*) + \sum_{i=p_1+1}^{p_2} Var(E(X_i^*|\theta_i)) \tag{6}$$
$$+ \sum_{i=1}^{p} \sum_{j(\neq i)=1}^{p} Cov(E(X_i^*|\theta_i), E(X_j^*|\theta_j))$$

and

$$V(R^*) = \sum_{i=p_1+1}^{p_2} Var(X_i^*) + \sum_{i=p_2+1}^{p} E(Var(X_i^*|\theta_i))$$
$$+ \sum_{i=1}^{p} \sum_{j(\neq i)=1}^{p} E(Cov(X_i^*, X_j^*|\theta_{ij})). \tag{7}$$

One further decomposition of (6) and (7) is needed to determine the degree to which variables that are subject to both uncertainty and variability contribute to the uncertainty in X_i separately from the variability in X_i. For $X_1, \ldots, X_p$, let $U_i(R^*)$ and $V_i(R^*)$ denote the contribution of X_i to the uncertainty in R^* due to the uncertainty and to the variability in X_i, respectively. Then,

$$U_i(R^*) = Var(E(X_i^*|\theta_i^*)) + \sum_{j(\neq i)=1}^{p} Cov(E(X_i^*|\theta_i), E(X_j^*|\theta_j)) \tag{8}$$

and

$$V_i(R^*) = E(Var(X_i^*|\theta_i^*)) + \sum_{j(\neq i)=1}^{p} E(Cov(X_i^*, X_j^*|\theta_{ij})). \tag{9}$$

When the risk factors $X_1, \ldots, X_p$ are independent, the covariance terms in (6)–(9) vanish. In this case, the total uncertainty/variability in R^* due to X_i partitions into two components:

$$W_i(R^*) = U_i(R^*) + V_i(R^*), \tag{10}$$

the first due to uncertainty in X_i and the second due to variability in X_i.

Risk Distributions

In order to provide the fullest possible characterization of risk, consider the distribution of $R^* = \sum_{i=1}^{p} X_i^*$. Allowing for both uncertainty and variability in risk, the distribution of R^* is given by

$$H^*(R^* \leq r^*) = \int_{x_1^* + \ldots + x_p^* \leq r^*} \int h(X_1, \ldots, X_p|\theta^0) dX_p \ldots dX_1$$
$$= \int_{x_1^* + \ldots + x_p^* \leq r^*} \int f(X_1, \ldots, X_p|\theta) g(\theta|\theta^0) d\theta dX_p \ldots dX_1, \tag{11}$$

where $h(\cdot)$ is the joint density function of all the risk factors with the parameter θ^0. This joint density function $h(\cdot|\theta^0)$ can be partitioned into two parts: $f(\cdot|\theta)$ represents the joint density due to variability in the risk factors and $g(\cdot|\theta)$ represents the joint density function due to uncertainty in the risk factors. The distribution of R^* has mean $E(R^*)$ and variance $W(R^*)$.

If all of the risk factors in (1) are log-normally distributed, the distribution of R^* is normal with mean $E(R^*)$ and variance $W(R^*)$. If all of the risk factors are approximately log-normally distributed, the distribution of R^* can be approximated by a normal distribution. If one or more of the risk factors is not well approximated by a log-normal distribution, the distribution of R^* can be approximated by Monte Carlo simulation. Although straightforward, Monte Carlo simulation can become computationally intensive with a moderate number of risk factors.

To apply the Monte Carlo method, we simply draw a random sample of the values of the risk factors from the distribution $h(\cdot)$ and calculate the value of R^* based on this sample. Repetition of this procedure a sufficiently large number of times yields the Monte Carlo distribution of R^*. Note that when the $\{X_i\}$ are independent, values of the risk factors can be generated from the marginal distributions h_i.

In addition to examining the distribution of R^* taking into account both uncertainty and variability in the $\{X_i\}$, it is of interest to examine the distribution of R^* by considering only uncertainty in the $\{X_i\}$ or only variability in the $\{X_i\}$. By comparing the distributions of R^* allowing both uncertainty and variability, variability alone, and uncertainty alone, it is possible to gauge the relative contribution of uncertainty and variability to the overall uncertainty/variability in risk.

The density of R^* based only on uncertainty in the $\{X_i\}$ is the density of $\sum_{i=1}^{p} E_{f_i}(X_i^*)$, where

$$E_{f_i}(X_i^*) = \int_{-\infty}^{\infty} X_i^* f_i(X_i|\theta_i) dX_i. \quad (12)$$

This density can be approximated by a normal distribution with mean $E(R^*)$ and variance $U(R^*)$.

The density of R^* based on only variability in the $\{X_i\}$ is the density of $\sum_{i=1}^{p} \tilde{X}_i^*$, where $\tilde{X}_i^*$ has distribution f_i with known parameter

$$E_{g_i}(\theta_i) = \int_{-\infty}^{\infty} \theta_i g_i(\theta_i|\theta_i^0) d\theta_i. \quad (13)$$

This density can also be approximated by a normal distribution with mean $E(R^*)$ and variance $V(R^*)$.

CANCER RISK MODELS FOR RESIDENTIAL RADON EXPOSURE

In this section, we apply the methods described in the previous section to evaluate uncertainty and variability in estimates of lung cancer risk due to residential exposure to radon. A number of factors can contribute to uncertainty in radon risk estimates. If the uncertainty and variability in each of the risk factors can be specified, the overall impact of uncertainty and variability in risk can be evaluated. It is also possible to identify which risk factors contribute most to overall uncertainty and variability.

The U.S. National Research Council[7] recently conducted a comprehensive review of the potential health effects of residential exposure to radon. Of primary concern is the excess lung cancer risk demonstrated in 11 cohort studies of underground miners conducted in a number of countries around the world. Since radon appears to exert its carcinogenic effects through DNA damage to lung tissue caused by alpha particles emitted by radon daughters, it is thought that even low levels of exposure to radon confer some increase in risk. After considering different possible approaches to risk estimation, the BEIR VI Committee elected to base its risk models on epidemiological data derived from studies of the mortality experience of miners. The committee conducted a combined analysis of updated data from the 11 miner cohorts, and developed two models for projecting lung cancer risks to the general population. These two models are referred to as the exposure-age-concentration and exposure-age-duration models, based on the major risk factors included in the models.

If e_t denotes the excess relative risk at age t, these two models are expressed by

$$e_t = \beta \times \omega(t) \times \phi(t) \times \gamma_{wl}(\omega) \times K \tag{14}$$

and

$$e_t = \beta \times \omega(t) \times \phi(t) \times \gamma_{dur}(t) \times K . \tag{15}$$

The factor β ($[Bq/m^3]^{-1}$) reflects the carcinogenic potency of radon, as modified by the other risk factors in models (14) and (15). The last term in these models is the dosimetric K-factor (dimensionless), used to extrapolate from occupational to environmental exposure conditions. The factor $\omega(t)$ represents a time-weighted average exposure to radon, expressed in Bq/m^3, within exposure-time windows 5–14, 15–25, and 25+ years prior to disease diagnosis. The factor $\omega(t)$ can be expressed as

$$\begin{aligned}\omega(t) &= \omega \times [\Delta_{[5, 14]}(t) + \vartheta_2 \Delta_{[15, 24]}(t) + \vartheta_3 \Delta_{[25, \infty]}(t)] \\ &= \omega \times \eta_t ,\end{aligned} \tag{16}$$

where

$$\Delta_{[a, b]}(t) = \begin{cases} 10 & \text{for } t > b \\ t - a & \text{for } a \leq t \leq b \\ 0 & \text{otherwise} . \end{cases} \tag{17}$$

The factor $\phi(t)(y^{-1})$ indicates the effects of attained age, categorized into four broad age groups:

$$\phi(t) = \begin{cases} \phi_1 & \text{for } t \leq 54 \\ \phi_2 & \text{for } 55 \leq t \leq 64 \\ \phi_3 & \text{for } 65 \leq t \leq 74 \\ \phi_4 & \text{for } t \geq 75 . \end{cases} \tag{18}$$

The factors $\gamma_{wl}(\omega)$ (WL^{-1}) and $\gamma_{dur}(\omega)$ (y^{-1}) reflect the effects of radon concentration (in working levels) and the duration of exposure to radon (in years), corresponding to the exposure-age-concentration and exposure-age-duration models, respectively. These two factors are categorized as follows:

$$\gamma_{wl}(\omega) = \begin{cases} \gamma_{w1} & \text{for } \omega < 0.5 \\ \gamma_{w2} & \text{for } 0.5 \leq \omega < 1.0 \\ \gamma_{w3} & \text{for } 1.0 \leq \omega < 3.0 \\ \gamma_{w4} & \text{for } 3.0 \leq \omega < 5.0 \\ \gamma_{w5} & \text{for } 5.0 \leq \omega < 15.0 \\ \gamma_{w6} & \text{for } \omega \geq 15.0 \end{cases} \quad (19)$$

and

$$\gamma_{dur}(\omega) = \begin{cases} \gamma_{d1} & \text{for } t < 10 \\ \gamma_{d2} & \text{for } 10 \leq t < 20 \\ \gamma_{d3} & \text{for } 20 \leq t < 30 \\ \gamma_{d4} & \text{for } 30 \leq t < 40 \\ \gamma_{d5} & \text{for } t \geq 40 \, . \end{cases} \quad (20)$$

Our interest is in risks associated with low (residential) radon exposures. We demonstrate our methods for uncertainty analysis only for the exposure-age-concentration model at exposures less than 0.5 WL and the exposure-age-duration model for individuals that are at least 40 years old, for which $\gamma_{wl} = 1$ and $\gamma_{d5} = 10.18$, respectively.

In this analysis, the risk function (1) represents the age specific excess relative risk (ERR) as a product of four factors: the carcinogenic potency of radon $\beta = X_1$, the exposure to radon $\omega\eta_t = X_2$, the effect of age $\phi = X_3$, and $K = X_4$. Thus,

$$ERR = X_1 \times X_2 \times X_3 \times X_4 \times \gamma, \quad (21)$$

where $\gamma = 1$ or 10.18 for the exposure-age-concentration model or the exposure-age-duration model, respectively. For simplicity, we assume that γ is a constant, exhibiting neither uncertainty nor variability. In this application, X_1 and X_3 are assumed to be subject only to uncertainty, and X_2 and X_4, are assumed to be subject to both variability and uncertainty.

TABLES 1a and 1b summarize the basic distributional assumptions about uncertainty and variability in the risk factors $X_1, \ldots, X_4$ in equation (21). The carcinogenic potency of radon X_1 is assumed not to vary among individuals, reflecting constant susceptibility within the general population. Uncertainty in X_1 is characterized by a log-normal distribution, with known geometric mean and geometric standard deviation, The level of radon $\omega = X_2/\eta_t$ is assumed to vary among homes in accordance with a log-normal distribution. Uncertainty in radon levels is described by means of log-normal distributions for both the geometric mean and geometric standard deviation of the distribution of radon levels. Although the modifying effect of age (X_3) is assumed not to vary among individuals within a given age group, uncertainty is de-

TABLE 1a. Uncertainty and variability distributions for the risk factors in the exposure-age-concentration model[a]

Risk factor	Variability	Uncertainty
Potency ($\beta = X_1$)	constant	$\beta \sim LN\ (gm = 0.08,\ gsd = 1.36)$
Exposure ($\omega_{\eta_t} = X_2$)	$LN\ (gm,\ gsd)$	$gm \sim LN\ (0.1,\ 1.12);\ gsd \sim LN\ (3.1,\ 1.12)$
Age ($\phi = X_3$)	constant	
$X_3 \leq 54$ years		$\phi_1 \sim LN\ (1.00,\ 1.10)$
$55 \leq X_3 \leq 64$ years		$\phi_2 \sim LN\ (0.57,\ 1.27)$
$65 \leq X_3 \leq 74$ years		$\phi_3 \sim LN\ (0.29,\ 1.39)$
$X_3 \geq 75$ years		$\phi_4 \sim LN\ (0.09,\ 2.55)$
K-factor ($K = X_4$)	$LN\ (gm,\ gsd)$	$gm = 1.00;\ gsd \sim LU\ (1.2,\ 2.2)$

[a]LN, log-normal; gm, geometric mean; gsd, geometric standard deviation; LU, log-uniform.

scribed by means of a log-normal distribution. Variability in the K-factor (X_4) is characterized by a log-normal distribution; uncertainty is described by a log-uniform distribution for the geometric standard deviation. This description of uncertainty and variability was guided by both empirical data and expert judgement on the part of the BEIR VI committee.

Our analysis allows for correlation among the risk factors in the multiplicative model (21). (Note that the risk factors X_1, X_2, and X_3 are correlated). The covariance structure used to define the correlation matrix is given in TABLE 2a for the exposure-age-concentration model and in TABLE 2b for the exposure-age-duration model. This correlation structure is based on the covariance matrix obtained when estimating the model parameters. Other than statistical correlation between X_1 and X_3 induced due to the estimation procedure, the risk factors are assumed to be independent.

TABLE 1b. Uncertainty and variability distributions for the risk factors in the exposure-age-duration model[a]

Risk factor	Variability	Uncertainty
Potency ($\beta = X_1$)	constant	$\beta \sim LN\ (gm = 0.0055,\ gsd = 1.326)$
Exposure ($\omega_{\eta_t} = X_2$)	$LN\ (gm,\ gsd)$	$gm \sim LN\ (0.1,\ 1.12);\ gsd \sim LN\ (3.1,\ 1.12)$
Age ($\phi = X_3$)	constant	
$X_3 \leq 54$ years		$\phi_1 \sim LN\ (1.00,\ 1.10)$
$55 \leq X_3 \leq 64$ years		$\phi_2 \sim LN\ (0.52,\ 1.23)$
$65 \leq X_3 \leq 74$ years		$\phi_3 \sim LN\ (0.28,\ 1.36)$
$X_3 \geq 75$ years		$\phi_4 \sim LN\ (0.13,\ 2.66)$
K-factor ($K = X_4$)	$LN\ (gm,\ gsd)$	$gm = 1.00;\ gsd \sim LU\ (1.2,\ 2.2)$

[a]LN, log-normal; gm, geometric mean; gsd, geometric standard deviation; LU, log-uniform.

TABLE 2a. Parameter estimates for the exposure-age-concentration model

	I. Estimated Values of Parameters[a]									
	β	ϑ_2	ϑ_3	ϕ_2	ϕ_3	ϕ_4	$\gamma_{\omega 2}$	$\gamma_{\omega 3}$	$\gamma_{\omega 4}$	$\gamma_{\omega 5}$	$\gamma_{\omega 6}$
	−2.57	0.77	0.51	−0.56	−1.23	−2.38	−0.72	−0.98	−1.13	−1.80	−2.21

	II. Covariance Matrix[b]										
β	9.47										
ϑ_2	−0.36	0.77									
ϑ_3	−0.04	0.24	0.42								
ϕ_2	−2.87	−0.10	−0.15	5.71							
ϕ_3	−3.18	−0.17	−0.33	2.85	10.87						
ϕ_4	−3.44	−0.19	−0.54	2.90	3.20	87.65					
$\gamma_{\omega 2}$	−5.57	−0.10	−0.02	0.14	0.42	0.83	8.24				
$\gamma_{\omega 3}$	−6.36	−0.12	−0.11	0.15	0.53	0.97	5.88	6.93			
$\gamma_{\omega 4}$	−6.58	−0.16	−0.10	0.18	0.59	1.08	5.83	6.69	7.30		
$\gamma_{\omega 5}$	−6.90	−0.05	−0.09	0.26	0.61	0.81	5.69	6.51	6.67	7.84	
$\gamma_{\omega 6}$	−7.04	−0.02	−0.08	0.27	0.54	0.50	5.63	6.44	6.64	7.33	8.59

[a]Except for ϑ_2 and ϑ_3 values are $\log_e$ scale.
[b]Except for ϑ_2 and ϑ_3 values are $\log_e$ scale; all values multiplied by 100.

TABLE 2b. Parameter estimates for the exposure-age-duration model

	I. Estimated Values of Parameters[a]								
	β	ϑ_2	ϑ_3	ϕ_2	ϕ_3	ϕ_4	γ_{d2}	γ_{d3}	γ_{d4}	γ_{d5}
	−5.20	0.72	0.44	−0.65	−1.29	−2.07	1.02	1.49	1.89	2.32

	II. Covariance Matrix[b]									
β	7.98									
ϑ_2	−0.30	0.98								
ϑ_3	−0.01	0.25	0.44							
ϕ_2	−2.07	−0.11	−0.21	4.32						
ϕ_3	−2.16	−0.20	−0.39	2.10	9.60					
ϕ_4	−2.43	−0.24	−0.59	2.15	2.43	95.37				
γ_{d2}	−5.06	−0.21	−0.14	0.31	0.37	0.54	4.60			
γ_{d3}	−5.66	−0.39	−0.23	0.31	0.54	0.93	4.67	5.94		
γ_{d4}	−6.58	−0.40	−0.15	0.20	0.45	0.83	4.73	5.60	6.75	
γ_{d5}	−5.65	−0.37	−0.12	−0.15	0.18	0.65	4.76	5.61	603	7.26

[a]Except for ϑ_2 and ϑ_3 values are $\log_e$ scale.
[b]Except for ϑ_2 and ϑ_3 values are $\log_e$ scale; all values multiplied by 100.

We note that the covariance matrices given in TABLES 2a and 2b are derived from an overall model fit to the data from 11 miner cohorts considered by the BEIR VI committee, using two-stage regression methods.[21] In this analysis, the effects of time since exposure, attained age, and either exposure-duration or exposure-concentration were considered to be the same in all cohorts. This assumption is generally consistent with the available data. The key parameter β was, however, considered to vary across cohorts.

UNCERTAINTY AND VARIABILITY IN EXCESS RELATIVE RISK

Measures of uncertainty and variability in the *ERR* are given in TABLES 3a and 3b. The first entry in columns 2 and 5 represent the percentage of the total uncertainty/variability in the *ERR* due to uncertainty and to variability, respectively, in X_1. The entries in column 3 represent the percentage of the total uncertainty in the *ERR* due to uncertainty only in specific risk factors. Similarly, the entries in column 6 represent the percentage of the total variability in the *ERR* due to variability in specific risk factors. Columns 4 and 7 of TABLES 3a and 3b reflect the relative contribution of uncertainty and variability to the total uncertainty/variability associated with a particular variable. (Note that these two columns sum to 100% for each risk factor.) The entries in columns 3 and 5 of the last row represent the percentage total uncertainty and total variability in the *ERR* relative to the total uncertainty/variability in the *ERR*, respectively. The entries in the last columns represent the percentage contribution to total uncertainty/variability in the *ERR* due to specific risk factors.

Several conclusions can be drawn from TABLES 3a and 3b. First, a comparison of these two tables indicates that the results for the exposure-age-concentration model (TABLE 3a) and the exposure-age-duration model (TABLE 3b) are quite similar. A comparison of columns 3 and 6 in the case of all risk factors $(X_1,...,X_4)$ indicates that variability tends to account for the majority of the total uncertainty/variability in the *ERR*. Whereas potency and age tend to be more uncertain than variable, exposure to radon and the *K*-factor are more variable than uncertain. The last column in these tables indicates that exposure is the most influential variable overall (contributing most to uncertainty and variability), followed by the *K*-factor, potency, and then age in all but the last age group, where age is the most influential factor.

The distributions of the ERR based on the log-normal and Monte Carlo approximations described above are presented in FIGURES 1 and 2 for an individual 50 years of age. These two approximations are in close agreement regardless of whether both uncertainty and variability, only uncertainty, or only variability in the *ERR* is considered. These results confirm the previous observation that inter-individual variability in the factors determining the *ERR* accounts for most of the uncertainty/variability in the *ERR*. Qualitatively similar results are found for individuals aged 40, 60, 70, or 80 (see FIGURES 3 and 4). These results indicate that, whereas uncertainty in the *ERR* for an individual of a given age precludes being able to determine the *ERR* to less than a 10-fold range, variability in the *ERR* exceeds 100-fold.

TABLE 3a. Components of uncertainty and variability in *ERR* based on the exposure-age-concentration model (×100%)

Risk factor	Uncertainty			Variability			Both
	U_i/W	U_i/U	U_i/W_i	V_i/W	U_i/V	V_i/W_i	W_i/W
I. age ≤ 54 years							
Potency (X_1)	4.8	60.2	100	0	0	0	4.8
Exposure (X_2)	0.8	9.7	1.0	77.9	84.6	99.0	78.6
Age (X_3)	0.5	6.9	100	0	0	0	0.5
K-factor (X_4)	1.8	23.2	11.5	14.2	15.4	88.5	16.0
All ($X_1,...,X_4$)	8.0	100	na	92.0	100	na	100
II. 55 ≤ age ≤ 64 years							
Potency (X_1)	3.6	47.3	100	0	0	0	3.6
Exposure (X_2)	0.8	10.3	1.0	78.2	84.6	99.0	79.0
Age (X_3)	1.3	17.8	100	0	0	0	1.3
K-factor (X_4)	1.9	24.6	11.5	14.3	15.4	88.5	16.1
All ($X_1,...,X_4$)	7.5	100	na	92.5	100	na	100
III. 65 ≤ age ≤ 74 years							
Potency (X_1)	3.4	33.3	100	0	0	0	3.4
Exposure (X_2)	0.8	7.4	1.0	75.9	84.6	99.0	76.7
Age (X_3)	4.3	41.8	100	0	0	0	4.3
K-factor (X_4)	1.8	17.5	11.5	13.8	15.4	88.5	15.6
All ($X_1,...,X_4$)	10.2	100	na	89.8	100	na	100
IV. age ≥ 75 years							
Potency (X_1)	2.2	5.4	100	0	0	0	2.2
Exposure (X_2)	0.5	1.2	1.0	50.5	84.6	99.0	51.0
Age (X_3)	36.4	90.4	100	0	0	0	36.4
K-factor (X_4)	1.2	3.0	11.5	9.2	15.4	88.5	10.4
All ($X_1,...,X_4$)	40.3	100	na	59.7	100	na	100

NOTE: na, not applicable.

TABLE 3b. Components of uncertainty and variability in *ERR* based on the exposure-age-duration model (×100%)

Risk factor	Uncertainty			Variability			Both
	U_i/W	U_i/U	U_i/W_i	V_i/W	U_i/V	V_i/W_i	W_i/W
			I. age $\leq$ 54 years				
Potency (X_1)	5.6	64.3	100	0	0	0	5.6
Exposure (X_2)	0.8	8.7	1.0	77.2	84.6	99.0	77.9
Age (X_3)	0.5	6.2	100	0	0	0	0.5
K-factor (X_4)	1.8	20.8	11.5	14.1	15.4	88.5	15.9
All ($X_1,...,X_4$)	8.8	100	na	91.2	100	na	100
			II. 55 $\leq$ age $\leq$ 64 years				
Potency (X_1)	3.9	39.6	100	0	0	0	3.9
Exposure (X_2)	0.8	10.3	1.0	78.2	84.6	99.0	79.0
Age (X_3)	3.4	34.3	100	0	0	0	3.4
K-factor (X_4)	1.8	18.4	11.5	13.9	15.4	88.5	15.7
All ($X_1,...,X_4$)	9.8	100	na	90.2	100	na	100
			III. 65 $\leq$ age $\leq$ 74 years				
Potency (X_1)	3.6	29.2	100	0	0	0	3.6
Exposure (X_2)	0.7	6.0	1.0	74.2	84.6	99.0	74.9
Age (X_3)	6.2	50.5	100	0	0	0	6.2
K-factor (X_4)	1.8	14.3	11.5	13.5	15.4	88.5	15.3
All ($X_1,...,X_4$)	12.3	100	na	87.7	100	na	100
			IV. age $\geq$ 75 years				
Potency (X_1)	2.4	6.1	100	0	0	0	2.4
Exposure (X_2)	0.5	1.3	1.0	51.5	84.6	99.0	52.1
Age (X_3)	34.9	89.4	100	0	0	0	34.9
K-factor (X_4)	1.2	3.1	11.5	9.4	15.4	88.5	10.6
All ($X_1,...,X_4$)	39.1	100	na	60.9	100	na	100

NOTE: na, not applicable.

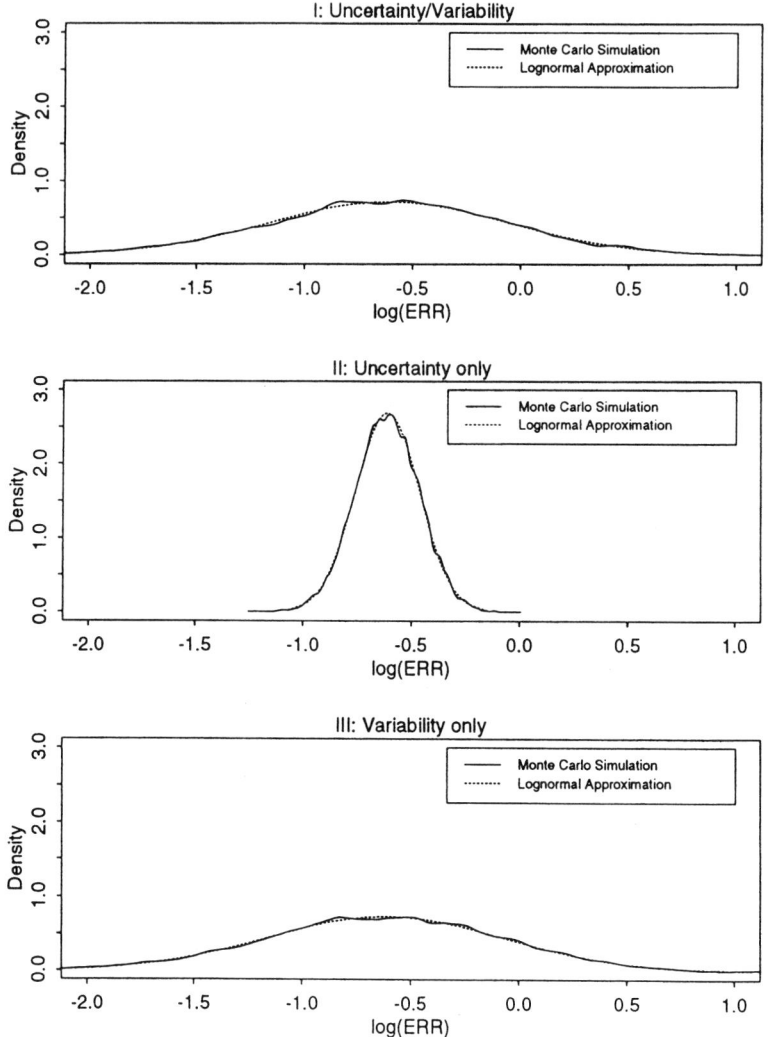

FIGURE 1. Distributions of *ERR* for the exposure-age-concentration model obtained by using Monte Carlo simulation and log-normal approximation for a representative person 50 years of age.

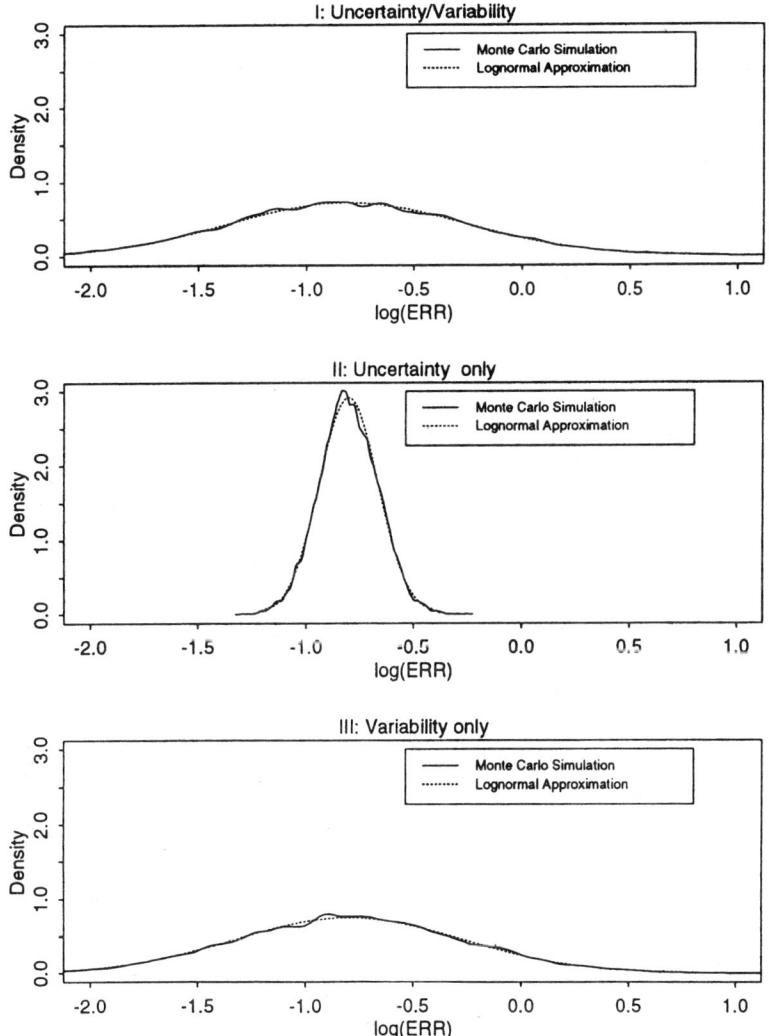

FIGURE 2. Distributions of *ERR* for the exposure-age-duration model obtained by using Monte Carlo simulation and log-normal approximation for a representative person 50 years of age.

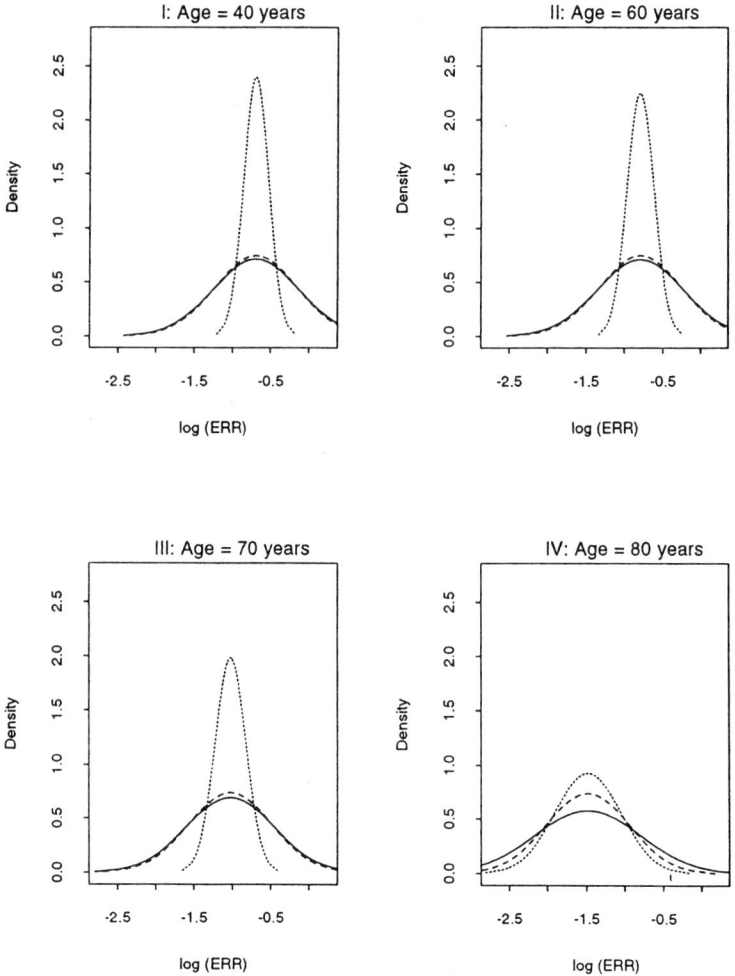

FIGURE 3. Distributions of *ERR* for the exposure-age-concentration model obtained by using a log-normal approximation: ····, uncertainty/variability; ——, uncertainty only; – –, variability only.

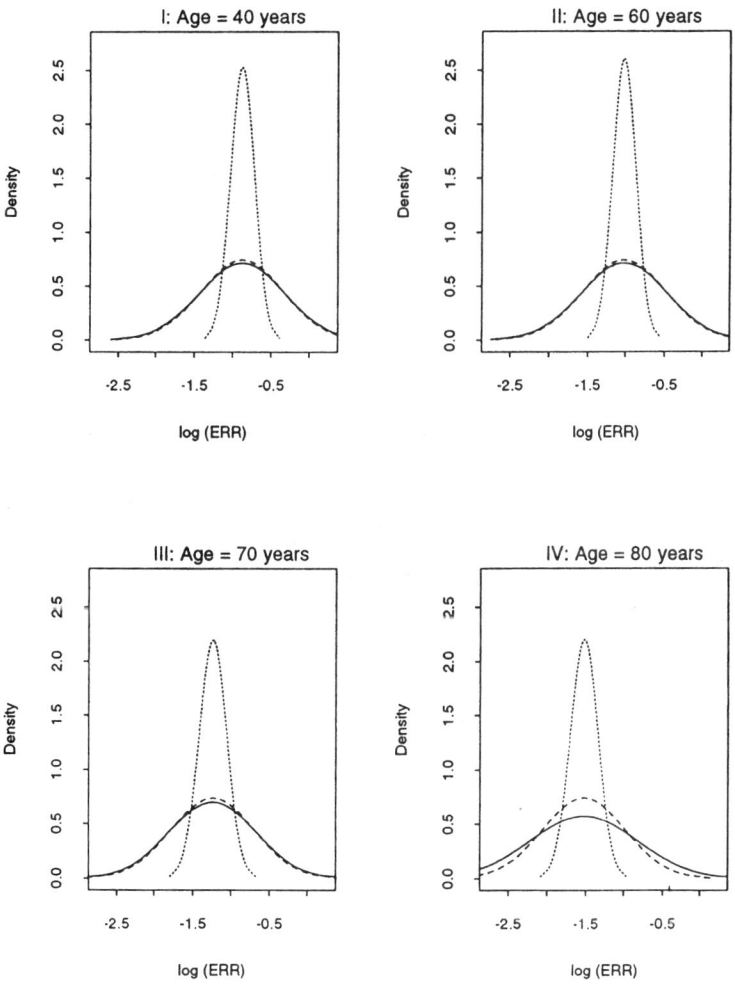

FIGURE 4. Distributions of *ERR* for the exposure-age-duration model obtained by using a log-normal approximation: ····, uncertainty/variability; ——, uncertainty only; – –, variability only.

UNCERTAINTY AND VARIABILITY IN LIFETIME RELATIVE RISK

To determine the lifetime relative risk of radon-induced lung cancer, we require the hazard function for the death rate in the general population. Deaths can be classified into two categories; those due to lung cancer and those due to other competing causes. Assume that the age at death T is a continuous random variable. Let $h(t)$ and $h^*(t)$ be the lung cancer and overall death rates at age $T = t$ in an unexposed population, respectively. Furthermore, let $e(t)$ be the excess relative risk in an exposed population. The lung cancer death rate in the exposed population at age t is $h(t) + h(t)e(t)$ and the overall death rate is $h^*(t) + h(t)e(t)$.

Let $R(t)$ be the probability of death due to lung cancer for a person of age t, and let $S(t)$ be the survival probability up to age t in the exposed population. Following Kalbfleisch and Prentice,[22] the survival function can be expressed as

$$S(t) = \Pr\{T \geq t\} = \exp\left\{-\int_0^t [h^*(u) + h(u)e(u)]du\right\}, \qquad (22)$$

and the probability of death due to lung cancer, $R(t)$, can be written as

$$R(t) = [h(t) + h(t)e(t)]\exp\left\{-\int_0^t [h^*(u) + h(u)e(u)]du\right\}. \qquad (23)$$

For simplicity, we assume that the death times are recorded in years and identify the range of T as $\{1, 2, \ldots, 110, \ldots\}$. Let h_t and h_t^* be the respective lung cancer and overall mortality rates for age group t in an unexposed population; and e_t be the excess relative risk for lung cancer mortality in an exposed population for age group t. Then, the death rates in the exposed population are given by $h_t + h_t e_t$ for lung cancer and $h_t^* + h_t e_t$, for all causes including lung cancer. The discrete-time versions of (22) and (23) are:

$$\begin{aligned} S_t = \Pr\{T \geq t\} &= \prod_{l=1}^{t-1} \{1 - (h_l^* + h_l e_l)\} \\ &\approx \exp\left\{-\sum_{l=1}^{t-1} (h_l^* + h_l e_l)\right\} \end{aligned} \qquad (24)$$

and

$$R_t = \Pr\{T = t\} = (h_t + h_t e_t)S_t. \qquad (25)$$

The approximation in (24) is highly accurate and will be treated as exact in what follows. Substituting (24) into (25), the age specific death rate due to lung cancer in the exposed population is given by

$$R_t = (h_t + h_t e_t)\exp\left\{-\sum_{l=1}^{t-1} (h_l^* + h_l e_l)\right\}. \qquad (26)$$

This differs slightly from the expression for R_t used by the BEIR IV committee.[7] In that report, R_t is multiplied by

$$\frac{1 - \exp\{-(h_t^* + h_t e_t)\}}{h_t^* + h_t e_t} \approx 1, \tag{27}$$

which is not required. Our expression for R_t is not only more accurate, but considerably simplifies the calculation of the lifetime relative risk and the population attributable risk.

Assuming a maximum life span 110 years, the lifetime lung-cancer risk is given by the sum of the annual risks:

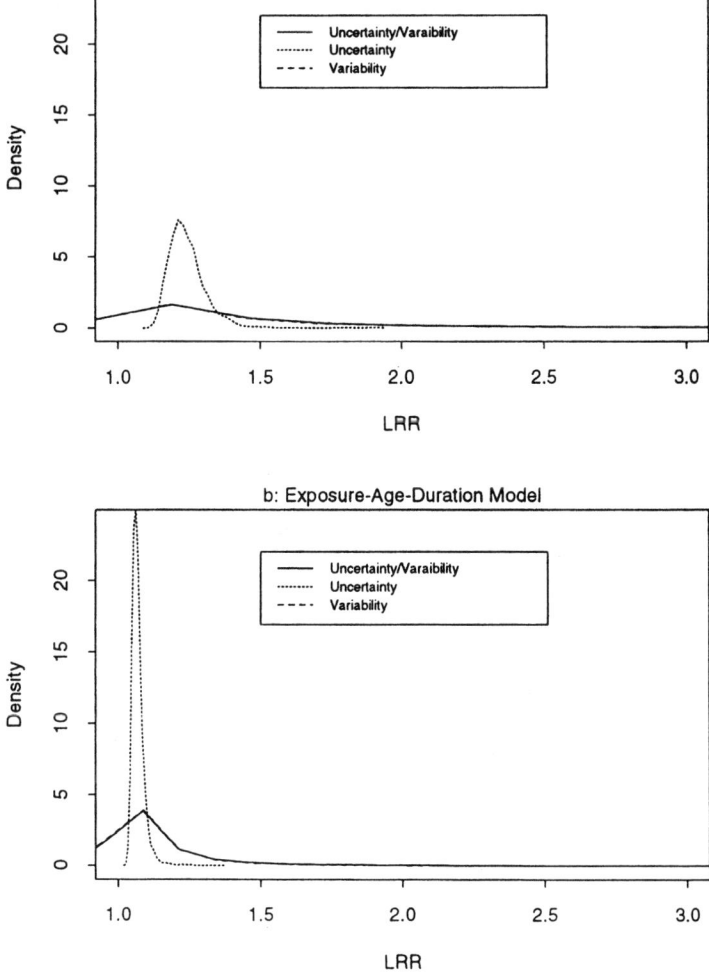

FIGURE 5. Distributions of *LRR* obtained by using Monte Carlo simulations.

TABLE 4a. Quantiles of the distribution of *LRR* based on the exposure-age-concentration model

Distribution	Min	Quantiles									Max	Mean
		2.5^a	5	10	25	50	75	90	95	97.5^b		
Uncertainty	1.113	1.151	1.160	1.172	1.198	1.231	1.273	1.323	1.363	1.397	1.914	1.243
Variability	1.002	1.018	1.027	1.043	1.097	1.220	1.508	2.067	2.684	3.372	13.278	1.461
Both	1.002	1.020	1.030	1.047	1.098	1.222	1.502	1.954	2.372	2.842	13.674	1.409

[a]Lower 95% limit.
[b]Upper 95% limit.

TABLE 4b. Quantiles of the distribution of *LRR* based on the exposure-age-duration model

Distribution	Min	Quantiles									Max	Mean
		2.5^a	5	10	25	50	75	90	95	97.5^b		
Uncertainty	1.029	1.014	1.045	1.048	1.055	1.065	1.078	1.094	1.107	1.123	1.365	1.069
Variability	1.001	1.006	1.008	1.013	1.028	1.062	1.144	1.296	1.470	1.673	6.895	1.133
Both	1.001	1.005	1.008	1.013	1.027	1.067	1.161	1.353	1.578	1.829	6.679	1.152

[a]Lower 95% limit.
[b]Upper 95% limit.

$$R = \sum_{i=1}^{110} R_i = \sum_{t=1}^{110} (h_t + h_t e_t) \exp\left\{ -\sum_{l=1}^{t-1} (h_l^* + h_l e_l) \right\}. \quad (28)$$

In the unexposed population, the $\{e_i\}$ are assumed to be zero, so that

$$R_0 = \sum_{t=1}^{110} h_t \exp\left\{ -\sum_{l=1}^{t-1} h_l^* \right\}. \quad (29)$$

Note that the evaluation the lifetime risk R in (28) depends on the excess relative lung cancer risks $\{e_i\}$ within each of the age groups.

The lifetime relative risk (LRR) is the ratio of the lifetime risk in the exposed population relation to that in the unexposed population:

$$LRR = R/R_0. \quad (30)$$

Like the ERR, the LRR is subject to both uncertainty and variability. Although the LRR is summed over all age groups, the uncertainty in the modifying effects of each age group in the sum is taken into account in our analysis.

Since the LRR is not in multiplicative form, however, the risk distributions for uncertainty/variability, uncertainty only, and variability only are obtained by Monte Carlo methods (see FIGURE 5 and TABLES 4a and 4b). These results indicate that the variability in the LRR (due to interindividual variation in the level of radon exposure and the dosimetric K-factor) is much greater than uncertainty in the LRR (due to the uncertainty in the model parameters, the level of radon exposure and the K-factor).

UNCERTAINTY IN POPULATION-ATTRIBUTABLE RISK

Following Lubin and Boice,[23] the attributable risk of lung cancer mortality due to exposure to radon is defined as the excess lung cancer risk in a population due to exposure as a fraction of total lung cancer risk. Thus, the population-attributable risk (PAR) is given by

$$PAR = \frac{E(R) - R_0}{E(R)} = \frac{\sum_{t=1}^{110} E(R_t) - R_0}{\sum_{t=1}^{110} E(R_t)}. \quad (31)$$

Here, $E(R)$ is the average value of R, the lifetime risk of death due to lung cancer across individuals in the exposed population. The quantity R_0 is the lifetime risk in an unexposed population.

As noted previously, the interindividual variability in LRR is due to variability in radon exposure and the dosimetric K-factor. In order to evaluate $E(R_t)$, we need to know the distribution of $b = K\omega$ for the exposure-age-duration model and $b = K\omega\gamma(\omega)$ for the exposure-age-concentration model. These distributions are derived in the Appendix.

Five different scenarios for the analysis of uncertainty in the PAR were considered, depending on whether variability (v) or uncertainty (u) (or both) in the K-factor and radon level ω was taken into account. In the first scenario, denoted by

$PAR(K=1,\omega^v)$, the K-factor was held fixed at unity, with variability, but not uncertainty, in residential radon levels considered. In the second scenario, $PAR(K^v, \omega^v)$, both K and ω are subject to variability, but not uncertainty. In scenario three, $PAR(K^{v,u}, \omega^v)$, uncertainty in the K-factor is introduced; uncertainty in ω is introduced in scenario four, $PAR(K^v, \omega^{v,u})$. Finally, the K-factor and radon level ω^v are subject to both variability and uncertainty in scenario five, $PAR(K^{v,u}, \omega^{v,u})$.

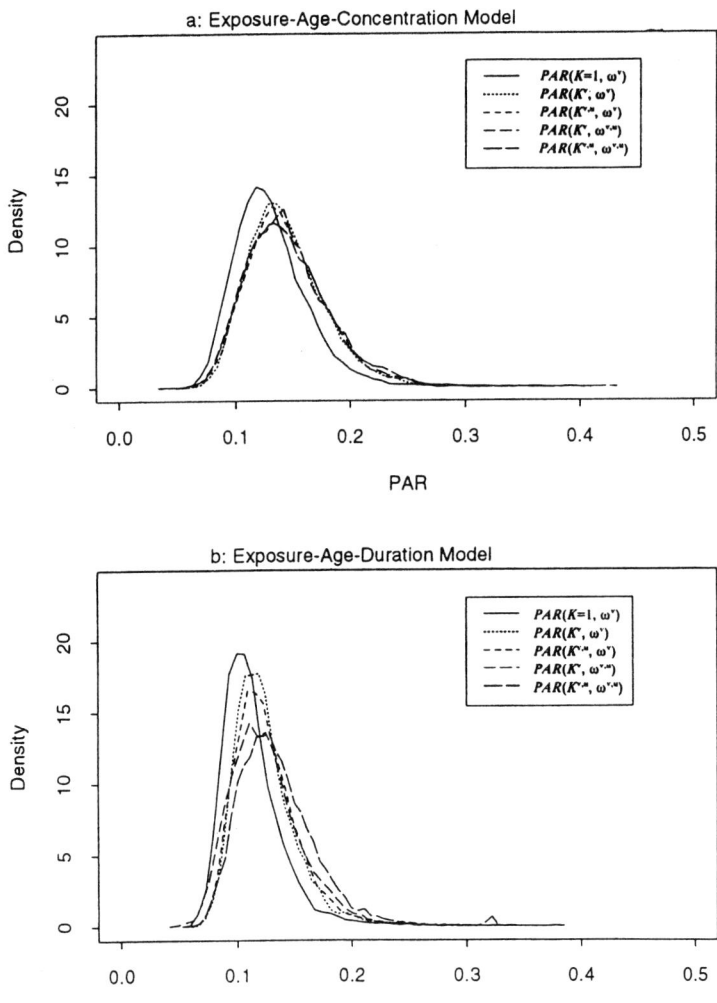

FIGURE 6. *PAR* distributions obtained by using Monte Carlo simulations.

TABLE 5a. Quantiles of the distribution of *PAR* based on the exposure-age-concentration model

Distribution	Quantiles											
	1	2.5[a]	5	10	25	50	75	90	95	97.5[b]	99	Mean
$PAR(K=1, \omega^v)$	0.075	0.082	0.087	0.094	0.109	0.126	0.148	0.172	0.189	0.205	0.226	0.131
$PAR(K^v, \omega^v)$	0.084	0.091	0.097	0.105	0.120	0.140	0.163	0.189	0.206	0.223	0.246	0.144
$PAR(K^{v,u}, \omega^v)$	0.082	0.089	0.096	0.105	0.121	0.141	0.166	0.192	0.211	0.228	0.254	0.146
$PAR(K^v, \omega^{v,u})$	0.080	0.087	0.094	0.102	0.118	0.140	0.164	0.191	0.210	0.230	0.250	0.145
$PAR(K^{v,u}, \omega^{v,u})$	0.080	0.087	0.094	0.103	0.120	0.141	0.168	0.196	0.217	0.235	0.255	0.147

[a]Lower 95% limit.
[b]Upper 95% limit.

TABLE 5a. Quantiles of the distribution of *PAR* based on the exposure-age-duration model

Distribution	Quantiles											
	1	2.5[a]	5	10	25	50	75	90	95	97.5[b]	99	Mean
$PAR(K=1, \omega^v)$	0.071	0.076	0.081	0.086	0.095	0.108	0.124	0.145	0.160	0.180	0.210	0.113
$PAR(K^v, \omega^v)$	0.079	0.085	0.089	0.095	0.106	0.120	0.137	0.159	0.175	0.196	0.227	0.125
$PAR(K^{v,u}, \omega^v)$	0.078	0.084	0.089	0.095	0.106	0.121	0.141	0.163	0.179	0.200	0.226	0.127
$PAR(K^v, \omega^{v,u})$	0.068	0.074	0.081	0.089	0.102	0.121	0.143	0.167	0.184	0.201	0.225	0.125
$PAR(K^{v,u}, \omega^{v,u})$	0.068	0.075	0.081	0.089	0.102	0.121	0.145	0.169	0.185	0.204	0.226	0.126

[a]Lower 95% limit.
[b]Upper 95% limit.

The resulting uncertainty distributions for the population attributable risk are shown in FIGURE 6a (exposure-age-concentration model) and FIGURE 6b (exposure-age-duration model). The uncertainty distributions are approximately centered on the best estimates of the *PAR* based on the fitted models: about 14% for the exposure-age-concentration model and 10% for the exposure-age-duration model. The uncertainty distribution for the *PAR* based on the exposure-age-concentration model is shifted to the right of the uncertainty distribution for the exposure-age-duration model, and demonstrates a heavier right tail.

The uncertainty distributions for the five scenarios considered here do not differ greatly. Allowing for variability in the K-factor does not appreciably increase the dispersion of the uncertainty distribution beyond that observed with $K = 1$. Furthermore, allowing for uncertainty in either the K-factor or radon level ω (or both) also does not appear to greatly increase the dispersion of the uncertainty distribution for the *PAR*.

The distributions in FIGURE 6 can be used to obtain uncertainty intervals for the *PAR* based on the selected quantiles of the uncertainty distributions given in TABLES 5a and 5b. For example, a 95% uncertainty interval may be constructed based on the central 95% of the mass of the uncertainty distribution. In the first scenario, in which $K = 1$ and ω is variable but not uncertain, the 95% limits for the *PAR* are 0.07–0.21 for the exposure-age-concentration model and 0.06–0.16 for the exposure-age-duration model. As additional variability and uncertainty are introduced, the 95% limits tend to shift slightly to the right and to expand slightly in length.

DISCUSSION

In this article, we have applied new methods for the analysis of uncertainty and variability to evaluate the lung cancer risks due the presence of radon gas in homes. This important population health issue was recently examined by the U.S. National Research Council.[7] The NRC evaluation included not only an assessment of the most likely risk estimates, but also an analysis of the uncertainties in such estimates. Such stochastic analyses take into account both uncertainty and variability in the risk factors affecting risk. In our analyses, each risk factor is assumed to follow a distribution with one or more parameters reflecting variability within the population of interest; uncertainty in the value of each risk factor is characterized by an appropriate distribution for the parameter values. Within this framework, overall measures of uncertainty and variability and relative contributions of individual risk factors to overall uncertainty and variability in lung cancer risk due to radon are computed. Influential factors that contribute most to uncertainty and variability may then be targeted for further study.

As noted by Rai and Krewski,[18] the analysis of uncertainty and variability is greatly simplified when risk can be expressed as multiplicative factors of the several risk factors. The age-specific *ERR* based on BEIR VI risk models is of this multiplicative form. However, the *LRR* cannot be expressed as a multiplicative risk model. In this case, Monte Carlo methods are needed to evaluate uncertainty and variability in risk.

The results of this analysis of uncertainty and variability are informative in several ways. Estimates of the age-specific excess relative risk of lung cancer are highly variable among individuals, largely due to the substantial variability in radon levels in U.S. homes. Indeed, radon exposure appears to be the most influential factor affecting individual risk among the four factors included in the BEIR VI risk models. Although uncertainty in these factors leads to about a 10-fold range in risk, variability in the *ERR* exceeds 100-fold. Our analysis indicates that like the *ERR*, the *LRR* is more variable than uncertain.

In contrast to such individual measures of risk, population-based measures of risk such as the population-attributable risk are subject to uncertainty but not variability. This is because variation in individual risk levels is effectively averaged out when calculating the *PAR*. The uncertainty analysis presented here extends the analysis conducted by the BEIR VI committee by allowing for uncertainty in residential radon levels, in addition to uncertainty in the *K*-factor. Allowing for uncertainty in both the *K*-factor and level of radon exposure did not dramatically increase uncertainty in the *PAR* beyond that due to statistical uncertainty in the model parameters. This observation suggests that uncertainty in the *PAR* can be achieved only if more reliable risk models can be developed.

The analysis of variability in radon lung cancer risks presented in this article assumes that individuals are exposed to the constant amount of radon throughout their lives. Warner *et al.*[24] note that ignoring normal patterns of residential mobility leads to considerable overestimation of the lung cancer risk associated with radon for the vast majority of people living in high-radon homes. Population mobility was not considered in the present analysis, in part because of the difficulty in identifying realistic mobility scenarios. In the limiting case of infinite mobility (in which each person would move at random to a new home at a short interval of time), all individuals in the population would be exposed to the average amount of radon in U.S. homes. Although this limiting case eliminates variability in the *ERR* and *LRR* due to variability in radon exposure, the assumption (calculation not shown) has relatively little impact on the distributions of uncertainty in the *PAR* shown in FIGURE 6.

A complete quantitative analysis of all sources of uncertainty and variability in factors affecting radon lung cancer is not feasible for two principle reasons. First, it is difficult to enumerate all of the factors that may influence, to some extent, the lung cancer risk associated with environmental exposures to radon. Second, characterization of the extent of both interindividual variability and uncertainty in some of these factors may not be possible based on existing information. In addition to the factors considered in the present quantitative analysis of uncertainty and variability, the BEIR VI committee discussed a number of other sources of uncertainty for which insufficient information was available to conduct a quantitative uncertainty analysis. One factor that may be amenable to quantitative analysis with additional effort is uncertainty about the degree of synergism between radon and tobacco smoking.

Methods for incorporating model uncertainty in future analyses also warrant attention. This has been addressed in part here by considering two plausible models, both of which are guided to a certain extent by radiobiological considerations relating to the shape of the exposure-response curve at low levels of exposure.[7] Nonetheless, a more structured approach to characterizing model uncertainty may be helpful.

Despite their limitations, these initial attempts at applying general methods for the analysis of uncertainty and variability in individual and population based measures of risk have proven useful in evaluating the reliability of radon risk estimates. These results may be refined as more information about uncertainty and variability the factors affecting radon related lung cancer risk becomes available.

APPENDIX: CALCULATION OF $E(R)$

Suppose b has a distribution $f_b(b)$. After some algebraic manipulation, it can be shown that

$$E(R_t) = h_t e^{-\sum_{i=1}^{t-1} h_i^*} \left\{ E(e^{-bn_t}) + \frac{m_t}{h_t} E(be^{-bn_t}) \right\}, \quad (A.1)$$

where $m_t = h_t \phi_t \eta_t \beta$ for the exposure-age-concentration model and $m_t = h_t \phi_t \eta_t \gamma_t \beta$ for the exposure-age-duration model, with $n_t = \sum_{i=1}^{t-1} m_i$. The expectation in (A.1) is taken with respect to the distribution $f_b(b)$.

Further simplification of (A.1) depends on the distributions of ω and K. Consider first the most general case, in which the distributions for these two risk factors are arbitrary. If these two risk factors are statistically independent, then it is straightforward to find $E(e^{-bn_t})$ and $E(be^{-bn_t})$, the former being the moment generating function at all values of $(-b)$ for which the expected value exists. Note that $E(be^{-bn_t}) = dE(e^{-bn_t})/db$ for the exponential family of distributions of b. Second, if these two factors are independent and log-normally distributed, computation of the moments is simplified since the product of two log-normally distributed variables has a log-normal distribution.

If there is no closed form expression for $E(e^{-bn_t})$, it can be approximated by

$$E(be^{-bn_t}) = \sum_{l=0}^{p} \frac{(-n_t)^l}{l!} E(b^l) + 10^{-\delta p}. \quad (A.2)$$

Note that the remainder term in the above expansion depends on the value of p. Substituting the values of $E(R_t)$ from (A.2) into (A.1) provides an estimate of the *PAR*.

To evaluate $E(b^l)$ in (A.2), we made use of the fact that $\log(b)$ has a normal distribution with mean μ and standard deviation σ. After some algebraic manipulation, it can be shown that

$$E(b^l) = \exp(l\mu + \tfrac{1}{2}l^2\sigma^2) \quad (A.3)$$

for the exposure-age-duration model and that

$$E(b^l) = \exp(l\mu + \tfrac{1}{2}l^2\sigma^2) \times \left[\sum_{p=1}^{6} \gamma_{wp}^l \{\Phi(A_p) - \Phi(A_{p-1})\} \right] \quad (A.4)$$

for the exposure-age-concentration model. Here, $\Phi(\cdot)$ stands for the standard normal cumulant with $A_0 = -\infty$, $A_6 = \infty$, and $A_j = \log WL_j/\sigma - l\sigma$ where $WL_j = 0.5$, 1.0, 3.0, 5.0, 15.0 ($j = 1, 2, 3, 4, 5, 6$).

REFERENCES

1. KREWSKI, D. *et al.* 1989. Managing environmental radon risks: a Canadian perspective. *In* Management of Risk from Genotoxic Substances Present in the Environment, F.L. Stockholm, Ed.: 242–257. Swedish National Chemicals Inspectorate.
2. LUBIN, J.H. *et al.* 1995. Lung cancer in radon-exposed miners and estimation of risk from indoor exposure. J. National Cancer Institute **87:** 817–827.
3. LUBIN, J.H. *et al.* 1997. Estimating lung cancer mortality from residential radon using data for low exposures in miners. Radiation Research **147:** 126–134.
4. ALAVANJA, C.R.M. *et al.* 1994. Residential radon exposure and lung cancer among nonsmoking women. J. National Cancer Institute **86:** 1829–1837.
5. LETOURNEAU, E.G. *et al.* 1994. Case-control study of lung cancer and residential radon exposure in Winnipeg, Manitoba, Canada. Am. J. Epidemiol. **140:** 310–322.
6. PERSHANGEN, G. *et al.* 1994. Residential radon exposure and lung cancer in Sweden. New Engl. J. Medicine **330:** 159–164.
7. U.S. NATIONAL RESEARCH COUNCIL. 1999. Health Effects of Exposure to Radon. BEIR VI. National Academy Press. Washington, DC.
8. BARTLETT, S. *et al.* 1996. Characterizing uncertainty in risk assessment—conclusions drawn from a workshop. Human and Ecological Risk Assessment **2:** 217–227.
9. LUBIN, J.H. *et al.* 1994. Radon and lung cancer risk: a joint analysis of 11 underground miners studies. National Institute of Health, National Cancer Institute. NIH Publication No. 94-3644. U.S. Department of Health and Human Services. Washington, DC.
10. MOOLGAVKAR, S.H. *et al.* 1993. Radon, cigarette smoke, and lung cancer. A reanalysis of the Colorado plateau uranium miners' data. Epidemiol. **4:** 204–217.
11. HOFFMAN, F.O. & J.S. HAMMONDS. 1994. Propagation of uncertainty in risk assessments: the need to distinguish between uncertainty due to lack of knowledge and uncertainty due to variability. Risk Analysis **14:** 707–712.
12. BOGEN, K.T. 1995. Methods to approximate joint uncertainty and variability in risk. Risk Analysis **15:** 411–419.
13. U.S. NATIONAL RESEARCH COUNCIL. 1994. Science and Judgment Risk Assessment. National Academy Press Washington, DC.
14. HATTIS, D. & D.E. BURMASTER. 1994. Assessment of variability and uncertainty distributions for practical risk analysis. Risk Analysis **14:** 713–730.
15. BAIRD, S.J.S. *el al.* 1996. Noncancer risk assessment: a probabilistic alternative to current practice. Human and Ecological Risk Assessment **2:** 79–102.
16. BURMASTER, D.E. & K.M. THOMPSON. 1996. Backcalculating cleanup targets in probabilistic risk assessments when the acceptability of cancer risk is defined under different risk management policies. Human and Ecological Risk Assessment **1:** 101–120.
17. RAI, S.N. *et al.* 1996. A general framework for the analysis of uncertainty and variability in risk assessment. Human and Ecological Risk Assessment **2:** 972–989.
18. RAI, S.N. & D. KREWSKI. 1998. Uncertainty and variability analysis in multiplicative risk models. Risk Analysis **18:** 37–45.
19. KREWSKI, D. *et al.* 1995. Uncertainty, variability and sensitivity analysis in physiologically based pharmacokinetic models. J. Biopharmaceutical Statistics **5:** 245–271.
20. RAI, S.N. *et al.* 1995. Analysis of short time series with an over-dispersion model. Communications in Statistics—Theory and Methods **24:** 335–348.
21. WANG, Y. *et al.* 1995. Meta analysis of multiple cohorts of underground miners exposed to radon. Proc. Statistics Canada Sympos. 95 From Data to Information—Methods and Systems. 21–28. Statistics Canada. Ottawa.
22. KALBFLEISCH, J.D. & R.L. PRENTICE. 1980. The Statistical Analysis of Failure Time Data. Wiley, New York.
23. LUBIN, J.H. & J.D. BOICE, JR. 1989. Estimating Rn-induced lung cancer in the United States. Health Physics **57:** 417–427.

24. WARNER, K.E. *et al.* 1996. Toward a more realistic appraisal of the lung cancer risk from radon: the effects of residential mobility. Am. J. Public Health **86:** 1222–1227.
25. U.S ENVIRONMENTAL PROTECTION AGENCY. Technical support document for the 1992 citizen's guide to radon. EPA 1992; 400-R-92-011.

Risk Assessment—the Mother of All Uncertainties

Disciplinary Perspectives on Uncertainty in Risk Assessment

JOHN C. BAILAR III[a] AND A. JOHN BAILER[b,c]

[a]*Department of Health Studies and Harris School of Public Policy, University of Chicago, 5841 South Maryland Avenue, MC 2007, Chicago, Illinois 60637, USA*

[b]*Department of Mathematics and Statistics, Miami University, Oxford, Ohio 45056, USA*

[c]*National Institute for Occupational Safety and Health, Education and Information Division, Risk Evaluation Branch, 4676 Columbia Parkway, Cincinnati, Ohio 45226, USA*

> ABSTRACT: Uncertainty in the detection and evaluation of chemical hazards to health leads to challenges when conducting risk assessments. Some of the uncertainty has to do with data, some with incomplete understanding of processes, and some with the most fundamental ways of viewing the questions. True variability—across space, in time, or among individuals—complicates the search for understanding many important aspects of risk. A few statistical and toxicologic tools are available to assess uncertainty. Three methods of classifying uncertainty are briefly discussed. In addition, our disciplinary background may influence how we view and discuss variability and uncertainty. We rarely know as much as we think we do (and not just in risk assessment). Great uncertainty is likely to remain an important part of risk assessment for some decades to come.

INTRODUCTION

Uncertainty in the detection and estimation of the impact of chemical hazards to health is extensive and difficult to deal with. Much of our presentation here is likely to be familiar; however, we hope to present familiar things in new contexts and to stimulate rethinking about their implications. Some of the uncertainty has to do with inaccurate and incomplete data, some with incomplete understanding of natural processes, and some with the most fundamental ways of viewing the matter. Uncertainty in risk assessment is commonly associated with issues such as the selection of concentration-response models, or extrapolating across exposure conditions, species, or routes of exposure. In contrast, variability is risk assessment usually relates to interindividual variation. Here we interweave general discussions of uncertainty and variability in risk assessment with disciplinary perspectives on these two topics.

Addresses for correspondence:
[a]John C. Bailar III: 773-834-1242 (voice); 773-702-1979 (fax); e-mail: jcbailar@midway.uchicago.edu
[b]A. John Bailer: 513-529-3538 (voice); 513-529-1493 (fax); e-mail: ajbailer@muohio.edu

TABLE 1. Measured responses in an experiment in which two chemicals were administered (hypothetical data)

		Chemical A dose (mg)		
		0	20	40
Chemical B dose (mg)	0	5 units	15	40
	300	10	30	70
	600	40	60	90

To motivate this discussion, consider a simple example of conceptual uncertainty that arises when statisticians, epidemiologists, and toxicologists encounter the same data set. In this example, we explore how synergy is to be defined, including negative synergy, or antagonism.

TABLE 1 shows hypothetical results from a study of the effects of giving two toxic agents, A and B, simultaneously. Nine tests were performed in a 3×3 factorial design. Assume that sample sizes are large enough and observations are accurate enough to take these figures at face value. Is there synergy at the central point in this table (20 mg A, 300 mg B)? The statistician, using a linear model, will note that the baseline response (untreated) is 5 units, that 20 mg of A, alone, increases the response by 10 units, and that 300 mg of agent B increases the response by 5 units, so that if the agents act independently the center point, with 20 mg of A and 300 mg of B, will be increased over background by $5 + 10 = 15$ units. However, the data show a larger increase, of 25 units. Thus, the statistician who uses the customary additive approach to the study of such data is likely to conclude that there is positive synergy between 20 mg of A and 300 mg of B. The epidemiologist may be more at ease with multiplicative models (e.g., relative risk or odds ratio models), and will see that 20 mg of A increases the response by a factor of three over background, 300 mg of B increases risk by a factor of two, so that the combination of independent effects would result a sixfold increase, and this is just what is observed. That is, the agents act independently on a multiplicative scale. Although these two views differ, both focus on the combination of response rates, and both depend on some assumption about the additivity of responses. The natural view of the toxicologist is quite different, because it focuses on additivity of doses rather than responses. If 40 mg of A alone produces a 40 unit response rate, and the same is true for 600 mg of B, one might expect a mixture of $x\%$ of A and $(100 - x)\%$ of B to have the same outcome. However, here half a dose of A (20 mg) plus half a dose of B (300 mg) produces only a 30 unit response, not 40 units, so that the agents do not just fail to be synergistic, they are in fact antagonistic. (As an aside, the three other non-central combination treatments might suggest synergy to the toxicologist, which further complicates this informal assessment.) TABLE 2 summarizes these results. Is there synergy? That depends on one's view of *synergy*, which may be related to intended uses of the concept, or may be simply a matter of custom within relevant disciplines. These differences are conceptual and not a matter of data, biologic process, or scientific understanding.

TABLE 2. Summary of the results of the disciplinary perspectives on synergy

Model type (scientist)	Joint action?
additive outcome (statistician)	synergy
multiplicative outcome (epidemiologist)	independence
additive dose (toxicologist/ pharmacologist)	antagonism

Although these three views are mathematically incompatible except under extreme conditions of little practical interest, each makes a great deal of sense in its own context, and the world would be poorer if we had to give up any of them. This example, used to illustrate these perspectives, is clearly contrived and selectively viewed to illustrate a point. As some of our toxicology colleagues have noted, the notion of synergy defined by dose additivity would not be immediately applied in a situation where the dose-response pattern for each chemical given separately was non-linear as we presented in our example. In reality, a toxicologist would consider the expected mechanism of action. For example, two chemicals competing for the same receptor site leads to predictions of antagonism, whereas independent sites of action would lead to dose additivity. Finally, we are not advocating the compartmentalizing of an individual approach by discipline. Our drawings of *statistician*, *epidemiologist*, and *toxicologist* are caricatures rather than portraits. We hope that these exaggerated disciplinary definitions will suggest how different training and experience may result in different evaluations of the same data pattern. This has clear implications for risk assessment, an interdisciplinary exercise of serious societal impact.

In the same manner, there may be substantial differences in the ways that statisticians and others view broader concepts of uncertainty. In fact, any discussion of risk assessment must examine bias, or nonrandom uncertainty. In many biological problems, questions of bias typically dominate the questions of randomness or variability that make up most of statistics. These questions of bias lead to the awkward, but common, result that two or more risk assessments of the same chemical hazard may result in wildly different conclusions. It is not uncommon to see risk estimates that differ by three orders of magnitude or more (that is, more than 10^3), and in the case of dioxin the variation among agencies of the U.S. federal government was at one time 14 orders of magnitude, although the subset used in regulation showed much less variation.[1] That is real uncertainty.

Another example is provided by the analysis of four separate risk assessments of the chemical Tris.[2] The risk assessments were for the use of Tris as a flame retardant in children's sleepwear. These risk assessments were made at about the same time (over a period of about three weeks) by investigators who knew each other and were in frequent contact by telephone and mail. They had access to the same databases and used similar procedures, and yet still reached the estimates shown in TABLE 3. Despite the close communication and the great overlap in both data and technical understanding, these estimates differ by almost three orders of magnitude. The primary differences were in the ways that human exposure were estimated and the ways that exposure was used to assess risk. Four estimates, if they were independently derived

TABLE 3. Added lifetime risk of kidney cancer per million children using Tris-treated sleepware

Author	Lifetime risk
Hooper and Ames	17,000
Bayard	180 (combined)
	300 (male)
	60 (female)
Schneiderman	52
Harris	≥ 7

and if each had a distribution with the correct median, would have one chance in eight of all falling on the same side of the true value. Of course, these four estimates used much of the same data and so are not independent. Thus, there is a large chance that even the range here might not include the true risk. Fortunately, in this case, the exact value did not matter. The Commissioners of the Consumer Product Safety Commission decided that even the lowest estimate of risk from Tris-treated sleepware was too high, and they acted promptly to ban Tris from the marketplace. As an aside, the manufacturers recognized the problem with equal clarity, and moved even faster, so that Tris was off the market even before the Commissioners could ban it.

Nonrandom uncertainty utterly swamps any contribution from randomness in risk assessment. In the case of a new chemical, for instance, we may need to extrapolate from animal studies to human outcomes, from high to low doses, from one route of administration to another, and from lifetime exposure to information on once-only exposures. In the face of such uncertainty, it hardly matters whether 3, or 8, or 20 animals from a total of 60 have some particular outcome. This is important because a false sense of security can be a result of a refusal to acknowledge (and attempt to quantify) the uncertainty in risk predictions. We have all heard of the call for one-handed risk assessors (to avoid "on one hand this, on the other hand that"), but a false sense of security can have major harmful effects on both governmental regulation and public acceptance of regulations. Since great uncertainty is always with us in this field, it is crucial that we learn how to conduct risk assessment in the face of it.

DISCIPLINARY PERSPECTIVES ON UNCERTAINTY

During the recent meetings of a committee that examined the foundations of risk assessment (primarily of chemical hazards),[3] with special reference to regulation by EPA but with much broader implications, the eminent scientists serving on the committee viewed uncertainty from a variety of different perspectives. The statistician's concepts of variance and bias, with some allowance for averaging over populations that reflect some true variability from one subject to another, was by no means a consensus. These different views are instructive, and worth understanding for effective communication across the different disciplines reflected in the risk assessment community. TABLE 4 highlights our perspective regarding how uncertainty in risk assessment is often considered and classified by statisticians, risk assessors, and toxicologists.

In general terms, disciplinary perspectives are influenced by background and training. (An implication of this observation is that our comments in this paper are *biased* by our own disciplinary training as statisticians. Note also that our TABLE 4 does not result in classifications that are either mutually exclusive or collectively exhaustive in defining these perspectives. With these caveats acknowledged, we boldly proceed.) The statistician tends to explore systems by the application of probability and statistical models. Variability is viewed in light of random departures from a specified model whereas all other uncertainty is typically viewed as a bias associated with differences between the model and the state of nature. Toxicologists often classify uncertainty as being associated with either a parameter or a model. To the toxicologist, parameter uncertainty (e.g., for some component of a physiologically-based pharmacokinetic model) is more likely to be viewed as mea-

TABLE 4. Uncertainty and variability as viewed by statisticians, risk assessors, and toxicologists

Statistician	Risk Assessor	Toxicologist
1. Variances and covariances are used to evaluate subject, technician, season, and other sources of variability (*true* variation).	1. Hazard identifications—are exposure E and disease D independent given characteristics and context C, where C represents confounders or other risk factors (gender, age, etc.) Is $f(E,D|C) = f(E|C) f(D|C)$?	1. Parameter uncertainty—measurement error (variance and bias) and surrogate data (species extrapolation, e.g., using effects in mice to estimate human risk).
2. Uncertainty is reflected in bias—unadjusted (or even unrecognized) confounders, miscalibration of instruments, etc.	2. Hazard characterization—examine the probability distribution of D given E and C [$f(D|E,C)$]—uncertainty rests in low dose extrapolation and species extrapolation.	2. Model uncertainty—gaps in understanding disease processes or the disposition of xenobiotics—e.g., linear nonthreshold model for carcinogenesis or the construction of physiologically-based pharmacokinetic models.
	3. Exposure characterization—the joint distribution of E and C [$f(E,C)$]—uncertainty arises from scant or absent information about the joint occurrence of E and C.	3. *True* variation—across space, time, individuals (e.g., biologic repair mechanisms) and concerns related to concurrent exposures (confounding, synergy, effect modification, etc.).
	4. Risk determination—can we determine the likelihood of adverse responses as a function of dose—$f(D)$. Note that other kinds of conceptual complexities and political imperatives occur when *integrating out* E and perhaps C.	

surement error, in contrast to the statistician's commonly employed construct of sampling variation. Most toxicologists would also be sensitive to the biological variability of the systems being modeled and they might worry about using a single set of parameter values for making statements about a population. The toxicologist's concern about model uncertainty are analogous to the statistician's concerns about bias in model selection. The statistician and toxicologist would agree that interindividual differences reflect variability, and they are likely to concur that differences in other factors (e.g., space or time) would also contribute to variation in outcome and should be incorporated in an analysis. Some important problems of exposure (confounding, effect modification, and synergy) would be described by a statistician as bias in model specification although the toxicologists might consider this as variation.

A risk assessor may see uncertainty and variability in light of the components of the risk assessment process. In our TABLE 4, we have discussed the risk assessor's considerations of uncertainty and variability in light of probability distributions (no real surprise, given the bias that we bring as statisticians to this discussion). Hazard identification involves evaluating whether hazard exposure (E) and disease (D) are independent given characteristics and context (C). In statistical terms, the question is whether $f(E, D|C) = f(E|C)f(D|C)$. This is a question of partial correlation (after removing the effects of C) in the relationships between E and D. Exposure characterization explores the joint distribution of E and C, $f(E,C)$, where uncertainty arises from scant or absent information about states of nature, expressed in the joint distribution of E and C. Hazard characterization examines the probability distribution of D given E and C, $f(D|E,C)$] with the greatest uncertainty often resting in low dose extrapolation and species extrapolation. Risk determination determines the value of $f(D)$, the frequency or severity of adverse responses, under the specified distribution of conditions as a function of dose, where the conceptual complexities and political imperatives expressed by E and C are integrated out. Note that other disciplines and perspectives could have been considered here. For example, a physician or an epidemiologist may work to a model more like those for infectious disease, where many individuals are exposed but individual factors determine who gets the disease.

REFLECTIONS ON UNCERTAINTY

Uncertainty can be defined as a lack of precise knowledge about the state of nature. This creates practical problems in determining how to assess and deal with, first, the uncertainty itself, and second, estimates of risk that necessarily embody great uncertainty. Since major uncertainty is always with us in this field, it is crucial to learn how to conduct risk assessment in the face of it.

EPA decision-makers have long recognized the usefulness of uncertainty analysis, but they have made only slow headway in replacing *ad hoc* procedures based on a few simple but sweeping assumptions with procedures based on information about the range of risk values consistent with biologic mechanisms of carcinogenic or other toxic effects, the current knowledge of biology and chemistry, or even actual exposures in some group. This is beginning to change as risk assessment based on understanding of biological mechanisms increases, but replacing a few heroic assumptions with a vast number of individually much smaller assumptions will not necessarily reduce uncertainty or get us any closer to true answers. For example, if there is uncertainty about which of the biologic models is correct, great refinement, in either—or even both—may do little to reduce uncertainty in the risk estimates.

One way to examine uncertainty in risk assessment is to classify sources of uncertainty according to the step in the risk assessment process in which they occur (see the *Risk Assessor* column in TABLE 4), including such matters as the failure to identify some hazards, incompatible results from different, but similar studies, estimation of parameters of biological response, the lack of some critical exposure data, and balancing the use of poor epidemiologic data against better but less relevant animal data. This is often done, and now commonly categorized under four headings that may be designated hazard identification, hazard characterization, exposure-response characterization, and risk determination.[4] (These terms vary a bit from author to author, though the four-way breakdown is widely used.) This still does not deal in a satisfactory way with all major uncertainties. For example,

- relating ambient exposures to internal tissue doses,
- extrapolation across mammalian models,
- extrapolation across different routes of exposure,
- extrapolation from lifetime exposure (of workers or animals) to intermittent, and usually lower, exposures of the general population,
- appropriate averaging times for exposure (instantaneous, day, year, etc., where the best answer may depend on biologic half-life).

Another approach, which the Committee[3] adopted, has already been developed as one basis for EPA regulations. This begins with three sets of terms, for parameter uncertainties, model uncertainties, and true variability. Each of these may include important aspects of the two schemes already mentioned—variance/bias and phase of analysis—but the basic approach is quite different. Uncertainties in parameter estimates may arise from measurement error (including such things as random errors in analytic devices, as well as systematic bias), the use of generic or surrogate data in lieu of direct analysis of the parameter to be estimated, misclassification of subjects, random sampling error, and other kinds of non-representativeness.

Model uncertainty arises because of gaps in the scientific theory that is needed to make predictions about risk on the basis of causal inferences. An example is provided by the controversy about whether the linear, non-threshold model for carcinogenesis is sufficiently accurate to be used in setting *conservative* limits to exposure to carcinogens. Evidence suggests that it is not.[5] Other kinds of model uncertainties include errors in understanding relationships and oversimplified models of reality. Important variables may be omitted or perhaps not even recognized as relevant at the time the model is used. The model may fail to account for nontrivial correlations, or miss potentially important confounders or effect modifiers. An important example has to do with the extent of aggregation used in the model; the modeler may either underaggregate (as in considering effects on separate cells or tissues rather than the body as a whole) or overaggregate (as in including persons with a variety of prior exposures that may affect their individual responses). Another example of model uncertainty arises in the use of physiologically-based pharmacokinetic (PBPK) models to relate exposure to internal doses.[6]

True variability—across space, in time, or among individuals—complicates the search for a single value that captures some important aspect of risk. Examples include changes over time in the emission of toxic agents and person-to-person differences in susceptibility. In addition, changes over time may occur in individual susceptibility due to age, diet, or other exposures.

Some scientists now believe that Monte Carlo methods offer a separate and special approach to uncertainty analysis. This is not true, of course; Monte Carlo methods are no more than a computational means to estimate outcomes of complex and mathematically intractable models developed in other ways, not a method in themselves.[7] However, it seems that this perspective is so deeply embedded in the culture of risk assessment that views, as well as terminology, about Monte Carlo methods will be difficult to change. This is not to suggest that Monte Carlo methods are not useful.

The need for Monte Carlo simulation is evident from the TABLE 5, taken from the Committee report.[3] It shows some of the key variables in risk assessment for which probability distributions might be needed. Although not all of these may be needed in every risk assessment, this is by no means a complete list. Furthermore, both distributional forms and parameters of these forms are not generally known, with some forms far from Gaussian, so that the convolutions become mathematically difficult and of unknown reliability. Clearly, computations in risk assessment may become very highly complex. A further problem is that the goal of some environmental regulatory agencies is to protect the most sensitive members of the most sensitive group with a high degree of certainty, with overall allowable risks not greater than, say, 1 in 100,000 or 1 in 1,000,000. This requires untestable assumptions regarding extrapolation from experiments with small numbers of animals, or even from epidemiologic studies with mere tens of thousands of persons. As a final observation on the use of Monte Carlo methods, sampling of different model variables (*parameters*) is often conducted by assuming that the variables are independent. Although this may be true for many variables, correlations clearly exist for others. For example, in physiologically-based pharmacokinetic models, volumes of compartments are probably positively correlated but partition coefficients are probably independent.

Bayesian methods of statistical analysis, which deal with subjective probabilities and the totality of relevant knowledge from *other* sources, have many attractions. There is some history of using subjective approaches to probability distributions in risk assessment, although this history seems to be focused on well-identified components of the risk assessment rather than on the outcome of the assessment as a whole. The NAS Committee Report[3] noted the following:

> Objective probabilities might seem inherently more accurate than subjective probabilities, but this is not always true. Formal methods (Bayesian statistics) exist to incorporate objective information into a subjective probability distribution that reflects other matters that might be relevant but difficult to quantify, such as knowledge about chemical structure, expectations of the effect of concurrent exposure (synergy), or the scope of plausible variations in exposure. The chief advantage of an objective probability distribution is, of course, its objectivity; right or wrong, it is less likely to be susceptible to major and perhaps undetectable bias on the part of the analyst; this has palpable benefits in defending a risk assessment and the decisions that follow. A second advantage is that objective probability distributions are often far easier to determine. However, there can be no rule that objective probability estimates are always preferred to subjective estimates, or vice versa. (NRC, 1994.)[3]

TABLE 5. Examples of variables in risk assessment for which probability distributions might be needed[a]

Model component	Output variable	Independent parameter variables
transport	air concentration	chemical emission rate; stack exit temperature; stack exit velocity; mixing heights
deposition	deposition rate	dry-deposition velocity; wet-deposition velocity; fraction of time with rain
overland	surface-water load	fraction of chemical in overload runoff
water	surface-water concentration	river discharge; chemical decay coefficient in rivers
soil	surface-soil concentration	surface-soil depth; exposure duration; exposure period; cation-exchange capacity; decay coefficient in soil
food chain	fish concentration	water-to-fish bioconcentration factor
	plant concentration	plant interception factors; weathering elimination rate; crop density; soil-to-plant bioconcentration factor
dose	inhalation dose	inhalation rate/body weight
	ingestion dose	plant/soil ingestion rates
	dermal-absorption dose	exposed skin surface area; soil absorption factor; exposure frequency; body weight
risk	total carcinogenic risk	inhalation/ingestion carcinogenic potency factors; dermal-absorption carcinogenic potency factors

[a]Modified from TABLE 6 in Reference 3.

The report noted that there are substantial differences between these approaches, particularly the inability to include aspects of certainty for which there is no quantitative measure, or even to include an extra *fudge factor* to allow for sources of uncertainty not yet thought of. Overall, to explore the difference between parameter uncertainty and model uncertainty, consider the following example in which cancer risk is treated as a parameter to be estimated. In situation A, 3 of 60 animals in a test group develop cancer. This outcome may be regarded as having a distribution very close to Poisson, and the observed frequency of 5% (3/60), has ordinary 95% confidence bounds of 1.03% to 14.6%. Larger samples will ordinarily lead to narrower confidence bounds. In situation B, the chemical under test is thought to follow one of six well-identified chemical pathways, but it is not known which, and these are considered to be about equally likely. The pathways have different means, but the sum of the probability distributions of risk is close to that for the single Gaussian distribution in situation A. Even if sample sizes in B are very much larger than in A, major uncertainty will remain because the level of risk is determined almost exclusively by the biologic situation, and we do not know which biologic model is correct. In more familiar terms, if risk depends on gender, any single population-risk estimate will refer to a hypothetical person who is unknown and will not provide an accurate estimate for any population member. In either situation A or B, it would be mathematically correct to say something like the following: "The expected value of the estimate of the number of annual excess cancer deaths nationwide caused by exposure to this substance is five per million persons; the lower and upper confidence bounds on this estimate are 1.03 per million and 14.6 per million." However, the risk manager who is developing regulations to protect the public health might respond to these situations in quite different ways because of the difference in the source of the uncertainty. The problem is that the summary statement in Situation B, dominated by model uncertainty, obscures important information about the state of scientific knowledge.

In a more extreme example, every knowledgeable scientist may agree that some substance is likely to pose no risk to a population, but that there is one chance in a thousand that it will cause a major disaster. The mode, the median, the 99-percentile are all quite firmly at zero risk. How should the risk regulator respond? Risk managers and the public should be given an opportunity to understand the sources of the controversy, to appreciate why the subjective weights assigned to each model have their given values, and to judge for themselves what action is appropriate when the various theories, of which at most one can be correct, predict such different outcomes. Simply put, it is not in the best interest of either the decision maker or society to treat fundamentally different kinds of predictions as quantities that can be averaged and compared directly without considering the effects of each prediction on the decision it leads to. There may also be quite profound impacts on needs for further information; in one case, one needs a substantially larger sample size, and in the other, one needs additional fundamental research on the mechanisms involved.

There is still another fundamental issue to deal with here. Philosophers, including philosophers of statistics, have noted that the probability of any unobserved event must be either zero or one; the problem is that we do not know which. This is of course built into the foundations of statistics, whether one's basic approach begins with concepts of relative frequencies, or strength of belief, or axioms of probability. The calculated probability is thus a measure of our ignorance. However, this matter is not well understood by the public, and it seems that large numbers of people do not look on probabilities in the same way that statisticians do. This has led to a large literature on risk perception and risk communication, matters that should be well understood by any statistician who may want to enter this field.[8]

Finally, it is quite fair to say that we rarely know as much as we think we do. We observe our data, go through our statistical computations, and find confidence bounds; we then add uncertainty for this, that, and the other thing; to come up with wider limits for plausible risks, but even then it seems that we fail to account for how little we truly know about the world around us. Recall that the four estimates of risk associated with Tris exposures ranged over nearly three orders of magnitude. Each of the four reports on these risk assessments included extensive discussion about the uncertainties, with an estimate of how far off the final assessment might be. Each of these statements of uncertainty was on the order of a factor of ten. Since orders of magnitude are multiplicative, even these four experienced and knowledgeable risk assessors, working from much the same data base, differed by close to one hundredfold more than any one of them thought plausible in terms of his own analysis. This situation is not at all uncommon. (The observation that we never know as much as we think we do is most certainly not limited to risk assessment. It seems to be pervasive throughout science and throughout our daily lives. The discrepancy between what is known and what is thought to be known probably varies with investigator as well.) This subjectivity allows for investigator bias, whether conscious or subconscious, to enter into analyses.[9]

When uncertainty is great, it is important to devise philosophies, political agendas, computational procedures, and regulations that accommodate this uncertainty. An approach at one extreme would be to assume that regulations should not deal with any risk until it has been adequately demonstrated to be present. (*Adequate* is of course subjective.) This puts the focus on the lower end of the range of uncertainty. This has been described as the "wait for dead bodies" method. Another approach is to focus on the high end, and regulate and otherwise treat the risk as if it were at the greatest level not excluded by a generous interpretation of present information. (This could be a counsel of paralysis—progress would be much slower, but we would be safe from the possible hazards of innovation and risk would simply vanish—except perhaps, the risk of death from boredom.) It might be argued that excessive risk regulation may increase the costs of doing business for some industries which, in turn, may in turn decrease productivity and even lead to economic conditions under which workers lose jobs. Unemployed workers may then be at greater risk of adverse health outcomes. Thus, overly conservative assumptions in risk assessment may result in increasing other risks.

A third approach would be to pick some measure of central tendency. For this, the mean might be preferred over the median, because the median might often be zero though there is an appreciable likelihood of a very substantial harmful effect. For example, in Bailer and Dankovic,[6] the distribution of risks from a Monte Carlo simulation of methylene chloride was bimodal where the two modes differed by three orders of magnitude. (The different modes corresponded to different simulated patterns of cancer response data. One pattern suggested a linear component of dose-response was possible and the other was strictly nonlinear.) In this example, the estimated median risk was significantly less than the estimated mean risk. It is likely that no measure of central tendency is uniformly best for all contexts. This matter requires considerably more public discussion. In this discussion, however, we would strongly discourage the use of logarithmic or geometric distributions, orders of magnitude, and the like for communicating risk. The reason is that many people tend to equate an order of magnitude at one point of the scale with an order of magnitude elsewhere, whereas the difference in their practical effects may be immense—in fact, orders of magnitude. Furthermore, using logarithmic or similar distributions for the purpose of stabilizing variance and/or making observed distributions more tractable may lead to unwarranted confidence in results. The practical effects of such steps are to substantially reduce the impact of high observations, whereas those high observations are arguably of most concern to us. They ought to be studied in detail and have a major impact on the result.

We all deplore the great uncertainty in risk assessment, yet there seems to be little careful analysis of how much certainty is needed. Does it matter if we are off by a factor of two? A factor of 10? Or 100 or more? We do seem to find value in what we do now, which may be off by a factor of 1,000. In the face of this great uncertainty, the approach that has generally been used by the EPA and other regulatory agencies is to develop *default options* for model uncertainty. These are assumptions that certain approaches to modeling will be used and taken to be correct unless there is evidence to the contrary. Examples are, to assume that the dose-response relation is linear down to a dose of zero, that extrapolations from small rodents to humans should be on the basis of surface area or body weight raised to a specified exponent, and that an agent toxic by one route of administration is toxic by another. In practice, however, it has been extremely difficult to persuade any agency that the evidence is strong enough to overturn any default option; default options are generally considered *conservative*, in that their results are thought to indicate more toxicity than is likely (though not the most extreme results). The effect of this is that the actual level of public protection may often be somewhat higher than the formal estimates would indicate, though the default options may sometimes be quite seriously in error in the other direction.[5] Another effect of reliance on default options may be to reduce the appearance of uncertainty in the risk estimate. If default options are treated as having no uncertainty whereas real data always include uncertainty, then increasing the number or scope of default options might appear to make the answer more and more precise (less variable). Thus, the use of default values, if not accompanied by associated uncertainty, may have the effect of masking much of the nonrandom uncertainty. Returning to our consideration of disciplinary perspectives, not every discipline will necessarily see this as bad. From a legal standpoint, and perhaps from a risk management standpoint, it is easier to make a case for regulating a hazard that is assumed to be precisely known (even if it is a biased estimate) than for regulating a hazard with a very uncertain risk. From either a mechanistic (toxicologic) point of view, or from a statistical point of view, we tend to see a realistic appraisal of the true uncertainty as a good thing. It is not clear that the entire risk assessment community would agree.

Although safety above the estimated level may be most prudent, many people, particularly those allied with chemical manufacturers and users, often complain that we should instead be using our best estimates. It is not clear what *best estimate* means, especially in the face of serious model uncertainty. If knowledgeable scientists are 99% sure that the risk from some exposure is zero, but believe there is a 1% chance that it may be as high as one in one thousand persons, should we assume that the risk is nil? We think not. Even at this point, debate still remains. One response in one thousand exposed individuals is assumed to represent significant impact. Additionally, can risk be reduced in light of feasibility constraints (economic and technological) without inducing other outcomes that may effect health adversely (e.g., unemployment, or substituting an untested alternative).

Risk assessment is a process of analysis, not a specific kind of research and not a result, and it must be viewed as a process that is subject to much uncertainty. Our objective in this paper has been to consider uncertainty and variability in risk assessment from the perspective of the different disciplines and actors involved in the process. After this discussion, we further explored how uncertainty and variability are reflected in typical risk assessments. We closed our reflections with observations on how these risk assessment uncertainties should be communicated to risk managers and the public alike. Although we are encouraged with advances in mechanistic understanding in disease processes and in statistical methods for incorporating uncertainty in risk assessments, we believe that the evaluation and exploration of uncertainty are likely to remain an important part of risk assessment for some decades to come.

ACKNOWLEDGMENTS

The authors thank Drs. James Deddens, David Dankovic, and Eileen Kuempel, whose critiques, comments, and suggestions have led to improvements in the presentation in this paper.

REFERENCES

1. ANDERSON, P.D. 1988. Scientific origins of incompatibility in risk assessment. Stat. Sci. **3**: 320–327.
2. BAILAR, J.C., J. NEEDLEMAN, B. BERNEY & J.M. MCGINNIS. 1993. Assessing Risks to Health: Methodologic Approaches. Auburn House, Westport.
3. NATIONAL RESEARCH COUNCIL, COMMITTEE ON RISK ASSESSMENT OF HAZARDOUS AIR POLLUTANTS. 1994. Science and Judgment in Risk Assessment. National Academy Press, Washington, D.C.
4. MCGINNIS, J.M., J.C. BAILAR & R.G. TARDIFF. 1986. Determining Risks to Health: Federal Policy and Practice. Auburn House, Westport.
5. BAILAR, J.C., E.D.C. CROUCH, R. SHAIKH & D. SPIEGELMAN. 1988. One-hit models of carcinogenesis: conservative or not? Risk Analysis **8**: 485–497.
6. BAILER, A.J. & D.A. DANKOVIC. 1997. An introduction to the use of physiologically-based pharmacokinetic models in risk assessment. Statistical Methods in Medical Research **6**: 341–358.
7. SPECIAL ISSUE. 1996. Commemoration of the 50th Anniversary of Monte Carlo. Human and Ecological Risk Assessment **2**(4).
8. NATIONAL RESEARCH COUNCIL, COMMITTEE ON RISK PERCEPTION AND COMMUNICATION. 1989. Improving Risk Communication. National Academy Press, Washington, D.C.
9. KOZLOWSKI, L.T. *et al.* 1996. Smokers are unaware of the filter vents now on cigarettes: results of a national survey. Tobacco Control **5**: 265–270.

Distributions of Individual Susceptibility among Humans for Toxic Effects

How Much Protection Does the Traditional Tenfold Factor Provide for What Fraction of Which Kinds of Chemicals and Effects?

DALE HATTIS,[a] PRERNA BANATI, AND ROBERT GOBLE

Center for Technology, Environment, and Development, George Perkins Marsh Institute, Clark University, Worcester, Massachusetts, USA

ABSTRACT: A significant data base has been assembled on human variability in parameters representing a series of steps in the pathway from external exposure to the production of biological responses: contact rate (e.g., breathing rates/body weight, fish consumption/body weight); uptake or absorption (mg/kg)/intake or contact rate; general systemic availability net of first pass elimination and dilution; systemic elimination or half-life; active site availability/general systemic availability; physiological parameter change/active site availability; functional reserve capacity—change in baseline physiological parameter needed to pass a criterion of abnormal function or exhibit a response. This paper discusses the current results of analyzing these data to derive estimates for distributions of human susceptibility to different routes of exposure and types of adverse effects. The degree of protection is tentatively evaluated by projecting the incidences of effects that would be expected for a tenfold lowering of exposure from a 5% incidence level if the population distribution of susceptibility were truly log-normal out to the extreme tails, and if the populations, chemicals, and responses that gave rise to the underlying data were representative of the cases to which traditional uncertainty factor is applied. The results indicate that, acting by itself, a tenfold reduction in dose from a 5% effect level is associated with effect incidences ranging from slightly less than one in ten thousand, for a median chemical/response, to a few per thousand, for chemicals and responses that have greater human interindividual variability than 19 out of 20 typical chemicals/responses. In practice, for many of the cases where the traditional tenfold factor is applied, additional protection is provided by other uncertainty factors. Nevertheless, the results generate some reason for concern that current application of traditional safety or uncertainty factor approaches may allow appreciable incidences of responses in some cases.

---

[a]Address for correspondence: Center for Technology, Environment, and Development, George Perkins Marsh Institute, Clark University, 950 Main Street, Worcester, MA 01610, USA. 508-751-4603 (voice); 508-751-4600 (fax).
e-mail: dhattis@clarku.edu

INTRODUCTION

This paper is one of several efforts[1–7] that are attempting to help build the basis for improved quantitative assessment of the noncancer effects of chemicals. Much has changed since the landmark paper of Lehman and Fitzhugh[8] in 1954, which set the paradigm for traditional analyses with the original *100-fold safety factor* (of which 1/10 is allocated to possible differences in sensitivity among people). Today we have the experience and the computational capabilities to employ distributional approaches in place of simple rule-of-thumb formulæ. We also have the benefit of an enormous flowering of biomedical science over the last few decades from which we can draw helpful data (although many of the data are not ideal for our purposes). Finally, we live in an age where the questions for analysis have broadened beyond the main issues confronting the U.S. Food and Drug Administration of 1954. In contexts as diverse as occupational safety and health, general community air pollution, drinking water contaminants, and community exposures from waste sites decision makers and the public ask questions like "does exposure to X at fraction Y of an estimated no-adverse-effect level really pose enough of a risk of harm as to merit directing major resources to prevention?" On the other hand, are questions such as "would it not be more prudent to build in additional safety factors to protect against effects to people who may be more sensitive than most because of young or old age, particular pathologies, or other causes of special vulnerability?" In the U.S., the Occupational Safety and Health Administration may only promulgate a new permissible exposure level for a chemical if can produce a credible estimate that the risk under the pre-existing standard is *significant* by some broadly defined quantitative criteria. To address these questions, we need to make at least quantitative estimates of the risks that result from current approaches.

One basic concept that lies at the heart of this analysis has not changed from the time of Lehman and Fitzhugh; the idea that many toxic effects result from placing a chemically-induced stress on an organism that exceeds some homeostatic buffering capacity. From this follows an expectation that there should be individual thresholds for such effects. An individual will show a particular response (or a response at a specific level of severity) only when the individual threshold exposure level for the chemical in question has been exceeded.

Now consider a population of individuals, each of whom has a different threshold for a particular response. How many people in a mixed group are affected depends on the fraction of people whose individual thresholds are exceeded at each exposure level. The broader the distribution of thresholds in the population—the greater the individual variability of the thresholds—the more gradual will be the decrease in the proportion of people showing a specific response as dose is lowered below the levels where effects can be readily observed in small test populations. For this reason, quantifying the functional form and degree of spread (interindividual variability) for individual threshold exposure levels is a key issue in quantitative risk assessment for this kind of biological response.[3]

Imagine, for purposes of illustration, that the distribution is log-normal; that is, that the logarithms of the individual thresholds have a normal Gaussian distribution. (This is the standard assumption that we use in our analysis below. Such a distribution would be expected if there are many factors, each contributing modestly to the individual variability in threshold doses, and if each factor tends to act multiplicatively to affect individual thresholds. This assumption of log-normality of population distributions of thresholds is by no means new—it is the basis for traditional probit analysis of toxicological data that predates Lehman and Fitzhugh.[9]) For example, consider a log-normal distribution with a Log_{10}(geometric standard deviation) of 0.5. (We abbreviate variability estimates in this form to Log(GSD).) This means that one standard deviation of the threshold dose population distribution corresponds to $10^{0.5}$ or just over a threefold change in dosage, and of course two standard deviations would correspond to a tenfold change in dosage. If 1 mg/kg of such a chemical causes an effect in 5% of the population (corresponding to a point in a cumulative log-normal distribution that is 1.645 standard deviations below the mean) then a tenfold reduction in dosage to 0.1 mg/kg would place us at a point $1.645 + 2 = 3.645$ standard deviations below the mean. From normal curve area tables (or, in Microsoft Excel, by using the *normsdist* function) one can easily determine that in this case the 0.1-mg/kg dose would be expected to affect about one in ten thousand of the population—again assuming that the distribution of thresholds is log-normal. If there were much less variability than this, a Log(GSD) of 0.25, the same tenfold reduction in dose to 0.1 mg/kg would yield a $1/0.25 = 4$ standard deviation difference in the population distribution, to a point 5.645 standard deviations below the mean. In this case the calculated risk would be very small; much less than one in a million. By a similar calculation, a higher Log(GSD) of 0.75 would imply a risk of 1.4 per thousand at 0.1 mg/kg.

To further illustrate the significance of log-normal variability, TABLE 1 shows the implications of various Log(GSD) variability values for the multiplicative difference

TABLE 1. A scale for understanding log-normal variability differences between particular percentiles of log-normal distributions[a]

Log_{10}(GSD)	Probit slope $1/\text{Log}_{10}$(GSD)	Geometric standard deviation	5%–95% Range (3.3 standard deviations)	1%–99% Range (4.6 standard deviations)
0.1	10	1.26	2.1-fold	2.9-fold
0.2	5	1.58	4.5-fold	8.5-fold
0.3	3.33	2.0	10-fold	25-fold
0.4	2.5	2.5	21-fold	73-fold
0.5	2	3.2	44-fold	210-fold
0.6	1.67	4.0	94-fold	620-fold
0.7	1.43	5.0	200-fold	1800-fold
0.8	1.25	6.3	430-fold	5,300-fold
0.9	1.11	7.9	910-fold	15,000-fold
1	1.0	10.0	1,900-fold	45,000-fold
1.1	0.91	12.6	4,200-fold	130,000-fold
1.2	0.83	15.8	8,900-fold	380,000-fold

[a]Adapted from Hattis.[10]

spanned by 3.3 standard deviations. If human susceptibility distributions were truly log-normal out to the extreme tails, then 3.4 standard deviations would be expected to be the difference between 20% and a 10^{-5} incidence of effect; 3.1 standard deviations would be expected to be the difference between a 5% and a 10^{-6} incidence of effect. Thus, the dosage spreads shown in TABLE 1 can be used as a crude first guess at the dose reduction that would be needed to take a typical LOAEL or NOAEL effect incidence (not incompatible with a 5% incidence of effect in typical cases) down close to or into the frequency region that has been considered *acceptable* for some general population exposures for the serious outcome of cancer.

Making calculations of this type, of course, begs the question of how well log-normal distributions actually describe real variability distributions out to the extreme tails. In this paper we do not examine the possible effects of departures from log-normality. However FIGURE 1A shows a comparison of 2700 individual data points from our pharmacokinetic data base with expectations under a log-normal distribution. In this figure, the *ordinal Z-score* is the inverse of the cumulative normal distribution calculated solely from the order statistics of the data using the formula of Cunane.[10]

$$\frac{i - 3/8}{N + 1/4}$$

where N is the number of data points in the data set, and i is the order of each data point in the data set (1 for the lowest and N for the highest). The log-normal Z-score for each data point is

$$\frac{\text{Log(data value)} - \text{mean of all Log(data values)}}{\text{standard deviation of all Log(data values)}}.$$

In all cases shown in FIGURE 1 the data points have been arranged so that the points to the right indicate relatively greater potential for toxicity (e.g., longer half-lives, smaller distribution volumes). FIGURE 1B shows an analogous comparison under the hypothesis that the data are normally distributed. It can be seen that the log-normal distribution provides a much better description of the data than does a normal distribution. Nevertheless, there appears to be some tendency for the data points at the extreme right of FIGURE 1A to be above, rather than below the line, indicating the log-normal expectation. This suggests that there may be some tendency toward bimodality, or other departures from log-normality for the larger data sets in the direction of having somewhat larger numbers of high risk values than would be expected. The statistical significance of this apparent tendency and possible implications for risk will be explored in future work. It is clear, however, that these data exhibit no apparent tendency for the distributions to be truncated at the high risk end, as might be expected if the variability in susceptibility due to these parameters were to be constrained to a defined upper limit.

We first briefly describe our data base of variability observations. Then we give our approaches for estimating the statistical uncertainties in our estimates of variability from individual data sets. These estimates of uncertainty are used in the following section to develop a set of statistically weighted estimates of the median amounts of variability associated with various steps in the causal pathway from external exposure to end-effects. From these estimates we derive estimates for the overall variability in susceptibility for median chemicals, with responses of different types and with different modes of exposure. Subsequently, we assess the spread of variability values for individual chemicals from the median-chemical predictions, after control for toxicity type, route of exposure, and statistical uncertainties in the derivation of the Log(GSD) estimates. Finally, based on the spread of likely Log(GSD) variability among chemicals/responses of a given type, we draw inferences about the degree of protection likely to be provided by the standard tenfold uncertainty factor, and arithmetic mean *expected value* estimates of risk at various fractions of a dose that produces a 5% response in a mixed human population. These results update those in a previous report[11] to the U.S. Occupational Safety and Health Administration based on unweighted analyses of a portion of the present data base.

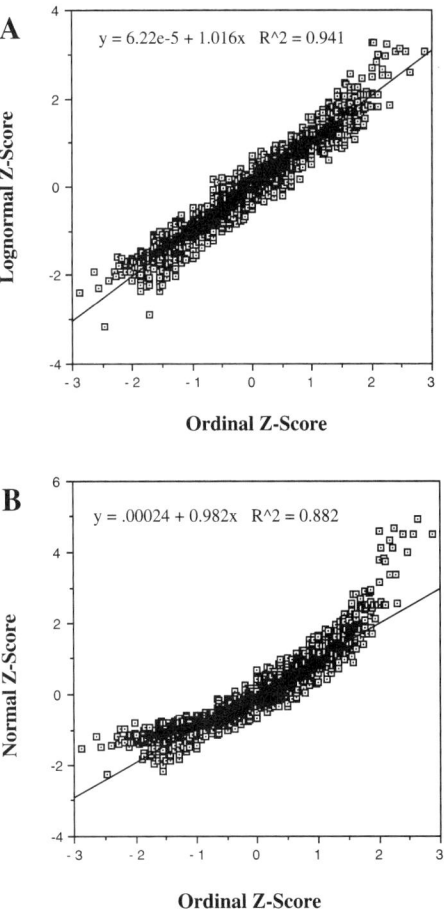

FIGURE 1. Comparison of 2700 pharmacokinetic data points with expectations: **A.** log-normal distribution; **B.** normal distribution.

DESCRIPTION OF THE DATA BASE

Screening criteria and basic approaches for analyzing many of the individual observations of variability have been described in previous papers,[2–4,11–16] of which the most comprehensive and recent summary can be found in Reference 16. By an *observation* of variability, we do not mean a single measurement of a relevant parameter in an individual, but the variability within a data set of separate values for at least five people, summarized by a Log(GSD) value. The full data base, including detailed analyses and references, is available in the form of Microsoft Excel spreadsheets from the first author of this paper. Documentation can also be obtained via our website, www.clarku.edu/~dhattis.

For cases for which the data were in the form of individual measurements of a continuous parameter, Log(GSD) values were calculated directly as the standard deviations of the Log_{10}-transformed parameter values. This was done for all the pharmacokinetic data and for a few cases where parameters with pharmacodynamic information were presented in the form of continuous parameter values (e.g., internal concentrations causing 50% of some specified maximal effect). Additionally, for pharmacokinetic observations where the same parameter had been measured in more than one independent study for a particular chemical, we pooled the observed within-study variances to derive a combined estimate of a Log(GSD). Thus, some of the individual *observations* reflect information from several different data sets.

For the great majority of observations of pharmacodynamic variability, the data were given in the form of the fraction of an exposed group that met some criterion of physiological parameter change or response. In these cases we used a spreadsheet system described by Haas[17] to make maximum likelihood Log(GSD) estimates from a probit[4,9] population dose-response model. Where the data included a control group with a finite incidence of the effect being studied, the models included a background term whose value was also estimated by likelihood maximization. In addition, where age-related information was given that seemed to be important in determining the response, the background response term was made dependent on the average age of each group in the analysis. Finally, for some large data sets of the variability of contact rates (e.g., breathing rates and tap water ingestion rates), where the original data were presented as the values at various percentiles of a population distribution, Log(GSD) values were calculated as the slopes of regression lines from probability plots.[16]

The different parameters whose variability has been measured incorporate variability for different portions of the pathway, from external exposure to end effects. Therefore each parameter is assigned a set of *dummy*-variable classifications of (0 or 1) that indicate the kinds of variability that are included. For example, measurement of the integrated area under the curve (AUC)—the product of internal concentration and time per mg/kg of administered dose, includes variability in steps #2-#5 in the following schema:

1. Contact rate: breathing rates/body weight; fish consumption/body weight (subclassified by oral, inhalation, or other route).
2. Uptake or absorption (mg/kg)/intake or contact rate (subclassified by oral, inhalation, or other route).

3. General systemic availability net of first pass elimination and dilution via distribution volume (subclassified by oral versus inhalation/other route).
4. Dilution via distribution volume.
5. Systemic elimination/clearance or half-life.
6. Active site availability/general systemic availability.
7. Physiological parameter change/active site availability.
8. Functional reserve capacity: change in baseline physiological parameter needed to pass a criterion of abnormal function.

Measurements of the fraction of people who experience a given percentage change in the amount of air they can exhale in one second (FEV_1) in relation to an exposure to ozone in external air, are classified as having variability types 1–7; whereas, measurements of the fraction of patients who suffer dose-limiting toxic symptoms in relation to plasma concentrations of an administered drug, are considered to include variability types 6–8.

In addition to these sources of real variability in items that are relevant to susceptibility distributions, some data sets implicitly included variability and/or uncertainty of other types. Four observations resulted from epidemiological studies of occupational or community groups for which there was considerable uncertainty about individual exposure levels. For these cases we included a dummy variable, indicating the additional source of apparent variability in order to isolate uncertainty in individual dosimetry from the estimates of real variability affecting estimates of risk. In a few other cases, C_{max} (maximum blood or plasma concentrations) and AUC pharmacokinetic parameters were measured after administering a dose of a drug expressed in weight units (e.g., a 200 mg pill), but there was no accompanying information about individual body weights to permit normalization of the results per dose in mg/kg body weight. In these cases we included an additional dummy variable to represent the fact that the data set included variability in body weights in the test population. Although this variable is needed to help explain the aggregate variability seen in some of the observations, it is not relevant to the variability in susceptibility per unit mg/kg dose and will not be included in later summary calculations of risks related to the usual application of the tenfold uncertainty factor.

Given this classification, TABLE 2 offers a simple unweighted summary of the variability data for pharmacokinetic and contact rate parameters. TABLE 3 does the same for parameters that include pharmacodynamic variability. As noted in the table footnotes, the 10%–90% ranges in each cell are calculated by assuming that the Log(GSD) observations within each grouping are themselves log-normally distributed. FIGURES 2–4 show probability plots that indicate rough correspondence of the distributions of LogLog(GSD) values to regression lines for log-normal expectations.

Of these types, pharmacodynamic variability data are by far the most difficult to find. To convey a clearer impression of the nature of pharmacodynamic observations, TABLES 4 and 5 list the individual measurements included in this group. TABLE 4 gives observations of variability in parameter change and response susceptibility at sites of direct contact with an agent (e.g., eye, skin, and respiratory system irritation). TABLE 5 shows cases where the toxicant travels systematically before reaching the site of action. (Derivation of the confidence limits for individual data points is described in the next section.) It can be seen that the pharmacodynamic observations

TABLE 2. Summary of unweighted Log(GSD) variability observations for different types of uptake and pharmacokinetic parameters in adults (data for groups including children under 12 excluded)

Parameter type	Oral	Intravenous	Inhalation	Other routes	All routes + route-nonspecific data
Blood concentration for toxicant delivered mainly by indicated route	0.322[a] (3) 0.295–0.351				0.322 (3) 0.295–0.351
Body weight (adults only)					0.086 (2) 0.065–0.113
Contact rate/body weight	0.257 (1—tap water daily intake)		0.108 (2—daily) 0.094–0.125	0.168 (1) (time showering)	0.150 (4) 0.088–0.256
Volume of distribution/body weight					0.128 (16) 0.058–0.284
Volume of distribution with no control for body weight					0.092 (1)
C_{max}/(dose/body weight)	0.147 (20) 0.059–0.367	0.154 (1)	0.071 (1)	0.224 (1)	0.145 (23) 0.060–0.350
C_{max}/dose with no control for body weight	0.225 (2) 0.133–0.379	0.177 (1)		0.238 (3) 0.169–0.334	0.222 (6) 0.156–0.315
Elimination half-life or clearance/body weight					0.112 (70) 0.058–0.214
Clearance with no control for body weight					0.116 (2) 0.046–0.289
AUC/(dose/body weight)	0.147 (20) 0.072–0.301	0.118 (9) 0.071–0.197	0.149 (1)	0.132 (4) 0.052–0.336	0.137 (34) 0.070–0.269
AUC/dose with no control for body weight	0.187 (11) 0.107–0.326	0.073 (1)		0.271 (2) 0.200–0.367	0.184 (14) 0.099–0.344
Total adult uptake and pharmacokinetic observations	(57)	(12)	(4)	(11)	(175)

[a]Within each cell of this table, the geometric mean of the Log(GSD) observations is given on the first line, the number of observations appears on the second line, and the third line gives a 10%–90% range of the observations calculated assuming that the Log(GSD) values themselves are log-normally distributed. Each *observation* consists of one or more data sets where the variability of a particular parameter was measured. In cases where the same pharmacokinetic parameter was measured for the same chemical in different groups of people, the variance was pooled to form a single *observation*.

TABLE 3. Summary of unweighted Log(GSD) variability observations for different types of pharmacodynamic parameters

	GI Tract	Nervous system	Respiratory system	Cardiovascular renal system + receptor-based effects	Other (e.g., eye, skin irritation)	All effects
Local (contact site) parameter change/external exposure or dose			0.357 (4) 0.272–0.468			0.357 (4) 0.272–0.468
Local (contact site) response/external exposure or dose	0.325 (1—stomach pH)		0.475 (7) 0.208–1.087		0.481 (6) 0.238–0.972	0.465 (14) 0.226–0.959
Physiological parameter change/internal concentration after systemic delivery		0.252 (5) 0.191–0.331		0.056 (2—Na$^+$ or K$^+$ excret./drug excret.) 0.042–0.075		0.164 (7) 0.062–0.434
Physiological parameter change/external (IV) systemic dose		0.195 (1—cisplatin *significant* hearing loss)				0.195 (1)
Response/blood level or internal concentration after systemic delivery		0.206 (7) 0.103–0.412		0.519 (3) 0.375–0.720	0.502 (1— cataracts)	0.288 (11) 0.128–0.647
Response/external dose (IV or oral admin.) without large dosimetric uncertainty		0.497 (1—haloperidol dose limiting tox)		0.546 (1—ibuprophen dental pain analgesia)		0.521 (2) 0.479–0.568
Response/external dose with large dosimetric uncertainty (e.g., workplace epidemiology)			1.33 (1—talc lung disease)	0.684 (3) 0.430–1.09		0.807 (4) 0.456–1.43
Total observations including pharmacodynamic variability	(1)	(14)	(12)	(9)	(7)	(43)

NOTE: Within each cell of this table, the geometric mean of the Log(GSD) observations is given on the first line, the number of observations appears on the second line, and the third line gives a 10%–90% range of the observations calculated assuming that the Log(GSD) values themselves are log-normally distributed. For example, differences in the internal concentration needed to produce a specific fraction of an individual's maximal response in a measured parameter, such as specific changes on an electroencephalograph.

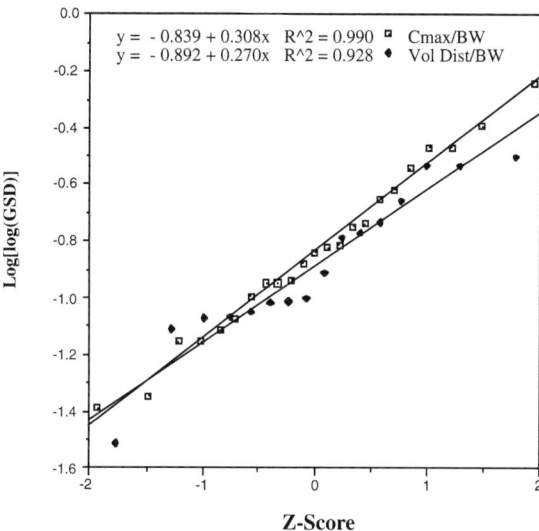

FIGURE 2. Log-normal plots of 23 C_{max}/body weight and 16 volume of distribution/body weight interindividual variability observations.

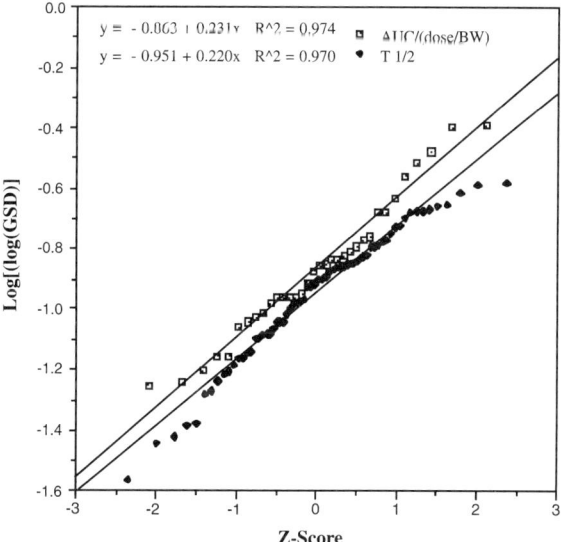

FIGURE 3. Log-normal plots of 34 AUC/body weight and 70 T1/2 or clearance/body weight interindividual variability observations.

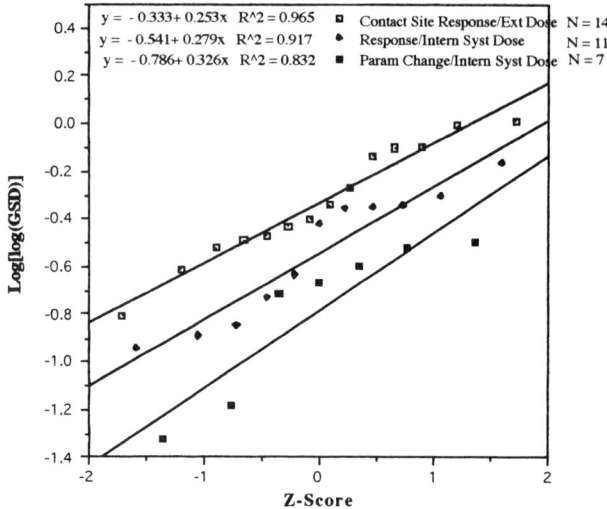

FIGURE 4. Log-normal plots of Log(GSD) values for three types of parameters that include pharmacodynamic variability.

tend to include much larger estimates of interindividual variability than the pharmacokinetic observations. Furthermore, among the pharmacodynamic observations, cases for which *response* is measured tend to show more variability than do cases for which the endpoint is some degree of change in a physiological parameter. In our schema, this difference is interpreted as indicating variability among people in functional reserve capacity; the amount of change in a physiologic parameter needed to cause different individuals to show a response—Step 8 in the outline given above.

STATISTICAL UNCERTAINTY IN THE ESTIMATES OF INTERINDIVIDUAL VARIABILITY

For continuous parameters, a standard statistical text[33] gives a formula for 95% confidence limits on the variance, σ^2, of a normally distributed parameter as:

$$\frac{(n-1)\hat{S}^2}{a} \text{ and } \frac{(n-1)\hat{S}^2}{b},$$

where n is the number of data points, a and b are the 0.025 and 0.975 fractiles, respectively, of a chi-squared distribution with $n-1$ degrees of freedom, and $\hat{S}^2$ is the observed unbiased estimator of the variance—the square of the ordinary standard deviation with $n-1$ weighting. In general, any fractile of the confidence distribution for σ^2 can be calculated similarly by adjusting the fractile of the chi-squared distribution.

TABLE 4. Detailed listing of pharmacodynamic variability observations at sites of direct contact with the toxicant

Parameter and reference	Chemical	Route	Log(GSD)	5%–95% conf. limits on Log(GSD)	Statistical weight = 1/variance of Log Log(GSD)
Long term FEV1 change/pack-year of smoking[3]	cigarette smoking	inhalation	0.279	0.25–0.31	1101
Specific airway resistance—conc. needed for 100% increase in individual baseline value[18]	methacholine	inhalation	0.421	0.39–0.46	1986
FEV1 change in relation to CXT of ozone exposure (clinical)[4]	ozone	inhalation	0.321	0.28–0.37	761
FEV1 increase by antiasthmatic[15]	salbutamol	inhalation	0.431	0.31–0.61	120
Lowering of gastric pH below 2[19]	pantoprazole	oral	0.325	0.09–1.20	8
Nasal dryness[20]	ammonia	inhalation	0.340	0.18–0.64	36
Throat irritation[20]	ammonia	inhalation	0.156	0.10–0.25	67
Olfactory cognition—air concentrations needed to produce three levels of smell perception[21]	diallylamine	inhalation	0.369	0.27–0.51	142
Nose irritation—slight or moderate[21]	diallylamine	inhalation	0.803	0.49–1.33	57
Nose irritation—slight or moderate[21]	mono-allylamine	inhalation	0.459	0.26–0.82	42
Nose irritation—slight or moderate[21]	triallylamine	inhalation	0.735	0.59–0.91	310
Pulmonary discomfort—*slight* and *moderate* or more[21]	triallylamine	inhalation	1.038	0.78–1.38	180
Eye irritation—external air concentration causing four levels[21]	acrolein	air—direct contact	0.301	0.23–0.39	229
Eye irritation[20]	ammonia	air—direct contact	0.243	0.13–0.45	39
Skin hypersensitivity to chromium (VI)[3]	chromium VI	skin	0.989	0.84–1.17	511
Eye irritation—slight or moderate and above[21]	diallylamine	air—direct contact	0.398	0.28–0.56	122
Skin irritation response to sodium laurel sulfate applied via skin patch[22]	sodium lauryl sulfate	skin	0.797	0.53–1.20	87
Eye irritation—slight or moderate and above[21]	triallylamine	air—direct contact	0.539	0.48–0.60	1228
Pneumoconiosis (two levels) in relation to cumulative talc air exposure (inc. dosimetry)[23]	talc	inhalation	1.330	0.78–2.25	52

TABLE 5. Detailed listing of observations of systemic pharmacodynamic variability

Parameter and reference	Chemical	Route	Log(GSD)	5%–95% conf. limits on Log(GSD)	Statistical weight = 1/variance of LogLog(GSD)
Diuretic efficiency (ml/µg) (Drug induced urine flow/drug excretion rate)[24]	furosemide	IV	0.048	0.03–0.07	74
Natriuretic efficiency (ml/µg) (drug induced response/drug excretion rate)[24]	furosemide	IV	0.066	0.04–0.10	74
EC50-effect site concentration producing 50% of predetermined maximal EEG changes[25]	alfentanil	IV	0.214	0.12–0.38	43
EC50-concentration producing 50% max. monoamine oxidase-A inhibition[26]	befloxatone	oral	0.194	0.14–0.28	117
EC50-effect site concentration producing 50% of a predetermined maximal EEG change[25]	fentanyl	IV	0.302	0.17–0.54	43
Proportion of patients receiving more than 95% of their individual maximal response in relation to plasma conc.[15]	imiprimine	oral	0.253	0.20–0.33	224
EC50-effect site concentration producing 50% of a predetermined maximal EEG change[25]	trefentanil	IV	0.319	0.20–0.51	64
Significant hearing loss/one dose of cisplatin[15]	cisplatin	IV	0.195	0.13–0.29	99
Haloperidol toxicity (minimum of four other signs mostly neurological)[27]	haloperidol	oral	0.115	0.06–0.22	36
Ataxia/blood level[28]	MeHg	diet	0.232	0.16–0.34	99
Deaths/blood level[28]	MeHg	diet	0.128	0.06–0.28	24
Disarthria/blood level[28]	MeHg	diet	0.186	0.08–0.45	19
Hearing defects/blood level[28]	MeHg	diet	0.143	0.09–0.23	60
Paresthesia/blood level[28]	MeHg	diet	0.382	0.27–0.53	127
Visual effects/blood level[28]	MeHg	diet	0.458	0.33–0.63	135
High β2M urinary excretion vs. occupational blood conc X time[4]	cadmium	inhalation	0.697	0.50–0.97	129
High β2M urinary excretion vs. urinary Cd[4]	cadmium	diet	0.445	0.37–0.53	442
High β2M urinary excretion vs. urinary Cd[4]	cadmium	diet	0.452	0.37–0.55	353
Cataracts in relation to TNT hemoglobin adducts[4]	trinitro-toluene	inhalation	0.502	0.37–0.69	144
Dose-limiting toxicity including malaise, neurotoxicity, pericardial effusion[29]	suramin	IV	0.497	0.19–1.27	16
Analgesia from dental pain (not taking medication at three and six hours after procedure)[30]	ibuprofen	oral	0.546	0.36–0.82	85
High β2M urinary excretion in relation to diet, controlling for age (inc. dosimetry)[31,32]	cadmium	diet, females	0.499	0.37–0.66	175
High β2M urinary excretion in relation to diet, controlling for age (inc. dosimetry)[31,32]	cadmium	diet, males	0.631	0.42–0.95	86
High β2M urinary excretion vs. occupational air conc X time (inc. dosimetry)[4]	cadmium	inhalation	1.016	0.73–1.42	129

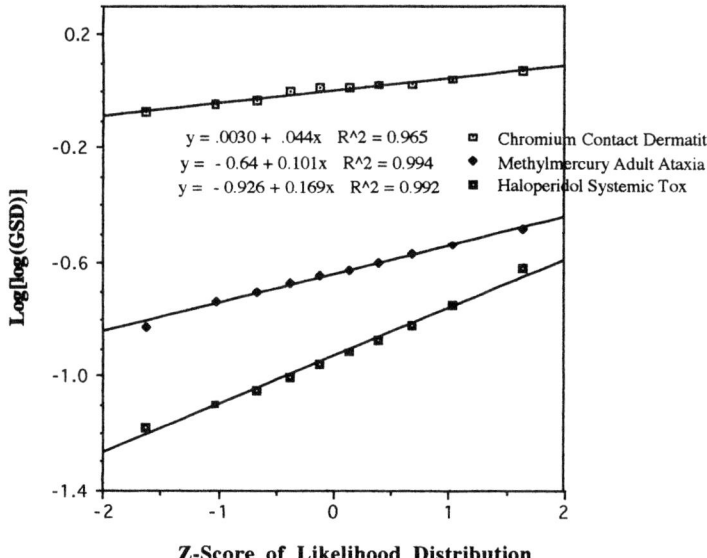

FIGURE 5. Log-normal probability plots of the likelihood distributions for quantal pharmacodynamic interindividual variability observations.

In model calculations we computed a large number of points on confidence distributions for log-normal distributions with different absolute values of Log(GSD) and n. We found that the desirable *statistical weight* for our analysis, the reciprocal of the variance of the LogLog(GSD) for each data set, was not affected by the absolute value of the Log(GSD) estimates but could be simply described by an empirical formula depending only on n:

$$\text{Weight} = 10.6n - 10.33$$

(approximately proportional to $n - 1$).

For quantal response parameters we used the Haas[17] spreadsheet-based likelihood fitting system cited earlier to calculate ten equally spaced fractiles (from 0.05 through 0.95) of the confidence distribution for each Log(GSD). As can be seen in the examples plotted in FIGURE 5, these confidence distributions appear to be well described as log-normal. We simply used these values to derive the variance of the corresponding LogLog(GSD) values. As for the continuous parameters, the reciprocal of this variance was used as the statistical weight in our later modeling.

MODELING THE COMBINED SUSCEPTIBILITY VARIABILITY FOR MEDIAN CHEMICALS—DEPENDENCE ON TYPES OF TOXICITY AND ROUTE OF EXPOSURE

If we assume that the interindividual variability, for each of several different steps in the causal sequence, from contact rate to effect, is independent and log-normal, then the population distribution of the overall variability in susceptibility can be described simply as a log-normal distribution with variance equal to the sum of the lognormal variances at the component steps. For example, for an inhaled chronic systemic toxicant,

$$\text{Log(GSD)}_{\text{total}} = \sqrt{\begin{array}{c}(\text{Log(GSD)}_{\text{total}})^2 + (\text{Log(GSD)}_{\text{fraction absorb}})^2 \\ + \ldots + (\text{Log(GSD)}_{\text{functional reserve}})^2\end{array}}$$

Based on this approach, we have developed a simple spreadsheet optimization model to estimate the median-chemical Log(GSD) values for each causal step, from external exposure to end response, that best correspond to our 226 observations. Given a set of starting values for the median-chemical Log(GSD) values for each causal step, and the set of dummy variables assigned to characterize which kinds of variability are included in each observation, the model makes a *prediction* of the expected median-chemical Log(GSD) for that observation. Then, in a series of iterative trials, the system calculates the set of median-chemical Log(GSD) values for each causal step that minimize the sum of the squares of the observed versus the predicted LogLog(GSD) values for all observations combined. This quantity is chosen for minimization because of the earlier finding that both the variability (FIGS. 2–4) and the uncertainty (FIG. 5) in Log(GSD) values appear to be reasonably described as log-normal. Parallel analyses are conducted by minimizing the sum of squares with and without the statistical weights derived in the previous section. In all cases the Log(GSD) values for each step are constrained to be nonnegative, because a negative values for a step-specific estimate of variability would be meaningless. TABLES 6–8 show the median-chemical Log(GSD) values for individual steps between contact rate and end effects that result from our model. For each table, the individual steps representing specific types of variability are shown in the first column. Each subsequent column represents a set of median-chemical Log(GSD) estimates that results from a progressive series of selections from the data base of variability observations. For comparison, the second column in each table gives results from a previous unweighted analysis[11] of the 126 variability observations that were available as of May, 1997. TABLE 6 shows results of analyses that only include physiological parameter changes and responses at sites of direct contact with external agents (i.e., those observations that were individually listed in TABLE 4). TABLES 7 and 8 show analyses of the full data base with progressive exclusions so that the final three columns combine the contact-rate and pharmacokinetic observations only with pharmacodynamic data on systemic toxic responses (excluding the direct-contact observations). TABLE 7 and the upper part of TABLE 6 show the results of unweighted analyses, in which each observation is treated equally in the optimization process. TABLE 8 and the lower part of TABLE 6 show the results using the statistical weights, in which the deviation of each observation from the corresponding model prediction is weighted in proportion to the inverse of the variance of the primary observation in the optimization.

Comparing the first numerical column with the subsequent columns in these tables, it can be seen that the expansion of the data base from 126 to 226 observations has not, in itself, given rise to major changes in the overall picture of step-specific

TABLE 6. Summary of median variability for specific steps for direct contact physiological parameter change and response

	Previous unweighted results[11]	Data only including direct contact observations	Data only including direct contact respiratory system observations	Direct contact observations for non-respiratory responses
A. Unweighted Analysis				
Number of observations	6	18	11	7
All steps up through physiological parameter change/active site availability	0.393	0.357	0.357	allocation not meaningful—all observations are responses
Functional reserve capacity—change in baseline physiological parameter needed to pass a criterion of abnormal function	0.499	0.298	0.314	allocation not meaningful—all observations are responses
Summary Log(GSD) for direct contact effects	0.635	0.465	0.475	0.455
B. Weighted Analysis				
Number of observations	6	18	11	7
All steps up through physiological parameter change/active site availability	0.393	0.357	0.357	allocation not meaningful—all observations are responses
Functional reserve capacity—change in baseline physiological parameter needed to pass a criterion of abnormal function	0.499	0.455	0.470	allocation not meaningful—all observations are responses
Summary Log(GSD) for direct contact effects	0.635	**0.578**	**0.590**	**0.574**

NOTE: The bold-face numbers are used for subsequent risk calculations in TABLE 11.

TABLE 7. Unweighted analysis: summary of median estimates of human interindividual variability for various steps in the pathway from external exposure to response

			Data Inclusions/Exclusions				
	Previous unweighted results[11]	All data, incl children and var. inflation	All adult data, including var. inflation	All adult data excluding var. inflation	Uptake, PK and 21 systemic PD obs. excluding direct contact PD obs.	Uptake, PK and only 14 systemic neurological PD obs.	Uptake, PK and 7 systemic non-neurological PD obs.
Number of variability observations included	126	226	218	214	196	189	182
Oral contact rate (tap water, fish consumpt/Kg BW)	0.286	0.275	0.257	0.266	0.264	0.264	0.264
Inhalation contact rate (breathing rate/Kg BW)	0.286	0.103	0.174	0.170	0.108	0.108	0.108
Other contact rate	0.286	0.168	0.168	0.168	0.168	0.168	0.168
Oral uptake or absorption (mg/Kg)/intake or contact rate	0.117	0.000	0.000	0.000	0.000	0.000	0.000
Inhalation fraction absorbed	0.117	0.103	0.000	0.000	0.000	0.000	0.000
Other route fraction absorbed	0.117	0.113	0.113	0.112	0.000	0.000	0.000
Oral systemic availability net of local or first pass liver metabolism	0.000	0.057	0.073	0.073	0.080	0.080	0.080
Systemic availability after absorption by inhalation or other route	0.000	0.000	0.000	0.000	0.000	0.000	0.000
Body weight correction	not included	0.083	0.083	0.083	0.089	0.089	0.089
Dilution via distribution volume/BW	0.075	0.121	0.113	0.113	0.113	0.113	0.113
Systemic elimination half life or clearance/BW	0.110	0.110	0.107	0.107	0.107	0.107	0.107
Active site availability/general systemic availability	0.000	0.000	0.000	0.000	0.071	0.000	0.347
Physiological parameter change/active site availability	0.079	0.186	0.179	0.180	0.158	0.227	0.056
Functional reserve capacity—change in physiological parameter needed for effect	0.338	0.316	0.316	0.316	0.252	0.000	0.445
Likely inflated variability— imperfect epidemiological estimation of exposure/dose	0.753	0.691	0.688				

TABLE 8. Weighted analysis: summary of median estimates of human interindividual variability for various steps in the pathway from external exposure to response

	Previous unweighted results[11]	Data Inclusions/Exclusions					
		All data, inc. children and var. inflation	All adult data, including var. inlation	All adult data excluding var. inflation	Uptake, PK and 21 systemic PD obs. excluding direct contact PD obs.	Uptake, PK and only 14 systemic neurological PD obs.	Uptake, PK and 7 systemic non-neurological PD obs.
Number of variability observations included	126	226	218	214	196	189	182
Oral contact rate (tap water, fish consumpt/Kg BW)	0.286	0.261	0.261	0.261	0.261	0.261	0.261
Inhalation contact rate (breathing rate/Kg BW)	0.286	0.090	0.117	0.117	0.117	0.117	0.117
Other contact rate	0.286	0.168	0.168	0.168	0.168	0.168	0.168
Oral uptake or absorption(mg/Kg)/intake or contact rate	0.117	0.000	0.000	0.000	0.000	0.000	0.000
Inhalation fraction absorbed	0.117	0.276	0.263	0.259	0.000	0.000	0.000
Other route fraction absorbed	0.117	0.072	0.068	0.068	0.000	0.000	0.000
Oral systemic availability net of local or first pass liver metabolism	0.000	0.091	0.107	0.107	0.110	0.110	0.109
Systemic availability after absorption by inhalation or other route	0.000	0.000	0.000	0.000	0.000	0.000	0.000
Body weight correction	not included	0.087	0.087	0.087	0.087	0.087	0.087
Dilution via distribution volume/BW	0.075	0.124	0.113	0.113	0.112	0.112	0.112
Systemic elimination half life or clearance/BW	0.110	0.136	0.135	0.135	0.135	0.135	0.135
Active site availability/general systemic availability	0.000	0.087	0.082	0.080	0.145	0.000	0.350
Physiological parameter change/active site availability	0.079	0.175	0.177	0.180	0.146	0.233	0.056
Functional reserve capacity—change in physiological parameter needed for effect	0.338	0.461	0.460	0.460	0.367	0.149	0.444
Likely inflated variability— imperfect epidemiological estimation of exposure/dose	0.753	0.405	0.408				

variabilities. The largest single contributor to overall variability is the last step or two in the process, representing pharmacodynamic variability (2–4 lines from the bottom in TABLES 7 and 8). What is somewhat different is that the weighted analyses, done here for the first time (TABLE 8), indicate somewhat larger variability than the unweighted analyses. Evidently the statistically stronger data sets happened to indicate larger amounts of variability than some of the statistically weaker data sets.

Progressing to the third numerical column in TABLES 7 and 8, it can be seen that excluding the very small number of data sets that have values for young children does not materially change the overall results. Furthermore, excluding the four data points that are likely to include substantial uncertainty in individual dosimetry (fourth numerical column) results in very little difference in the estimates. By contrast, excluding the direct contact observations, moving from the fourth to the fifth numerical columns in these tables, does cause a noticeable change in the variability allocated to the final three steps. A modest increase in variability for active site availability/general systemic availability is more than offset by reductions in the two last steps. This is further modified when systemic neurological and non-neurological observations of pharmacodynamic observations are segregated in the final two columns (although it should be stressed that the data are too few at this stage for us to be confident that the suggestion that non-neurological endpoints are more variable will survive as additional information accumulates).

One advantage of having these variability results disaggregated by causal steps in the pathway from contact to effect, is that one can recombine the step-specific results to estimate overall variability in susceptibility for different types of toxicants presented to people in different media. This is done by simply combining the logarithmic variances for the relevant steps, as illustrated in the previous section with the equation for the overall variability of an inhaled chronic systemic toxicant. TABLES 9 and 10 show the overall Log(GSD) values that result from a variety of such combinations in the same format that was previously used for TABLES 7 and 8. The aggregate Log(GSD) values for agents causing effects at the sites of direct contact with external agents were given previously in TABLE 6.

The bold face entries in TABLES 6 and 10 represent the *bottom line* results that we believe are most salient as points of departure for estimating risks for different categories of toxicants. These are used in later risk calculations. Of these, the results in the second line of TABLE 10 (for an oral agent whose dose is expressed in mg/kg, without allowing for contract rate variability) provide the single most relevant set of variability estimates for comparison with expectations for the original Lehman-Fitzhugh food additive/pesticide residue context. Without further calculation, however, it can be seen that, because most of the interindividual variability indicated by the present data base is associated with the pharmacodynamic steps, the details of route of exposure for systemic toxicants exert mainly second-order effects. Comparing TABLE 6 with TABLE 10, however, it can be seen that there is an appreciable tendency for the direct-contact responses to be associated with greater overall variability than the systemic toxic responses.

TABLE 9. Unweighted analysis: summary aggregate Log(GSD) estimates for different types of toxicants delivered in different ways

Type of agent and mode of administration	Previous unweighted results[11]	All data, incl. children and var. inflation	All adult data, including var. inflation	All adult data, excluding var. inflation	Uptake, PK and 21 systemic PD obs. excluding direct contact PD obs.	Uptake, PK and only 14 systemic neurological PD obs.	Uptake, PK and 7 systemic non-neurological PD obs.
Ingested systemic chronic toxicant (including variability in ingestion behavior)	0.483	0.489	0.477	0.482	0.441	0.400	0.656
Chronic toxicity from an orally administered drug with perfect compliance (no contact rate variability)		0.405	0.402	0.402	0.353	0.287	0.593
Inhaled chronic systemic toxicant		0.427	0.431	0.430	0.360	0.296	0.598
Chronic systemic toxicant delivered by other route		0.449	0.444	0.444	0.382	0.323	0.611
Ingested systemic acute toxicant (no elimination rate variability)		0.477	0.465	0.470	0.428	0.375	0.641
Acute toxicity from an orally administered drug with perfect compliance (no contact or elim. rate variability)		0.390	0.387	0.388	0.336	0.266	0.584
Inhaled systemic acute toxicant		0.412	0.418	0.417	0.344	0.276	0.588
Systemic acute toxicant delivered by other route		0.435	0.430	0.431	0.367	0.304	0.602

TABLE 10. Weighted analysis: summary aggregate Log(GSD) estimates for different types of toxicants delivered in different ways

Type of agent and mode of administration	Previous unweighted results[11]	All data, incl. children and var. inflation	All adult data, including var. inlation	All adult data, excluding var. inflation	Uptake, PK and 21 systemic PD obs. excluding direct contact PD obs.	Uptake, PK and only 14 systemic neurological PD obs.	Uptake, PK and 7 systemic non-neurological PD obs.
Ingested systemic chronic toxicant (including variability in ingestion behavior)	0.483	0.601	0.600	0.600	**0.536**	0.441	0.664
Chronic toxicity from an orally administered drug with perfect compliance (no contact rate variability)		0.541	0.541	0.541	0.469	**0.345**	**0.605**
Inhaled chronic systemic toxicant		0.607	0.603	0.602	**0.470**	**0.347**	**0.606**
Chronic systemic toxicant delivered by other route		0.564	0.560	0.560	**0.485**	0.368	0.618
Ingested systemic acute toxicant (no elimination rate variability)		0.585	0.585	0.585	**0.519**	0.411	0.645
Acute toxicity from an orally administered drug with perfect compliance (no contact or elim. rate variability)		0.524	0.524	0.524	**0.449**	0.318	0.590
Inhaled systemic acute toxicant		0.592	0.588	0.586	**0.451**	0.320	0.591
Systemic acute toxicant delivered by other route		0.547	0.544	0.544	**0.466**	0.342	0.603

NOTE: The bold-face numbers are used for subsequent risk calculations in TABLE 11.

ASSESSING THE SPREAD OF VARIABILITY VALUES AMONG CHEMICALS

Policies that utilize safety/uncertainty factors as a guide to risk management do so repeatedly for many chemicals with different toxic effects. Each risk management choice under such a system essentially makes a random draw from a group of chemicals and effects for which the mixed human population is likely to have different amounts of real interindividual variability in susceptibility. It is therefore important to assess the extent of real variation among chemicals/effects in the Log(GSD) values for human susceptibility.

One indicator of the possible extent of this variation is the spread of Log(GSD) values for similar types of parameters, such as the distributions plotted in FIGURES 2-4. The slopes of the regression lines in these figures indicate LogLog(GSD) standard deviations within different parameter types in the range of 0.22–0.33. Unfortunately, these spreads include both real Log(GSD) variability among chemicals and additional spread due to uncertainties in the estimation of the individual Log(GSD) values from the samples of people studied. The real variability is, therefore, likely to be somewhat smaller.

To distinguish real variability among chemicals from uncertainties in the estimation of the individual Log(GSD) values we borrow a technique from meta analyses and array the observed minus model predicted Log(Log(GSD) value deviations by the statistical strength of the individual data points, in the form of *funnel* plots.[34] The

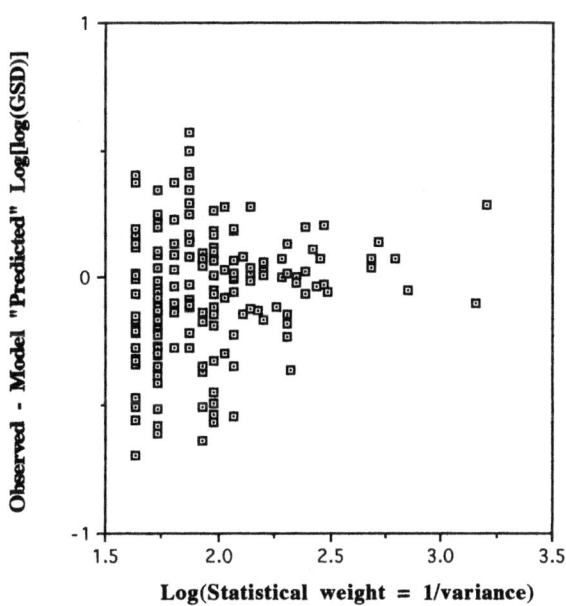

FIGURE 6. Funnel plot for pharmacokinetic interindividual variability observations.

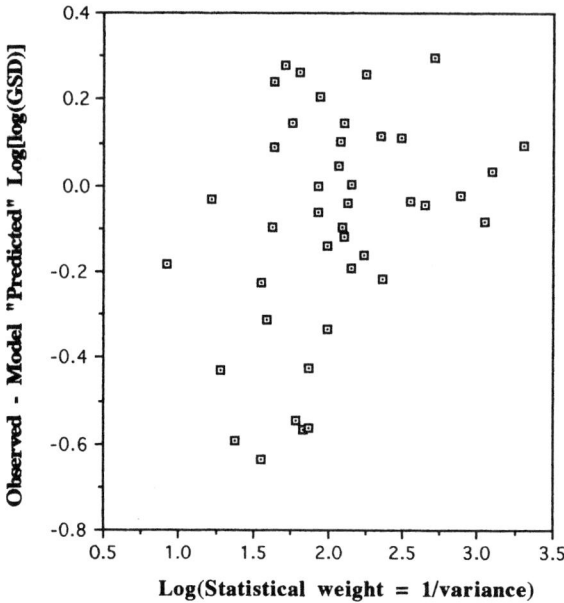

FIGURE 7. Funnel plot for pharmacodynamic interindividual variability observations.

expectation here is that the points will form a funnel shape with a wider variation in observed minus predicted results for the weaker data points on the left side of these plots, narrowing to a smaller residual variation (small part of the funnel) for the stronger points at the right. The basic idea is that the spread at the wider end of the funnel includes both real and chemical variation in Log(GSD) for a given parameter and measurement errors. At the narrower end of the funnel, however, the statistically stronger data points may have measurement errors that are small relative to the real variability among chemicals. FIGURES 6 and 7 show such plots for the individual pharmacokinetic and pharmacodynamic observations, respectively. FIGURES 8 and 9 show the observations grouped together to better reveal numerical trends in the spread among chemicals, quantified as the root mean square error (equivalent to a standard deviation) of the observed minus predicted LogLog(GSD) values. It can be seen that in each case the plots appear to converge on the right to a between-chemical standard deviation of about 0.14 (the weighted average of all the data in the indicated regions from both plots is 0.138). This number is considerably less than the 0.22–0.32 range for the raw standard deviation of all the LogLog(GSD) values within various parameter types. In subsequent risk calculations we will therefore assume that the susceptibility Log(GSD) values for different chemicals are characterized by log-normal distributions with geometric means equal to the bold face values in TABLES 6 and 10, and a geometric standard deviation equal to $10^{0.138} = 1.37$.

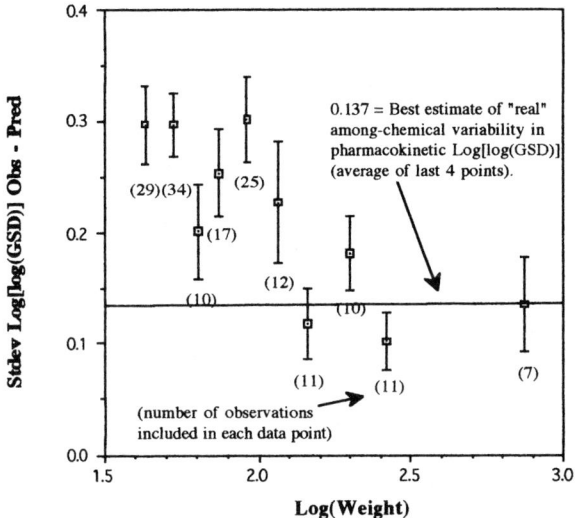

FIGURE 8. Relationship between root mean square prediction error and Log(statistical weight) for pharmacokinetic interindividual variability observations.

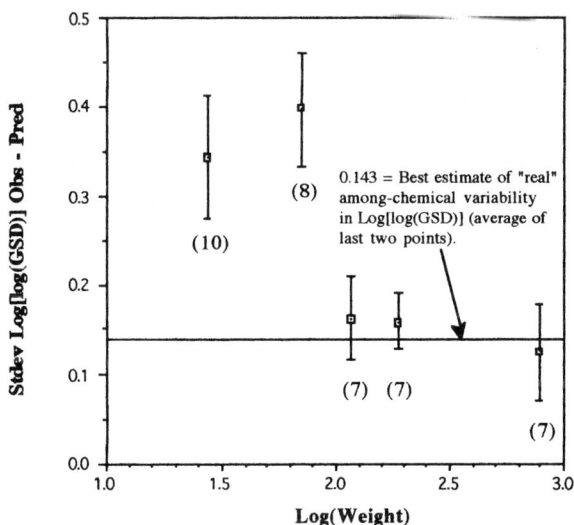

FIGURE 9. Relationship between root mean square prediction error and Log(statistical weight) for observations with pharmacodynamic interindividual variability.

TABLE 11. Weighted analysis: implications of the spread of variability results among chemicals; expected fraction of people showing a response at one tenth of the dose that produces the response in 5% of exposed people

	50% confidence (median chemical) risk	Arithmetic mean (expected value)	95th percentile chemical risk
Ingested systemic chronic toxicant (including variability in ingestion behavior)	2.2E–04	6.8E–04	3.0E–03
Chronic toxicity from an orally administered drug with perfect compliance (no contact rate variabity)	7.9E–05	3.7E–04	1.8E–03
Inhaled chronic systemic toxicant	8.1E–05	3.8E–04	1.8E–03
Chronic systemic toxicant delivered by other route	1.1E–04	4.4E–04	2.1E–03
Ingested systemic acute toxicant (no elimination rate variability)	1.8E–04	5.9E–04	2.7E–03
Acute toxicity from an orally administered drug with perfect compliance (no contact or elim. rate variabity)	5.4E–05	3.0E–04	1.5E–03
Inhaled systemic acute toxicant (no elimination rate variability)	5.6E–05	3.1E–04	1.5E–03
Systemic acute toxicant delivered by other route	7.6E–05	3.6E–04	1.8E–03
Chronic systemic neurological toxicity for an ingested drug with perfect compliance	2.8E–06	7.0E–05	3.9E–04
Chronic systemic non-neruological toxicity for an ingested drug with perfect compliance	4.9E–04	1.1E–03	4.3E–03
Chronic systemic neurological toxicity for an inhaled toxicant	3.1E–06	7.3E–05	4.1E–04
Chronic systemic non-neurological toxicity for an inhaled toxicant	4.9E–04	1.1E–03	4.4E–03
Acute systemic neurological toxicity for an inhaled toxicant	9.4E–07	4.3E–05	2.4E–04
Acute systemic non-neurological toxicity for an inhaled toxicant	4.2E–04	1.0E–03	4.1E–03
All direct contact effects	3.7E–04	9.2E–04	3.8E–03
Direct-contact respiratory effects	4.2E–04	1.0E–03	4.0E–03
Direct-contact non-respiratory effects	3.5E–04	8.9E–04	3.7E–03

IMPLICATIONS FOR RISK AT ONE TENTH OF AN ED05 DOSE

On this basis, TABLE 11 shows the incidences of response that are expected for exposure of populations at one tenth of an ED05 dose for different chemicals/responses within and among different exposure and toxicity types. For the second line of the table, the case that most resembles the original Lehman-Fitzhugh context of an orally-administered drug or food additive that causes chronic systemic toxicity after presentation at a defined mg/kg dose, the risk for a median chemical is expected to be slightly less than one in 10,000; but a chemical that has more variability than 95% of other chemicals would be expected to cause an incidence of effect exceeding one in 1,000. Risks for some other categories of exposure mode and response extend up to several per 1,000 at the 95% confidence level. Thus, if the underlying estimates of the extent of log-normal response variability are approximately correct, use of the traditional tenfold safety/uncertainty factor, without any other protective factors, would appear to run risks of response incidences that are large enough to be of some concern, although they would generally be difficult to detect directly at those exposure levels in any but the largest and best controlled epidemiological studies of effects with low background levels of response.

In general, however, the tenfold uncertainty factor for interindividual variability is not used in isolation, but is combined with other uncertainty factors (e.g., for interspecies projections or use of subchronic data to predict chronic response levels) many of which may tend to provide additional protection in the cases of typical chemicals.[1,7,35] Full quantitative assessments of the incidences of response expected in these cases must take the uncertainty distributions of these other factors into account.

IMPLICATIONS FOR MEAN EXPECTED VALUE INCIDENCES OF RESPONSE AT VARIOUS FRACTIONS OF ED05 EXPOSURES

In a number of cases, legislative and administrative authorities concerned with the economic impacts of measures intended to protect human health have requested that quantitative analyses be done that would facilitate juxtapositions of health and economic effects of proposed actions.[36] For such comparisons, it is desirable to have arithmetic mean *expected value* estimates of health response and health benefits of control, in addition to the *upper confidence limit* estimates that others may desire in order to make judgments of the equity of the risks imposed on protected parties.[37] FIGURE 10 shows log-log plots of the results of these arithmetic mean calculations for various exposure mode and response categories as a function of dose reductions below a defined 5% incidence level at the ED05. From the correspondence of the points to the straight lines, it can be seen that these risk versus dose functions are well described as power-law relationships with exponents ranging from about 1.6 to 3.2 for the different cases shown.

In conclusion, the generic analysis of the ensemble of all studied chemicals and toxic responses provided here permits preliminary pathway-specific estimates to be made of likely health benefits in the absence of detailed information about the Log(GSD) values associated with a particular chemical and toxic response.

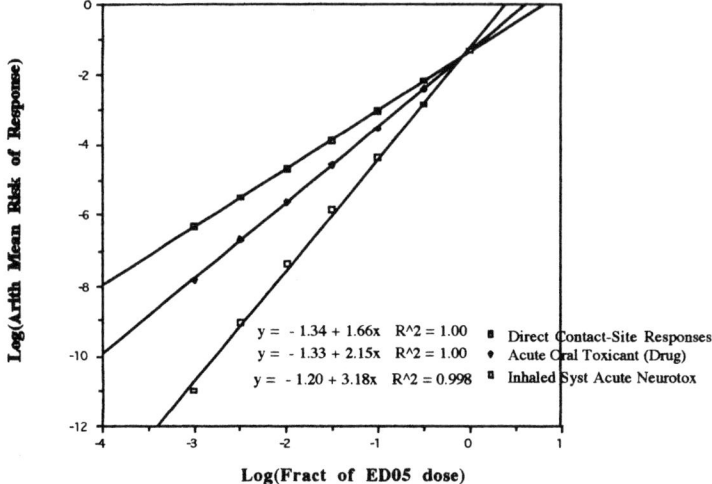

FIGURE 10. Log Log plots of model projections of the mean risk of toxicant exposures at various fractions of an ED05 dose or exposure level.

CAVEATS AND LIMITATIONS

This analysis should be understood as an early effort on the road toward quantitative analyses of effects that are produced by *threshold* (homeostatic system overwhelming) mechanisms. Not all non-cancer effects may be best treated in this way. Several other strategies for quantification dependent on different features of causal mechanisms were summarized in a previous paper.[4] Additionally, even within the context of effects whose mechanisms lend themselves to treatment as individual threshold responses, several notes of caution are in order:

- First, we have assumed that the data base of variability observations, for a highly diverse set of chemicals and toxic responses, is reasonably representative of the interindividual variability in cases that might be presented for evaluation by agencies charged with managing specific types of non-cancer risks. Some chemicals for which we have pharmacodynamic adverse effect information may have had that information collected and interindividual variability quantified just because there has been some visible toxic problem to be investigated by epidemiologists or toxicologists. The current data base may not be an unreasonable reflection of the spectrum of chemicals and effects encountered by an agency such as the U.S. Occupational Safety and Health Administration, which generally deals with problem chemicals for which toxicity of some sort has usually been noticed in human workers at not-uncommon exposure levels. However, these sets may not be entirely similar to the general purpose chemicals that are likely to be presented for decision-making by a regulator of food additives, for example; or even for the EPA Office of Toxic Substances, that evaluates new general industrial chemicals.

- Second, throughout this analysis we have assumed log-normal distributions of individual susceptibility in people, and, in the final analysis, log-normal distributions for the Log(GSD) values themselves. These assumptions appear to be generally compatible with the available data, but when projections are made to very low effect levels, the unsuspected presence of discrete subpopulations with unusual sensitivity could cause departures from population log-normality that would add uncertainty to the estimates of low dose risks.

- We have also implicitly assumed that each parameter included in our variability observations has a direct proportionate and independent effect on individual susceptibility (the dose at which an individual will experience a response), and that the combined effects of all the variability parameters are simply multiplicative. Correlations (positive or negative) between contact rate, pharmacokinetic, and pharmacodynamic variability parameters could appreciably modify the expected proportions of people who appear at the extreme tails of the population distribution of susceptibilities.

- Finally, we have not analyzed the measurement error and short term within-individual variability implicit in the individual estimates of human Log(GSD) values for various parameters. This could lead to a tendency to estimate higher risks than are actually likely to be present for chronic exposures. On the other hand, the populations studied for the original observations were generally less diverse than actual human populations likely to be exposed to toxicants. Investigators rarely include in their study groups very old or very young people, or people known to be suffering from serious pathologies that might make them specially vulnerable to the toxicants. This would be expected to result in understated risks relative to those likely to be experienced by more diverse groups of exposed people.

Nevertheless, recognizing these limitations, later efforts can strive to gather more extensive and better data, quantify as yet unanalyzed sources of uncertainty and variability, and eventually provide the foundation for risk analyses that can more frankly and fairly inform decision-makers, and the public, about the likely benefits of alternative policies to control exposures to chemicals posing toxic hazards.

ACKNOWLEDGMENTS

The analysis reported in this document was supported by a purchase order (#B9F74428) from the U.S. Occupational Safety and Health Administration. Construction of the underlying data base was supported by Grant # R825360 from the Office of Research and Development of the U.S. Environmental Protection Agency. The views expressed, however, are solely those of the authors and do not necessarily reflect either the technical or the policy judgments of either agency.

REFERENCES

1. BAIRD, S.J.S., J.T. COHEN, J.D. GRAHAM, A.I. SHLYAKHTER & J.S. EVANS. 1996. Noncancer risk assessment: A probabilistic alternative to current practice. Hum. Ecol. Risk Assess. **2:** 78–99.
2. HATTIS, D., L. ERDREICH & M. BALLEW. 1987. Human variability in susceptibility to toxic chemicals—a preliminary analysis of pharmacokinetic data from normal volunteers. Risk Analysis **7:** 415–426.
3. HATTIS, D. & K. SILVER. 1994. Human interindividual variability—a major source of uncertainty in assessing risks for non-cancer health effects. Risk Analysis **14:** 421–431.
4. HATTIS, D. 1998. Strategies for assessing human variability in susceptibility, and using variability to infer human risks. *In* Human Variability in Response to Chemical Exposure: Measures, Modeling, and Risk Assessment, D.A. Neumann and C.A. Kimmel, Eds.: 27–57. CRC Press, Boca Raton.
5. SWARTOUT, J.C., P.S. PRICE, M.L. DOURSON, H.L. CARLSON-LYNCH & R.E. KEENAN. 1998. A probabilistic framework for the reference dose (probabilistic RfD). Risk Anal. **18:** 271–282.
6. RENWICK, A.G. & N.R. LAZARUS. 1998. Human variability and noncancer risk assessment—an analysis of the default uncertainty factor. Regul. Toxicol. Pharmacol. **27:** 3–20.
7. RHOMBERG, L., S.J.S. BAIRD, G.M. GRAY, J.S. EVANS & J.T. COHEN. 1997. Framing for development of data-derived probability distributions in workshops of experts. Final Report for Health Canada, Priority Substances Section, Harvard Center for risk Analysis, Harvard School of Public Health, 718 Huntington Ave., Boston, MA.
8. LEHMAN, A.J. & O.G. FITZHUGH. 1954. 100-fold margin of safety. Assoc. Food Drug Off. U.S. Q. Bull. **18:** 33–35.
9. FINNEY, D.J. 1971. Probit Analysis, 3rd ed. Cambridge University Press, London.
10. CUNNANE, C. 1978. Unbiased plotting positions—a review. J. Hydrol. **37:** 205–222.
11. HATTIS, D., P. BANATI, I. SIROVIC & R. GOBLE. 1997. Preliminary analysis of a data base of human interindividual variability observations--implications for generic occupational health risk assessments for chronic toxic responses, Report to the Occupational Safety and Health Administration, Clark University, Worcester, MA.
12. HATTIS, D. 1997. Variability in susceptibility—how big, how often, for what responses to what agents? Environmental Toxicology and Pharmacology **4:** 195–208.
13. HATTIS, D. 1994. The importance of exposure measurements in risk assessment of drugs. Archives of Toxicology, Suppl. **16:** 201–210.
14. HATTIS, D. 1994. The use of well defined biomarkers (such as blood lead) in risk assessment. Environmental Geochemistry and Health **16:** 223–228.
15. HATTIS, D. 1996. Variability in susceptibility—how big, how often, for what responses to what agents? Environmental Toxicology and Pharmacology **2:** 135–145.
16. HATTIS, D., P. BANATI, R. GOBLE, & D. BURMASTER. 1999. Human interindividual variability in parameters related to health risks. Risk Analysis **19:** 711–726.
17. HAAS, C.N. 1994. Dose response analysis using spreadsheets. Risk Analysis **14:** 1097–1100.
18. BALMES, J.R., R.M. ARIS, L.L. CHEN, C. SCANNELL, I.B. TAGER, W. FINKBEINER, D. CHRISTIAN, T. KELLER, P.Q. HEARNE, R. FERRANDO & B. WELCH. 1997. Airway inflammation and responsiveness to ozone in normal and asthmatic subjects. *In* Effects of Ozone on Normal and Potentially Sensitive Subjects. Health Effects Institute Research Report Number 78, Cambridge, MA.

19. KOOP, H., S. KULY, M. FLUG, R. EISSELE, H. MONNIKES, K. ROSE, R. LUHMANN, A. SCHNEIDER, R. FISCHER & R. ARNOLD. 1996. Intragastric pH and serum gastrin during administration of different doses of pantoprazole in healthy subjects. Eur. J. Gastroenterol. Hepatol. **8:** 915–918.
20. INDUSTRIAL BIOTEST. 1973. International Institute of Ammonia Refrigeration irritation threshold evaluation study with ammonia. IBT Report No. 663-03161.
21. HINE, C.H., F.H. MEYERS, F. IVANHOE, S. WALKER & G.H. TAKAHASHI. 1961 Simple tests of respiratory function and study of sensory response in human subjects exposed to respiratory tract irritants. Fifth Air Pollution Medical Research Conference.
22. JUDGE, M.R., H.A. GRIFFITHS, D.A. BASKETTER, I.R. WHITE, R.J.G. RYECROFT & J.P. MCFADDEN. 1996. Variation in response of human skin to irritant challenge. Contact Dermatitis **34:** 115–117.
23. WILD, P., M. REFREGIER, G. AUBURTIN, B. CARTON & J. J. MOULIN. 1995. Survey of the respiratory health of the workers of a talc producing factory. Occup. Environ. Med. **52:** 470–477.
24. WALKELKAMP, M., G. ALVAN, J. GABRIELSSON & G. PAINTAUD. 1996. Pharmacodynamic modeling of furosemide tolerance after multiple intravenous administration. Clin. Pharmacol. Therapeut. **60:** 75–88.
25. LEMMENS, H.J.M., J. B. DYCK, S. L. SHAFER & D.R. STANSKI. 1994. Pharmacokinetic-pharmacokinetic modeling in drug development: application to the investigational opioid trefentanil. Clin. Pharm. Ther. **56:** 261–271.
26. PATAT, A., F. LECOZ, C. DUBRUC, J. GANDON, G. DURRIEU, I. CIMAROSTI, S. JEZEQUEL, O. CURET, I. ZIELENIUK, H. ALLAIN & P. ROSENZWEIG. 1996. Pharmacodynamics and pharmacokinetics of two dose regimens of befloxatone, a new reversible and selective monoamine oxidase inhibitor, at steady state in healthy volunteers, J. Clin. Pharmacol. **36:** 216–229.
27. DARBY, J.K., D.J. PASTA, L. DABIRI, L. CLARK & D. MOSBACHER. 1995. Haloperodol dose and blood level variability: toxicity and interindividual and intraindividual variability. J. Clin. Pharmacol. **15:** 334–340.
28. INSTITUTE OF MEDICINE. 1991. Seafood Safety Committee on the Evaluation of the Safety of Fishery Products, Food and Nutrition Board, Institute of Medicine. Farid E. Ahmed, Ed.: National Academy Press, Washington, D.C.
29. KOBAYASHI, K., E. VOKES, N. VOGELSANG, L. JANISCH, B. SOLIVEN & M. RATAIN. 1995. Phase I study of suramin given by intermittent infusion without adaptive control in patients with advanced cancer. J. Clin. Oncol. **13:** 2196–2207.
30. SCHOU, S., H. NIELSEN, A. NATTESTAD, S. HEILLERUP, M. RITZAU, P.E. BRANEBJERG, C. BUGGE & L.A. SKOGLUND. 1998. Analgesic dose-response relationship of ibuprofen 50, 100, 200, and 400 mg after surgical removal of third molars: a single-dose randomized placebo-controlled and double-blind study of 304 patients. J. Clin. Pharmacol. **38:** 447–454.
31. HOCHI, Y., T. KIDO, K. NOGAWA, H. KITO & Z. SHAIKH. 1995. Dose-response relationship between total cadmium intake and prevalence of renal dysfunction using general linear models. J. Appl. Toxicol. **15:** 109–116.
32. NOGAWA, K., R. HONDA, T. KIDO, I. TSURITANI, Y. YAMADA, M. ISHIZAKI & H. YAMAYA. 1989. A dose-response analysis of cadmium in the general environment with special reference to total cadmium intake limit. Environ. Res. **48:** 7–16.
33. WINKLER, R.L. & W.L. HAYS. 1975. Statistics: Probability, Inference, and Decision, second ed. 381–385, Holt, Rinehart and Winston, New York.
34. BHATIA, R., P. LOPIPERO & A.H. SMITH. 1998. Diesel exhaust exposure and lung cancer. Epidemiol. **9:** 84–91.

35. KODELL, R. 1999. Combining uncertainty factors in setting allowable exposure levels. Ann. N.Y. Acad. Sci. **895:** this volume.
36. HATTIS, D. & W.S. MINKOWITZ. 1996. Risk evaluation: criteria arising from legal traditions and experience with quantitative risk assessment in the United States. Environ. Toxicol. Pharmacol. **2:** 103–109.
37. HATTIS, D. & E. ANDERSON. 1998. What should be the implications of uncertainty, variability, and inherent 'biases'/'conservatism' for risk management decision making? Risk Analysis. **19:** 95–107.

Analysis of PBPK Models for Risk Characterization

FRÉDÉRIC YVES BOIS[a]

Lawrence Berkeley National Laboratory, USA

INERIS, Verneuil-en-Halatte, France.

ABSTRACT: Adoption of a Bayesian framework for risk characterization permits the seamless integration of different kinds of information available in order to choose and parameterize risk models. It also becomes easy to disentangle uncertainty from variability, through hierarchical statistical modeling. Appropriate numerical techniques can be found, for example, in the recently developed arsenal of Markov chain, Monte Carlo simulations. The developments in this area can actually be viewed as extensions of the *traditional* or standard Monte Carlo methods for uncertainty analysis. Following a brief review of the techniques, examples of Bayesian analyses of physiologically-based pharmacokinetic models are presented for tetrachloroethylene and dichloromethane. The discussion touches on some open problems and perspectives for the proposed methods.

INTRODUCTION

Physiologically-based pharmacokinetic (PBPK) models are increasingly used in risk characterization to perform rodent to human extrapolations of effective dose. PBPK models are mathematical representations of the animal or human body that group tissues or organs into compartments.[1,2] The characteristics of these compartments and the links between them are dictated by physiological and anatomical considerations (of organ sizes, blood flow, etc.) The time course of transport and transformations of a chemical through the various compartments can be simulated by resolving the set of equations belonging to the model.

Since PBPK models are by necessity incomplete representations of the underlying biology, some uncertainty is associated with their predictions. Such uncertainty is largely a consequence of potential error in model structure. It is also well known that physiological model parameters (e.g., organ volumes, blood flows, metabolic activity, or partition coefficients) exhibit biological heterogeneity.[3-8] Such variability in model parameter values is expected to result in variability of predictions. Finally, independently of variability, parameter values are known with only finite precision, if not with large uncertainty. The only way to quickly obtain the value of some parameters (without resorting to lengthy and specific experiments) is to adjust them statistically until the fit of the model to some toxicokinetic data is acceptable. Even if properly done, such statistical inference about parameter values results in a

---

[a]Address for correspondence: Dr. Frédéric Y. Bois, INERIS, Parc Alata, BP2, 60550 Verneuil-en-Halatte, France. (33) 44 55 6596 (voice); (33) 44 55 6899 (fax).
e-mail: frederic.bois@ineris.fr

certain amount of uncertainty. Neglecting the above sources of variability and uncertainty can lead to under- or overestimation of risks, and definitely to overconfidence in the results of risk assessments. Regulatory decision makers, considering use of PBPK models when setting regulatory standards, are understandably interested in good estimates of uncertainty in model predictions, so as to make motivated health-protective decisions. We present here a Bayesian approach to the treatment of uncertainty and variability in risk characterization, particularly for PBPK models. We use as examples, a toxicokinetic analysis of tetrachloroethylene disposition in humans, and an uncertainty analysis of the risk of dichloromethane-induced cancer in mice and humans.[9] The statistical framework invoked has also been applied to population PBPK modeling for benzene and trichloroethylene.[10–14]

INCORPORATING UNCERTAINTY IN RISK CHARACTERIZATION

PBPK models are becoming increasingly complex. This is also true of biologically-based cancer models. Uncertainty analyses for models of such complexity are difficult to apply by using analytical calculations. Stochastic simulation tools, in particular Monte Carlo (MC) simulations, have become popular for this purpose since they are quite transparent to the end-user.[15,16] For basic MC simulations, a distribution is assigned *a priori* to each input variable (e.g., dose) or model parameter (e.g., compartment volumes). Sets of input variables and parameter values are randomly sampled from these *prior* distributions, the model is run using these values, and its outputs are recorded. After many runs (the number of runs depends on the precision desired,) the accumulated output values can be used to form empirical distributions and to derive statistical moments or percentiles.[17] Sensitivity analyses can also be performed on the same collection of outputs by analyzing the relationships between sampled input values and resulting outputs.[2,12,18]

Simple MC simulations, as described above, have some limitations. An initial problem arises when assigning prior distributions for fitted parameters. This requires the fitting to be performed with appropriate statistical tools. Visual fitting does not achieve this purpose and is not acceptable for uncertainty analysis. The most natural framework for dealing with distributions is the Bayesian framework. Bayesian analysis permits a logical combination of two forms of information: *prior knowledge* about parameter values drawn from the scientific literature, separate measurements or *in vitro* experiments, and *data* from experimental whole animal or human studies. Clearly neither prior knowledge nor experimental data alone are capable of fully parameterizing a complex model. If prior information was sufficient, *in vivo* experiments would not be required. However, the available experimental data alone are insufficient to pin down all model parameters to reasonable values. By combining, through the use of Bayes' theorem, prior parameter distributions and data likelihood, the joint (multivariate) posterior distribution of all model parameters is obtained, including information about their full covariance structure.[19,20] In a sense, prior information is updated or *filtered* by the data into posterior distributions. Posterior parameter distributions are perfectly appropriate inputs for MC uncertainty analyses. Note that when fitting several parameters simultaneously, the joint posterior distribution of these parameters should be used (rather than their marginal distributions), since fitting usually induces covariance between parameter estimates. Failure to account for covariance when performing MC-sampling may overstate variance in model predictions by assuming independence where it does not exist.

This brings us to the subject of adjusting all model parameters, or only some of them. Clearly, we do not know exactly the values of organ volumes, blood flows, or partition coefficients for the animals or humans exposed during typical toxicokinetic studies. Fitting only two or three parameters (partial fitting) while holding others constant may lead to inconsistencies. In particular, the marginal variances of the fitted parameters are underestimated, since variability and uncertainty in the other model parameters is ignored.[10,21] Certainly, only *sensitive* parameters need to be adjusted: which parameters are sensitive remains to be defined. It is a common error, when justifying partial fitting, to assess sensitivity with respect to some model predictions of interest (e.g., number of metabolites formed). For fitting, sensitivity must be assessed with respect to the endpoint corresponding to the fitted data, and more precisely with respect with the likelihood function of the data (e.g., the least-squares criterion). Furthermore, to be correct, the assessment of sensitivity of the likelihood function should be performed in the maximum likelihood region, and this entails a preliminary global fitting. Thus, in order to prove that a partial fitting is adequate, a global fitting should first be made. It might be possible, in some cases, to perform a preliminary sensitivity analysis, adjust only the sensitive parameters, recheck for sensitivity of all parameters, and refit if necessary, iteratively. Such iterations, however, might not give the correct answer if there are multiple solutions to the fit. This is why we think it preferable to adjust all parameters globally. This is not an intractable problem if prior distributions are used to adequately constrain parameter values and if Markov chain Monte Carlo (MCMC) techniques are used to derive the joint posterior parameter distribution. MCMC sampling is a very powerful tool, that can be used for complex, nonlinear models. Details of the computational aspects of this method, including a summary of posterior distributions and tests for convergence of the algorithm are described in the statistical literature.[12,22–24]

Another problem is to disentangle variability (heterogeneity) from uncertainty. Separating these two sources of variance is important for a proper statistical analysis of toxicokinetic data (either for animals or humans) and for improved risk characterizations. For example, variability does not tend to decrease when larger populations are examined, whereas uncertainty (about the average) does. Furthermore, for most parameters, prior physiological information is about population averages and not about individual values (except when subject-specific measurements are made). The statistical concepts underlying current approaches to population toxicokinetics[10–12] were first laid out for drug pharmacokinetic studies.[25–28] The population approach is worth implementing even in cases that study small numbers of subjects.[29] In the case of animal experiments, this variability, although reduced for inbred strains, should also be considered. The current models are all hierarchical structures that consider individual parameters to be distributed around some population average value. Individual parameters, population averages, and population standard deviations are all inferred from data by model fitting (performed to obtain posterior parameter distributions, as described above). It is only recently, with the advance of computing power and the development of new algorithms, that we have been able to apply such techniques to complex (e.g., PBPK) models. Note, it is well known that naïve fitting of aggregate data (e.g., data averaged over all individuals) is at best undesirable, and at worse totally misleading.[25,26,29] Unfortunately, older data are often only available in aggregate form. A proper treatment of such data is difficult to implement. One solution would be to treat the individual data as *missing*,[20,30] but the computation power required to implement appropriate statistical techniques (e.g., imputation) is likely to be prohibitive, at least in the near future. For the present, the result of fitting aggregate data should be considered with caution, and we should insist that, for the experiments currently performed, individual data be collected and made available.

To summarize, FIGURE 1 depicts the first step of our proposed treatment of animal and human pharmacokinetic (PK) data for risk characterization. Species-specific population PBPK models (actually any reasonable model could be used) are first fitted to the data by using Bayesian updating. Various computational techniques, such as MCMC sampling can be used to derive fitted PBPK models. The fitted human and animal models consist of a model structure (unchanged in the process) together with a collection of parameter samples drawn from their joint posterior distribution.

The next step (see FIGURE 2) is to use the fitted animal PBPK model to predict, by straight MC simulations, the distribution of target dose for each animal group of the cancer bioassay. Although not shown explicitly here, it is possible at this step to use a hierarchical population structure to simulate separately variability and uncertainty. By means of these MC simulations, each sample of parameter values yields a numerical estimate of target dose. A cancer model is then fitted to the animal bioassay data in the same way that the PBPK model was fitted to PK data. Prior distributions can be assigned to the cancer model parameters, to take into account, for example, past experience of background cancer rates in similar lots of animals.[31] During the cancer model fitting process, target dose is treated as a random variable (using its previously obtained statistical distribution).

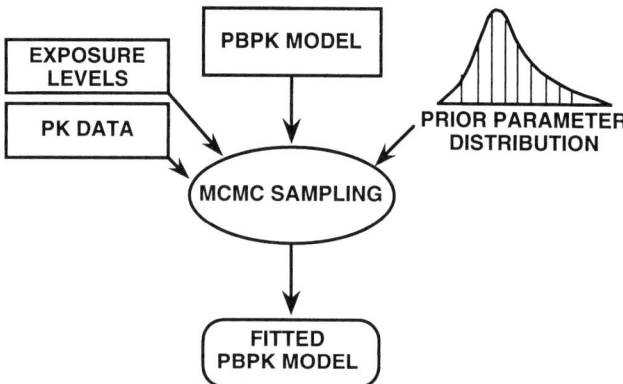

FIGURE 1. Flow chart for the first step of treatment of animal and human pharmacokinetic (PK) data in risk characterization. The models are fitted by using Bayesian techniques (see text).

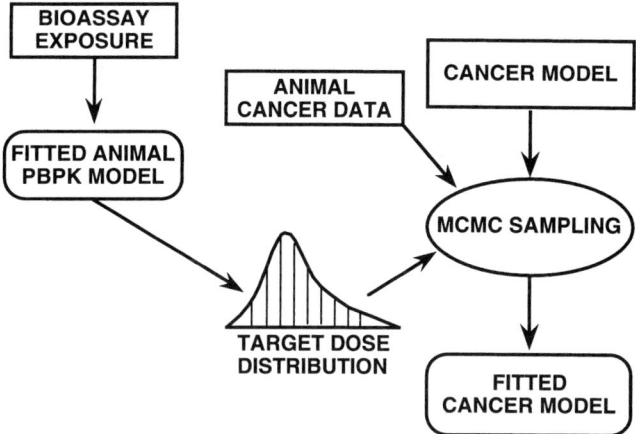

FIGURE 2. Flow chart for the second step of data treatment in risk characterization. The fitted animal PBPK model is used to predict a dose distribution and a cancer model is fitted to bioassay data using Bayesian techniques (see text).

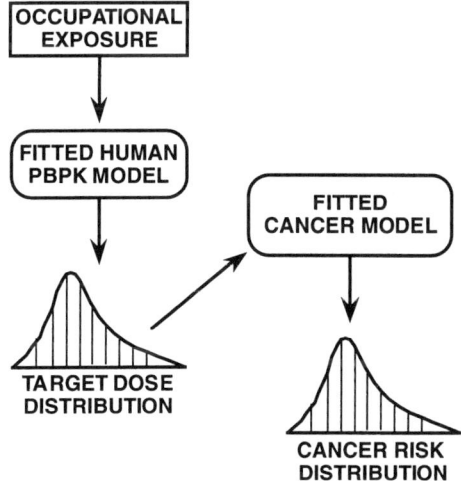

FIGURE 3. Flow chart for the third step of data treatment in risk characterization. Cancer risk for humans is obtained by estimating the statistical distribution of target dose exposure using the fitted human PBPK model. The fitted cancer model is finally used to predict the risk distribution.

Finally (see FIGURE 3), the cancer risk for humans is obtained by first estimating the statistical distribution of target dose exposure for a given external exposure. For this, MC simulations are performed with the fitted human PBPK model. Next, each estimate of target dose obtained is randomly associated with a set of cancer model parameter values obtained by the previous fitting, and the cancer model is then used to predict the corresponding risk. The complete collection of risk estimates gives an estimate of the distribution of risk. Since a physiological target dose is used, it can be argued that the cancer model parameters do not require conventional extrapolation to human values.

EXAMPLE OF POPULATION ANALYSIS TETRACHLOROETHYLENE (TETRA)

PBPK Model

FIGURE 4 illustrates a PBPK model, developed for TETRA.[10,12] In this standard model, exposure is supposed to be by inhalation and distribution limited by perfusion, as is often the case for apolar solvents. To take into account known physiological covariances between model parameters (e.g., between organ volumes and body weight, or alveolar ventilation rate and cardiac output) several of them are linked to the lean body mass or other parameter values, via scaling functions. It would be overly optimistic to hope that concentration-time profiles alone could carry enough information about these covariances to make them recoverable *a posteriori*. A solu-

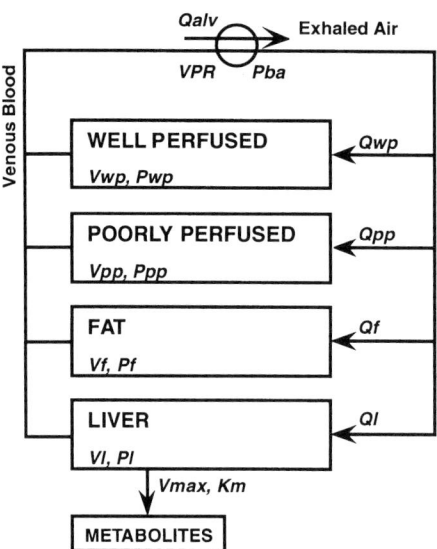

FIGURE 4. PBPK model developed for tetrachloroethylene in humans.[10,12] Symbols: *Q*, flow; *V*, volume; *P*, partition coefficient; *VPR*, ventilation over perfusion ratio; V_{max}, maximum rate of metabolism; and K_m, for Michaelis-Menten constant.

tion is therefore to implement an *a priori* deterministic model of physiological dependencies between parameters (not all parameters need to be scaled). Unfortunately, there is no unique way to implement scaling, and no rigorous foundation for the particular choices has been seen in the literature to date. Note that such a model does not concern the estimation covariance, induced by partial nonidentifiability (e.g., the posterior covariance between Michaelis-Menten parameters V_{max} and K_m). It is possible to parameterize the model so that the estimation covariances are minimized, but that is not required for the physiological relevance of the model.

Statistical Population Model

Dealing with the multilevel error structure of PK data requires the development of a *population* statistical model describing the links between the various sources of uncertainty (measurement errors, population variability, human heterogeneity). The physiological model then becomes a deterministic component of the statistical model. A simple population model, constructed around the above PBPK model, is illustrated graphically in FIGURE 5. The model has two major components: individual level and population level. At the individual level, for each subject, exhaled air and blood concentrations of TETRA (**y**) were measured experimentally. The expected value of **y** is a function (f) of exposure concentration (**E**), time (**t**), a set of physiological parameters with unknown values (**θ**), and a set of measured covariate param-

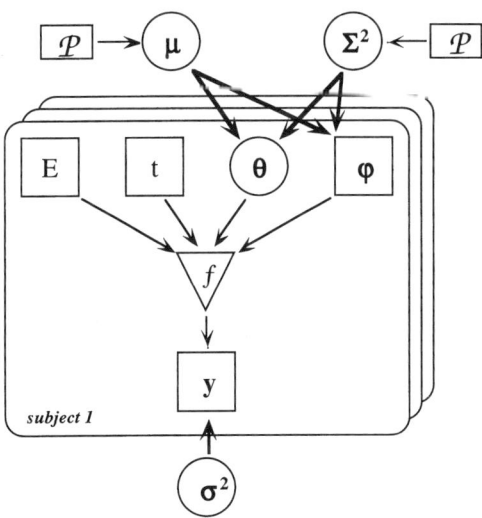

FIGURE 5. Graph of a statistical population model of tetrachloroethylene toxicokinetics. Symbols: $\mathcal{P}$, prior distribution; **μ**, mean population parameters; Σ^2, variances of the parameters in the population; **E**, toxicant exposure concentration; **t**, experimental sampling times; **θ**, unknown physiological parameters; **φ**, measured covariates; f, PBPK model; **y**, measured toxicant concentrations (e.g., in blood, exhaled air, or urine); σ^2, variance of the experimental measurements.

eters (φ) such as body weight or breathing rate. $\mathbf{E}$, $\mathbf{t}$, $\mathbf{q}$, and φ are subject-specific. The function f is the PBPK model. The TETRA concentrations actually observed in expired air and blood were also affected by measurement errors, which are assumed to be independent and log-normally distributed, with a mean of zero and a variance σ^2 (on a log scale). The variance vector σ^2 has two components, σ_1^2 for the measurements in blood, and σ_2^2 for the measurements in exhaled air, because these measurements had different experimental protocols and are likely to have different precision. Three types of nodes are featured in FIGURE 5:

- Square nodes represent variables for which the values are known by observation, such as $\mathbf{y}$ or φ; were fixed by the experimenters, such as $\mathbf{E}$ and $\mathbf{t}$; or were fixed by ourselves, such as the prior values on $\boldsymbol{\mu}$ and $\boldsymbol{\Sigma}^2$.
- Circle nodes represent unknown variables, such as $\boldsymbol{\theta}$, σ^2, $\boldsymbol{\mu}$, or $\boldsymbol{\Sigma}^2$.
- The triangle represents the deterministic PBPK model f.

An arrow between two nodes indicates a direct statistical dependence between the variables of those nodes. At the population level, we assumed that each component of the $\boldsymbol{\theta}$ parameter vector is distributed log-normally, with population averages $\boldsymbol{\mu}$ and variances $\boldsymbol{\Sigma}^2$ (in log scale). We have some *a priori* knowledge of $\boldsymbol{\mu}$ and $\boldsymbol{\Sigma}^2$—we assigned *a priori* truncated normal distributions to the population means $\boldsymbol{\mu}$ (with parameters $\mathbf{M}$ and $\mathbf{S}$), and inverse gamma distributions to the population variances $\boldsymbol{\Sigma}^2$, with parameters $\boldsymbol{\Sigma}_o$ and ν (set to 2 so as to correspond with a large degree of uncertainty about $\boldsymbol{\Sigma}^2$). Truncation is necessary to ensure that only physiologically meaningful values are used. In the next section we detail the setting of informative prior distributions for the TETRA model. In this model, information about the distribution of $\boldsymbol{\theta}$ and φ parameter values for an individual is given by the experimental data and by the population parameters.

Current standard practice in Bayesian statistics is to summarize a complicated high-dimensional posterior distribution by random draws of the vector of parameters, in this case, from the distribution $P(\boldsymbol{\theta}, \boldsymbol{\mu}, \boldsymbol{\Sigma}^2, \sigma^2 | \text{data})$. The simulations can then be used to compute posterior distributions of estimands of interest, including individual parameters, or derived (predicted) quantities such as the proportion of compound metabolized under specified conditions. Because $\boldsymbol{\theta}$ has many components, we used a combination of Gibbs sampling and Metropolis-Hasting sampling to perform a random walk through the posterior distribution. These MCMC samplings are iterative procedures that are particularly convenient in the case of hierarchical models.

Given the above statistical model, the conditional posterior density of σ^2 (sampled at each step of the sampler) is, for $m = 1$ or 2 (either blood or exhaled air):

σ_m^2 | all other parameters

$$\sim \text{Inverse} - \gamma\left((L_m, L_m^{-1})\sum_i\sum_j [\log(y_{ijm}) - \log(f_m(\boldsymbol{\theta}, \varphi, E_j, t_j))]^2\right) \quad (1)$$

where L_m is the total number of observations of type m for all measurements on all six subjects. For a given individual, i indexes the measurement time, and j the dose.

The conditional posterior density for any component of $\boldsymbol{\theta}$, θ_{kl}, is:

$P(\theta_{kl}|\mathbf{y}, \text{all other } \theta\text{s}, \varphi, \sigma^2, \mathbf{E}, \mathbf{t}, \mu, \Sigma^2)$

$$\propto \exp(-\tfrac{1}{2}\Sigma_l^{-2}[\theta_{kl}-\mu_l]^2) \cdot \prod_i \prod_j \prod_m \exp(-\tfrac{1}{2}\sigma_m^{-2}[\log(y_{ijm}) - \log(f_m(\theta, \varphi, E_j, t_j))]^2) \quad (2)$$

where $k = 1, \ldots, 6$ (six subjects), and $l = 1, \ldots, 18$ (18 model parameters). Because of f (the nonlinear PBPK model), this cannot be written in closed form as a function of θ. Instead of directly sampling θ_{kl} from this conditional distribution, we sampled a *proposal* value from $\mathcal{N}(\theta_{kl}, (S_{kl}/20)^2)$, that is, centered at the current value of θ_{kl}, and with a constant standard deviation proportional to S_{kl}. The proportionality factor 20 was set after preliminary runs. We then either updated the value of θ_{kl} to that new value, or left it unchanged, based on the Metropolis acceptance/rejection rule.

The conditional distributions of the population parameters μ_l and Σ_l^2 are normal. For each l:

$$\mu_l|\mathbf{y}, \text{all other parameters} \sim \mathcal{N}\left(\frac{M_l \Sigma_l^2 + S_l^2 \sum_k \theta_{kl}}{nS_l^2 + \Sigma_l^2}, \frac{\Sigma_l^2 S_l^2}{nS_l^2 + \Sigma_l^2}\right) \quad (3)$$

$$\Sigma_l^2|\mathbf{y}, \text{all other parameters} \sim \text{Inverse}-\gamma\left(n+\nu, \frac{1}{n+\nu}\left[\nu\Sigma_{0l}^2 + \sum_k(\theta_{kl}-\mu_l)^2\right]\right) \quad (4)$$

with $n = 6$.

All computer simulations were performed with the *MCSim* program.[32]

Defining Physiological Informative Priors

Defining prior distributions for the physiological parameters is somewhat difficult for reasons of data accessibility. Although it is well known that these parameters exhibit inter- or intraindividual variability in humans, the only values readily available, and those commonly used in physiological modeling, are *reference* values for young Caucasian males. Most of the time, information about population variance can only be found by going back to the original publications. Data about the shape of the distributions are even harder to find. A skewed, log-normal–like distribution is generally observed for biological parameters, but most, if not all, parameters are positive and have physiological bounds. Thus, we used truncated log-normal distributions. These do not differ appreciably from normal distributions for small values of the variance.

Prior values for the hyper-parameters **M**, **S**, and Σ_0 were set on the basis of the literature. In setting uncertainties, we tried to be conservative and set the prior variances higher rather than lower when there was ambiguity in the biological literature (for example, with the partition coefficients). Details can be found in.[10,12] As an example, let us examine the definition of the prior estimate for the maximum rate of metabolism, V_{max}. A prior estimate for the population V_{max} was obtained when fitting the model to animal data.[18] An extrapolation was performed by allometric scaling using body weight to the power 0.7. Independently, data from *in vitro* experiments indicated that V_{max} (in mg/min/kg) in humans is approximately 1/8 of that for the mouse and 2/5 of the rat value. This translates for humans into values of 1.4 mg/min and 0.64 mg/min from mouse and rat data, respectively. For humans, we adopted a geometric mean of 0.7 mg/min, bracketed by the extrapolated animal values. A large uncertainty is still associated with this number. The animal values are themselves uncertain and the agreement of the two extrapolation methods could be fortuitous. We chose a value of 10 for exp(S), and truncation at $\pm 2S$, in log space. This truncation corresponds to plus or minus two orders of magnitude around the geometric mean. Since *in vitro* human data indicated a population coefficient of variation of approximately two, we set exp(Σ_0) at that value. Thus, we believe this parameter to vary across study subjects by about a factor of two, but we are uncertain by a factor of ten as to its population mean. It would be difficult to express this sort of uncertainty without an explicit hierarchical model.

Some Results

The fits obtained by using the above approach can be quite good even for multiple endpoints, as shown in FIGURE 6 for human TETRA data. The predictions for this plot were produced by a random parameter vector drawn from the joint posterior parameter distribution. Using the population distributions obtained, parameter values for new *random subjects* can be simulated. It is possible in that case to let the body weight or breathing rate vary greatly, as in the general population, and much more than within the group of experimental subjects. This leads to population distributions for endpoints of toxicological interest. Random vectors of parameter values can also be used for simulations of the pharmacokinetic behavior of the individuals actually studied experimentally, under extrapolated scenarios. FIGURE 7 presents estimates of the fraction of TETRA metabolized after continuous inhalation at two concentra-

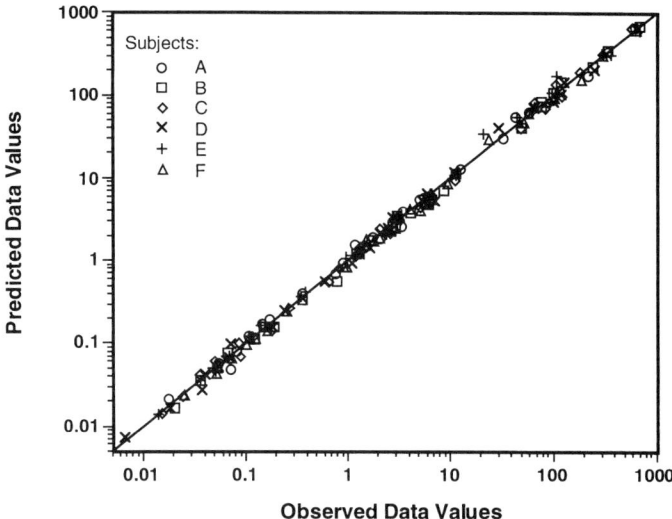

FIGURE 6. Predicted (by a random posterior parameter vector) versus observed blood and exhaled air concentrations for the human tetrachloroethylene data of Monster *et al.*[33] For a perfect adjustment (predicted equal to observed) all points would fall on the diagonal.

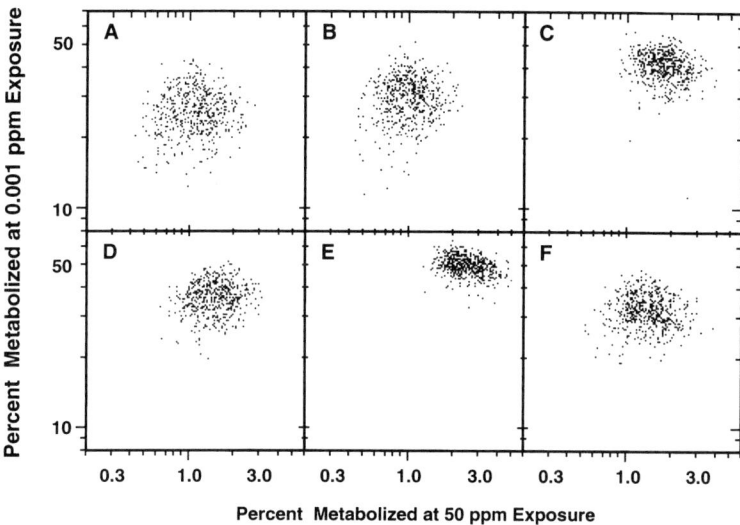

FIGURE 7. Estimates of the fraction of tetrachloroethylene metabolized per day during a continuous inhalation exposure to 50 ppm versus estimates at 0.001 ppm, for the subjects of the Monster et al. experiments.[33]

tions, for each of the six subjects studied by Monster et al.[33] In addition to a dose effect (higher fraction metabolized at low exposure compared to high exposure), an obvious inter-individual variability can be observed.

EXAMPLE OF RISK CHARACTERIZATION DICHLOROMETHANE (DCM)

Data

Data from 13 DCM uptake experiments with mice were provided to us by the US OSHA.[9] These experiments were performed with initial chamber concentrations ranging from 200 to 5200 ppm DCM (0.696 mg/l to 18.1 mg/l). Four additional experiments were performed with pretreatment by a mixed-function oxidase inhibitor, *trans*-dichloroethylene. For those, initial DCM concentrations ranged from 500 to 2000 ppm (1.74 to 6.96 mg/l). All the above gas uptake studies were performed with five female mice in a single chamber. Thus, measured observations of decline in chamber concentration of DCM with time represent the aggregate pharmacokinetic behavior of groups of five animals. There is no way to recover individual animal data with this experimental design.

For humans, we used the open chamber inhalation studies reported in Andersen et al.[34] These data consist in exhaled breath and venous blood DCM concentrations for six human male volunteers, exposed to concentrations of either 100 or 350 ppm

DCM (0.348 mg/l or 1.22 mg/l) for a period of six hours. These data have only been reported as means and standard deviations for the six subjects.

The NTP cancer bioassay data on DCM-induced lung tumor in B6C3F1 female mice[35] were used to adjust the cancer model. In the NTP studies, mice were exposed to either 0 (control), 2000 ppm (6.96 mg/l) or 4000 ppm (13.9 mg/l) dichloromethane for six hours per day, five days a week for 102 weeks. The number of animals bearing tumors at the end of the bioassay were 3/50, 30/48, and 41/48, respectively.

PBPK Model

The PBPK model used for DCM is based on Reference 36 (see Figure 8). DCM distributes in the various compartments and is metabolized in the lung and liver through a mixed-function oxidase (MFO) pathway, and a glutathione (GSH) conjugation pathway. MFO metabolic reactions were assumed to follow Michaelis-Menten kinetics, whereas GSH pathway metabolism was assumed to follow first-order kinetics. We made several structural modifications to the PBPK model:[36] (1) we added separate compartments representing the gastrointestinal tract and the bone marrow (as in Refs. 37 and 38); (2) the equations used to apportion MFO and GSH metabolism between liver and lung compartments were modified to account for differences in microsomal and cytosolic protein content; and (3) for humans, work intensity was allowed to vary and influence cardiac output, the ventilation-perfusion ratio, and fractional blood flows to compartments.

Estimates of the concentrations (in mg/day/L of lung tissue) of GSH pathway metabolites in mice exposed during the NTP bioassay were obtained by simulating 2000 ppm and 4000 ppm exposures with the PBPK model. When simulating the human data, the work load was assumed to be zero watts (i.e., rest) and the average body weight of the six subjects (86 kg) was assumed known with negligible error. For human cancer risk calculations, the PBPK model was used to compute the expected concentrations (in mg/day/L of lung tissue) of GSH pathway metabolites formed in human lung at a constant occupational exposure to 25 ppm DCM for eight hours per day, five days per week. Body weight and work load were varied in these simulation through Monte Carlo sampling to simulate their variability in a population of workers.

Statistical Model

The model adopted here is simpler than for TETRA. Experimental errors for the PK data were assumed to be log-normally distributed, without bias. The PBPK model was used to compute the expected geometric mean of the data. The standard deviation (in log space) of the experimental errors was estimated together with the model parameters for the case of mice data. For humans, rather than invoking an error model, we used the data-based standard errors of the mean responses (derived from the SDs reported by Andersen et al.[34]). In modeling the cancer bioassay response, the number of animals bearing tumors was, as usual, assumed to be binomially distributed. MCMC sampling was used to derive the joint posterior distribution of the parameters. Here also, all computer simulations were performed with the *MCSim* program.[32]

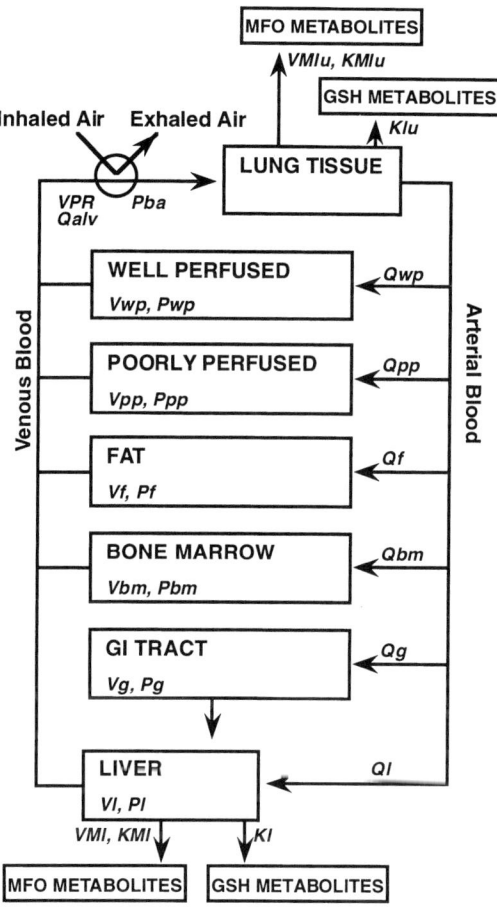

FIGURE 8. PBPK model for dichloromethane.[9] Symbols are the same as in FIGURE 4, with the addition of K_l and K_{lu}, first order rate constants for GSH pathway metabolism.

Prior Probability Distributions

Several sources of information were used as a basis for specifying the prior probability distributions of the DCM PBPK parameters—literature summaries for most physiologic and anatomic parameters, direct laboratory measurement of partition coefficients based on vial equilibration studies. Here also we used truncated lognormal distributions. In specifying prior probability distributions for model parameters, we also attempted to characterize variability in mean parameter values for small groups of rodents and humans, in order to make the prior values congruent with the data sets available. For example, the rodent gas uptake data represent the aggregate PK behavior of groups of five mice. Prior values were therefore constructed to reflect the degree of variability in mean physiological and anatomical PBPK parameters for groups of five mice. A similar approach was taken in defining prior values for human physiologic and anatomic parameters, since the available experimental data reflected the averaged PK behavior of six subjects.

Results

FIGURE 9 shows the fit to part of the animal data. The fit is reasonable, although improvements could certainly be achieved by considering the inter-lot variability (through a hierarchical model). The posterior distributions for mouse PBPK parameters obtained by Bayesian updating are not presented here for brevity, but can be found elsewhere.[9] Comparison of the prior and posterior probability distributions reveals that the gas uptake data contains considerable information about a number of PBPK model parameters: the coefficients of variation for nearly all posterior distributions were smaller than those of the prior distributions.

The fit to both exhaled air data (see FIGURE 10) and venous blood data (not shown) using the maximum posterior vector was quite good. The human *in vivo* data also contain considerable information about many of the model parameters, as evidenced by shifts in medians and tightening of posterior relative to the prior distributions (data not shown).

FIGURE 11 shows the posterior distributions for GSH metabolites in the mouse lung at 2,000 ppm exposure, six hours per day, five days per week. A similar distribution, but shifted to the right, is obtained for the 4,000 ppm exposure simulations

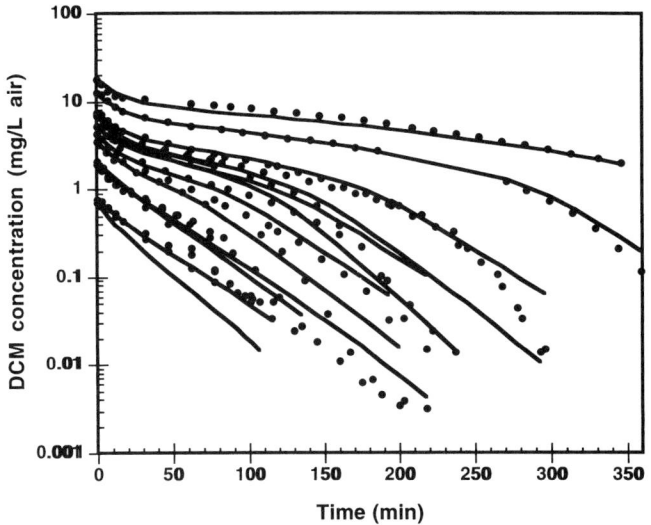

FIGURE 9. Maximum posterior fit of the PBPK model to the dichloromethane mouse chamber exposure data (without *trans*-dichloroethylene pretreatment). Initial gas chamber concentrations ranged from 200 to 5200 ppm dichloromethane.

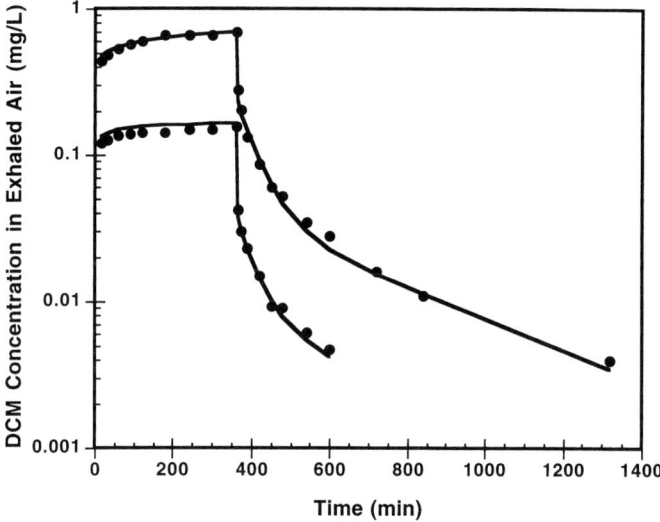

FIGURE 10. Maximum posterior fit of the model to the dichloromethane exhaled air concentrations data in humans.[34] Data points are averages from six human male volunteers, exposed to dichloromethane concentrations of either 100 or 350 ppm for six hours.

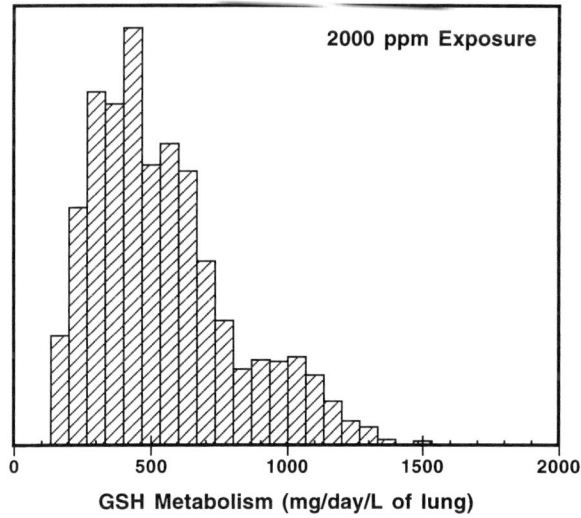

FIGURE 11. Posterior distribution of the amount of GSH pathway metabolites generated by mice during exposure to 2,000 ppm of dichloromethane, six hours per day, five days per week.

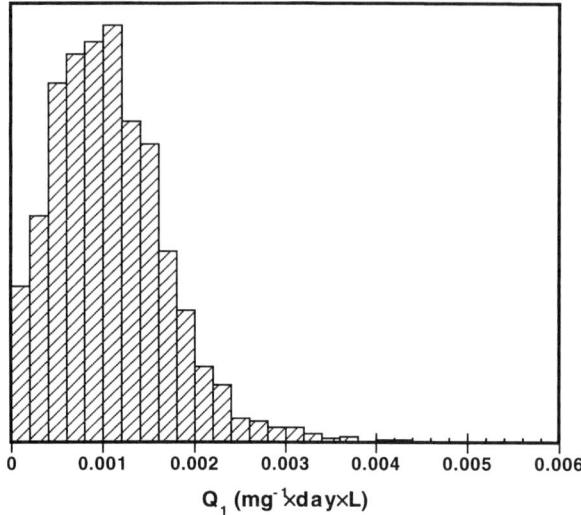

FIGURE 12. Posterior distribution of the linear parameter q_1 in the linear-quadratic multistage cancer model fitted to the NTP mouse dichloromethane cancer bioassay data.

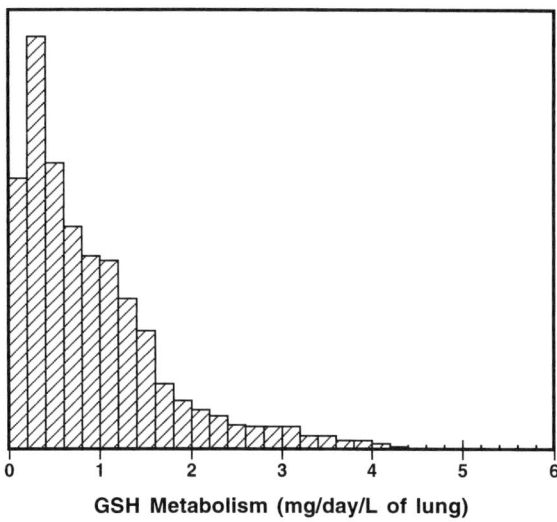

FIGURE 13. Posterior distribution of the amount of GSH pathway metabolites generated by humans during exposure to 25 ppm of dichloromethane, eight hours per day, five days per week.

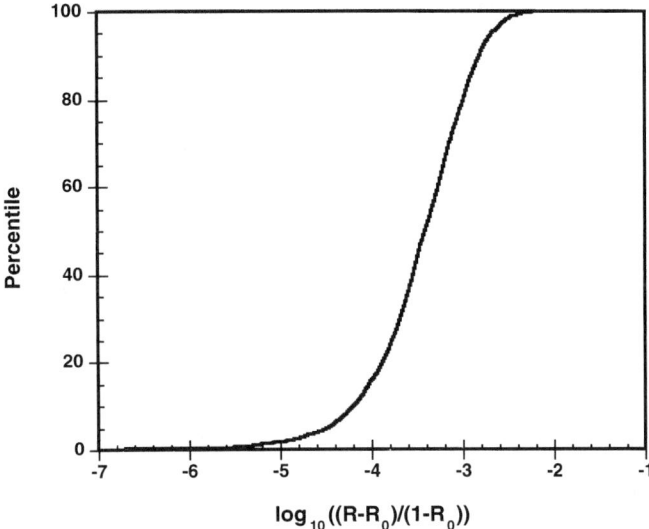

FIGURE 14. Estimated cumulative distribution of human cancer risk linked to a 45 year exposure to dichloromethane, at 25 ppm in the air, eight hours per day, five days per year (based on lung GSH metabolic pathway).

(data not shown). Both distributions were positively skewed, with CVs of 40 to 50%. For use as an input dose to the multistage model, these posterior distributions were approximated by truncated log-normals that were sampled independently for each simulated realization of the rodent bioassay. FIGURE 12 presents the posterior distribution of parameter q_1 of the multistage model, obtained from MCMC sampling. This distribution is conditional on the two rodent distributions of GSH lung metabolites (at 2,000 and 4,000 ppm exposures) and on the tumor incidence data for all three dose groups of 50 mice. FIGURE 13 gives the posterior distribution of GSH metabolites in the human lung when exposed to 25 ppm DCM, eight hours per day, five days per week. Comparison of this plot with FIGURE 11 shows that, at equal exposure, a human lung would form about 10 times fewer metabolites than mouse lung. FIGURE 14 shows the end result of this work: the estimated (based on GSH lung metabolic pathway) cumulative distribution of added cancer risk to humans from exposure to 25 ppm DCM, eight hours per day, five days per week, for 45 years.

DISCUSSION

PBPK models are essential tools in toxicokinetics and new approaches are needed for their validation. The most important applications of the Bayesian approach arise when informative (e.g., physiological or anatomical) prior distributions are available, in parallel with kinetic data. This is usually true for PBPK models. In this case, Bayesian updating results in all the information content of both prior distributions and data being transferred to the posterior distributions. Alternately, Bayesian updating of uniform prior distributions (i.e., feigning complete ignorance about plausible parameter values) with data leads to posterior distributions that are strictly proportional to the data likelihood —and this is asymptotically equivalent to the standard frequentist approach of maximum likelihood. Conversely, if the data do not convey information about some parameters (or, at the extreme, if no data are available), the corresponding posterior distributions are equal to the prior distributions. This approach then becomes equivalent to standard Monte Carlo sampling from the prior distributions.

Independently of its potential advantages, our proposed methodology is far from definitely established and several issues still need to be resolved. For example, a series of parametric assumptions is involved, particularly within the population model (e.g., the shape of the population distributions), and these should be further validated. Experience gained from population analyses using simpler models might be transposable to PBPK models, but not much has yet been done in this direction. Some questions about parameter identifiability are also open: What exactly happens in a population model when parameters are not identifiable for all subjects? Is estimation always satisfying in such a case? Another open question is intersubject or intrasubject covariance modeling. Within a subject we have seen that parameter scaling offers a way to model covariance; are there better approaches to covariance modeling? Should the population covariance matrix be systematically estimated? Model uncertainty also should be explored. Conceptually it is not too difficult to weight different models by their posterior probabilities or choose the *least wrong* among them,[19] but this can require a large amount of computer time.

In fact, to facilitate the testing of modeling alternatives, it is urgent to reduce the computational burden associated with MCMC sampling: for the population TETRA PBPK model presented above, the joint posterior distribution of about 140 parameters is required. On a standard UNIX workstation, running five independent Markov chains with 140 parameters until approximate convergence requires about five days. Faster samplers are being developed and should improve the situation, but it may still be necessary to reduce the complexity of the models when many subjects are involved. Hopefully, this can be done while retaining some of the advantages of PBPK models: we showed, for example, that a three-compartment *semi-physiological* model is a good alternative to a five-compartment PBPK model for benzene.[39] Obviously, minimal classical PK models can also be appropriate in cases where extrapolations needs are limited.

Other unresolved issues in the proposed framework concern interspecies and interpopulation transpositions. Interspecies transposition is conceptually resolved by allometric parameter scaling.[40] Assuming that the model structure is correct for two or more species (the above models, for example, are reasonable for any mammal), simply changing parameters to values specific to the species of interest realizes the transposition. This requires a value for each species or a validated transposition rule for each model parameter (these rules do no need to be the same as the scaling functions that describe parameter covariance within an individual). Too often, however, allometric rules are presented and used with a large degree of statistical naïveté: no measure of uncertainty is attached to the exponents and coefficients used, and they are usually rounded to nice rational numbers, such as 2/3 or 3/4, as if we were dealing with a well-defined mechanical system. The uncertainty about these coefficients (always obtained after some fitting) should be determined and taken into account, as for any other parameter.

The need for population transpositions stem from the fact that factors primarily affecting exposure (e.g., water consumption rate and length of exposure) are usually minimized in a controlled human study, however they may range widely in daily life. Similarly, the variability of internal human factors (e.g., genetics, disease states, and nutritional status) that affect toxicokinetic or toxicodynamic processes and result in a wide range of responses in the general population, is generally limited in controlled studies by the choice of few healthy young males of a particular ethnic group. Population transpositions can be accomplished if the factors responsible for heterogeneity (e.g., body weight, breathing rate, and metabolic constants) are among the list of model parameters. In this case, the population distributions obtained for these parameters, from fitting data sets with few volunteers, can be changed to reflect the range of values found in the general population. If these parameters have been measured for each volunteer and are introduced as fixed covariates during fitting, they can also be replaced by a distribution so as to make predictions for a large population.[10] For example, in the case of DCM we introduced extra-heterogeneity in body weight and work intensity (with concomitant effects on blood flows and the ventilation-perfusion ratio), when simulating a 25 ppm occupational exposure. However, changing the marginal distribution of some parameters, after fitting has been performed, can disrupt the estimation covariance structure. The consequences of this disruption can be difficult to estimate and further research is needed in this area.

To bypass the population transposition problem, we may want to consider toxicokinetic analyses of large cohorts of subjects, such as professional cohorts in occupational hygiene or epidemiology studies. A major challenge to modeling in toxicology is actually the exploitation of the numerous data sets collected during such studies, and generally in settings where exposure concentrations are unknown or estimated with nonnegligible uncertainty. Because, for such cohorts, exposure is usually indirectly measured, new estimation problems arise. Most of the time very simplistic analyses of such data are performed, for lack of experience in more powerful methodologies. Yet, there is no difficulty, in the above statistical framework, in considering exposure as one of the estimands. A problem, however, resides in fully accounting for the uncertainties stemming from unknown time-varying exposures.

Finally, for risk assessment, it seems somewhat vain to refine toxicokinetic modeling independently of the other parts of the risk characterization process. I think that we should focus our attention, for the sake of improved uncertainty analysis, on achieving a better integration of the exposure, toxicokinetic, and effect models used. It is obvious, for example, that cancer bioassay data may give information about effective dose (e.g., metabolite formation). Such information is now overlooked. Fitting a coupled toxicokinetic/dynamic model is the only way to recover that information. Attempts have been made in this direction, but with simplistic models.[41] We are now in a position to improve our analyses. Model integration would help solve the problems posed by the analysis of epidemiological cohort data and would also lead to an integrated modeling of biomarker data. We are confident that, as progress is made on such questions, uncertainty analysis will become a more powerful and widespread tool for risk assessment.

ACKNOWLEDGMENTS

This work was supported by the Association pour la Recherche contre le Cancer.

REFERENCES

1. BAILER, A.J. & D.A. DANKOVIC. 1997. An introduction to the use of physiologically based pharmacokinetic models in risk assessment. Stat. Method. Med. Res. **6:** 341–358.
2. SPEAR, R. & F. BOIS. 1994. Parameter variability and the interpretation of physiologically based pharmacokinetic modeling results. Environ. Health Perspect. **102** (Suppl. 11): 61–66.
3. DILLS, R.L. et al. 1994. Inter-individual variability in blood air partitioning of volatile organic compounds and correlation with blood chemistry. J. Exposure Anal. Environ. Epidemiol. **4:** 229–245.
4. FISEROVA-BERGEROVA, V. et al. 1980. Predictable "individual differences" in uptake and excretion of gases and lipid soluble vapour—simulation study. Brit. J. Ind. Med. **37:** 42–49.
5. DANKOVIC, D.A. & A.J. BAILER. 1994. The impact of exercise and intersubject variability on dose estimates for dichloromethane derived from a physiologically based pharmacokinetic model. Fund. Appl. Toxicol. **22:** 20–25.
6. SHIELDS, P.G. 1994. Pharmacogenetics - Detecting sensitive populations. Environ. Health Perspect. **102** (Suppl. 11): 81–87.
7. KALOW, W. 1982. Ethnic differences in drug metabolism. Clin. Pharmacokinet. **7:** 373–400.
8. CUDDIHY, R.G. et al. 1979. Variability in target organ deposition among individuals exposed to toxic substances. Toxicol. Appl. Pharmacol. **49:** 179–187.
9. UNITED STATES DEPARTMENT OF LABOR. 1997. 29 CFR Parts 1910, 1915, and 1926. Fed. Regist. January 10 1997.
10. BOIS, F.Y. et al. 1996. Population toxicokinetics of tetrachloroethylene. Arch. Toxicol. **70:** 347–355.
11. BOIS, F. et al. 1996. Population toxicokinetics of benzene. Environ. Health Perspect. **104** (Suppl. 6): 1405–1411.
12. GELMAN, A. et al. 1996. Physiological pharmacokinetic analysis using population modeling and informative prior distributions. J. Am. Stat. Assoc. **91:** 1400–1412.
13. BOIS, F. 1997. Statistical analysis of a PBPK model of trichloroethylene kinetics and metabolism in mice and humans. Report for the U.S. Environmental Protection Agency. Washington, DC.
14. BOIS, F. 1997. Statistical PBPK modeling of variability and uncertainty in trichloroethylene kinetics and metabolism in rodents and humans. Report for the U.S. Environmental Protection Agency. Washington, DC.
15. BOIS, F. et al. 1989. The use of pharmacokinetic models in the determination of risks for regulatory purposes. In Advances in Risk Analysis. Proc. 1987 Annual Meeting of the Society for Risk Analysis. J.J. Bonin and D.E. Stevenson, Eds. **7:** 573–583. Plenum Publishing Corporation, New York.
16. PORTIER, C.J. & N.L. KAPLAN. 1989. Variability of safe dose estimates when using complicated models of the carcinogenic process. Fund. Appl. Toxicol. **13:** 533–544.
17. HAMMERSLEY, J.M. & D.C. HANDSCOMB. 1964. Monte Carlo Methods. Chapman & Hall, London.
18. BOIS, F.Y. et al. 1990. Precision and sensitivity analysis of pharmacokinetic models for cancer risk assessment: tetrachloroethylene in mice, rats and humans. Toxicol. Appl. Pharmacol. **102:** 300–315.
19. BERNARDO, J.M. & A.F.M. SMITH. 1994. Bayesian Theory. Wiley, New York.

20. GELMAN, A. et al. 1995. Bayesian Data Analysis. Chapman & Hall, London.
21. WOODRUFF, T.J. & F.Y. BOIS. 1993. Optimization issues in physiological toxicokinetic modeling—a case study with benzene. Toxicol. Lett. **69:** 181–196.
22. GELFAND, A.E. & A.F.M. SMITH. 1990. Sampling-based approaches to calculating marginal densities. J. Am. Stat. Assoc. **85:** 398–409.
23. SMITH, A.F.M. 1991. Bayesian computational methods. Phil. Trans. Royal Soc. London, Series A. **337:** 369–386.
24. GELMAN, A. 1992. Iterative and non-iterative simulation algorithms. Computing Science and Statistics **24:** 433–438.
25. RACINE-POON, A. & A.F. SMITH. 1990. Population models. *In* Statistical Methodology in the Pharmaceutical Sciences. D.A. Berry Ed.: 139–162. Marcel Dekker, New York.
26. SHEINER, L.B. & T.M. LUDDEN. 1992. Population pharmacokinetics/dynamics. Annu. Rev. Pharmacol. Toxicol. **32:** 185–209.
27. SMITH, A.F.M. & J. WAKEFIELD. 1994. The hierarchical Bayesian approach to population pharmacokinetic modelling. Int. J. Bio-Med. Comput. **36:** 35–42.
28. WAKEFIELD, J.C. 1996. The Bayesian analysis of population pharmacokinetic models. J. Am. Stat. Assoc. **91:** 62–75.
29. SHEINER, L.B. 1984. The population approach to pharmacokinetic data analysis: rationale and standard data analysis methods. Drug Metab. Rev. **15:** 153–171.
30. KONG, A. et al. 1994. Sequential imputations and Bayesian missing data problems. J. Am. Stat. Assoc. **89:** 278–288.
31. DEMPSTER, A.P. et al. 1983. Combining historical and randomized controls for assessing trends in proportions. J. Am. Stat. Assoc. **76:** 221–227.
32. BOIS, F.Y. & D. MASZLE. 1997. MCSim: a simulation program. J. Stat. Software **2**(9): http://www.stat.ucla.edu/journals/jss/v02/i09 (also available at ftp://sparky.berkeley.edu/pub/mcsim).
33. MONSTER, A.C. et al. 1979. Kinetics of tetrachloroethylene in volunteers; Influence of exposure concentration and work load. Int. Arch. Occup. Environ. Health. **42:** 303–309.
34. ANDERSEN, M.E. et al. 1991. Physiologically based pharmacokinetics modeling with dichloromethane, its metabolite, carbon monoxide, and blood carboxyhemoglobin in rats and humans. Toxicol. Appl. Pharmacol. **108:** 14–27.
35. NATIONAL TOXICOLOGY PROGRAM (NTP). 1986. Toxicology and carcinogenesis studies of dichloromethane (methylene chloride) in F344/N rats and B6C3F1 mice. Technical Report Series No. 306 (NIH Publication No. 86-2562). NTP, Bethesda, MD.
36. ANDERSEN, M.E. et al. 1987. Physiologically based pharmacokinetics and the risk assessment process for methylene chloride. Toxicol. Appl. Pharmacol. **87:** 185–205.
37. DEDRICK, R.L. et al. 1972. *In vitro-in vivo* correlations of drug metabolism—deamination of 1-beta-D-arabinofuranosylcytosine. Biochem. Pharmacol. **21:** 1–16.
38. TRAVIS, C.C. et al. 1990. Pharmacokinetics of benzene. Toxicol. Appl. Pharmacol. **102:** 400–420.
39. WOODRUFF, T. et al. 1992. Structure and parametrization of toxicokinetic models: their impact on model predictions. Risk Anal. **12:** 189–201.
40. INGS, R.M. 1990. Interspecies scaling and comparisons in drug development and toxicokinetics. Xenobiotica **20:** 1201–1231.
41. VAN RYZIN, J. & K. RAI. 1987. A dose-response model incorporating nonlinear kinetics. Biometrics **43:** 95–105.

Uncertainty in Risk Characterization of Weak Carcinogens

NAOHITO YAMAGUCHI[a]

Cancer Information and Epidemiology Division,
National Cancer Center Research Institute,
5-1-1 Tsukiji, Chuo-ku, Tokyo, Japan

ABSTRACT: Epidemiologic inference is subject to uncertainty that is inherent to observational approaches. It was shown by the present analysis that an SMR of 1.4, as observed for 2,3,7,8-tetrachlorodibenzo-*para*-dioxin in the pooled analysis by IARC, would be observed in the absence of carcinogenic risk, if the smoking prevalence of cohort members was as low as 80%. It was also shown that a 1.4-fold increase in lung cancer risk among nonsmokers, which roughly corresponds to a daily consumption of one cigarette, might be extremely difficult to identify if the subjects are exposed to strong carcinogens such as those that result from cigarette smoking. On the other hand, a genotoxic agent that increases the lung cancer risk of smokers 1.4-fold, could increase the risk to nonsmokers by as much as 6.3-fold. In light of these uncertainties in epidemiologic inference, attempts to estimate the absolute risk in human populations by epidemiologic studies should be made with caution.

INTRODUCTION

Epidemiology has played a substantial role in identifying and assessing carcinogens, to which people are exposed in their daily life. As the focus shifts toward weaker carcinogens, however, an epidemiology study inevitably suffers from inadequate sensitivity in identifying an increased risk, and also from distortion of results by biases and confounding factors. The long-term rodent bioassay, when it is appropriately performed, also provides evidence that may be extrapolated to humans. However, it is not realistic to expect a rodent bioassay to cover thousands of agents that are potentially carcinogenic with weak potency. In light of these limitations, inherent to epidemiology and laboratory assays, the strengths and weaknesses of epidemiologic approaches should be studied in the context of risk assessment procedures.

Epidemiologic inference is subject to uncertainty that is inherent to observational approaches. The results obtained from epidemiologic studies can be extrapolated to humans as a whole in a more straightforward ways than can those of animal experiments, but the risk estimated by epidemiology is often distorted or biased from the true value of the study population, because of inappropriate study designs. The former is called the external validity and the latter is called the internal validity.[1] An

---

[a]Address for correspondence: Naohito Yamaguchi, M.D., Cancer Information and Epidemiology Division, National Cancer Center Research Institute, 5-1-1 Tsukiji, Chuo-ku, Tokyo 104-0045, Japan. +81-3-3542-2511 ext. 4250 (voice) +81-3-3546-0630 (fax).
 e-mail: nyamaguc@gan2.ncc.go.jp

epidemiologic study, when properly designed and conducted, is superior to animal experiments in terms of external validity, but animal experiments, or experimental approaches in general, are superior to epidemiology, or observational studies in general, in terms of internal validity.[2] Various methodologies have been proposed to guarantee internal validity. Among major methodology issues are selection avoidance and information bias, controlling the effects of confounding factors, and accounting for the existence of effect modifiers.

In this paper we discuss the role of epidemiology in the risk assessment of weak carcinogens, with special reference to the effects of confounding factors and effect modifiers. The lung cancer risk associated with exposure to dioxins is used for demonstrative purposes because the quantitative relationship between cigarette smoking and lung cancer risk has already been elucidated. This quantitative relationship will be used to characterize the combined effects of smoking and exposure to dioxins from epidemiologic viewpoints.

CUMULATIVE CIGARETTE CONSUMPTION AND LUNG CANCER MORTALITY IN JAPAN

Before dealing with the problem of dioxins, we describe the quantitative relationship between cigarette smoking and lung cancer mortality in Japan. In Japan, the lung cancer death rate has been increasing for both males and females, and this increase has previously been considered to be attributable to increased cigarette consumption. In an attempt to examine the quantitative relationship on a national level, trends in age-specific lung cancer death rates were analyzed, on a birth-cohort basis

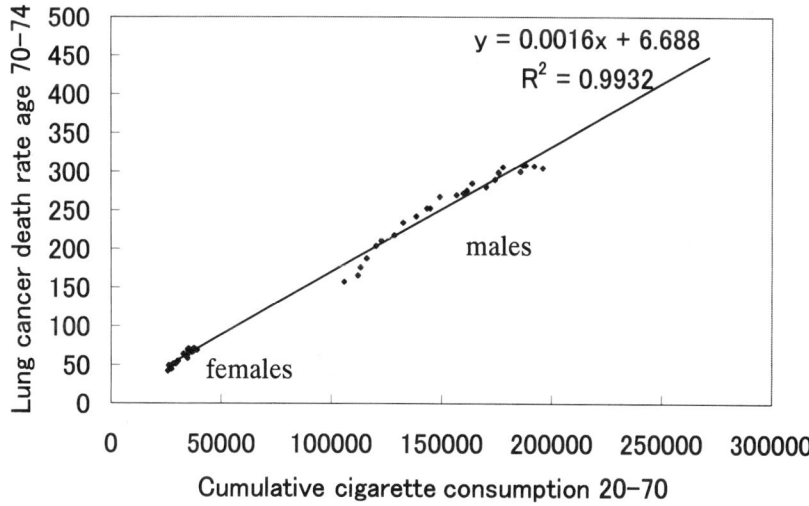

FIGURE 1. The linear relation between cumulative cigarette consumption during the period from age 20 to 70 and the lung cancer death rate for age 70–74 in Japan.

TABLE 1. Covariance analysis of age-specific lung cancer death rate in relation to cumulative cigarette consumption (CCC)

Age	Significance of effects			Intercept		Slope	
	sex	CCC	sex × CCC	males	females	males	females
25–29	ns	ns	ns	0.367	0.367	0	0
30–34	ns	ns	ns	0.817	0.817	0	0
35–39	ns	$p < 0.001$	ns	1.423	1.423	0.09457	0.09457
40–44	ns	$p < 0.001$	0.021	1.748	1.748	0.3421	0.8557
45–49	ns	$p < 0.001$	ns	4.372	4.372	0.5698	0.5698
50–54	$p < 0.001$	$p < 0.001$	ns	11.908	7.525	0.8548	0.8548
55–59	$p < 0.001$	$p < 0.001$	ns	18.573	10.266	2.132	2.132
60–64	0.001	$p < 0.001$	ns	20.837	11.562	4.913	4.913
65–69	0.006	$p < 0.001$	ns	24.680	12.243	9.019	9.019
70–74	ns	$p < 0.001$	ns	6.688	6.688	16.27	16.27

for males and females combined, in relation to cumulative cigarette consumption of the birth cohort prior to the observation of lung cancer deaths. Cumulative cigarette consumption of a birth cohort was estimated by summing, over age, the age-specific cigarette consumption, calculated by multiplying the average daily number of cigarettes consumed by a smoker of that age by the age-specific smoking prevalence. The results showed that the age-specific lung cancer death rate increases in proportion to

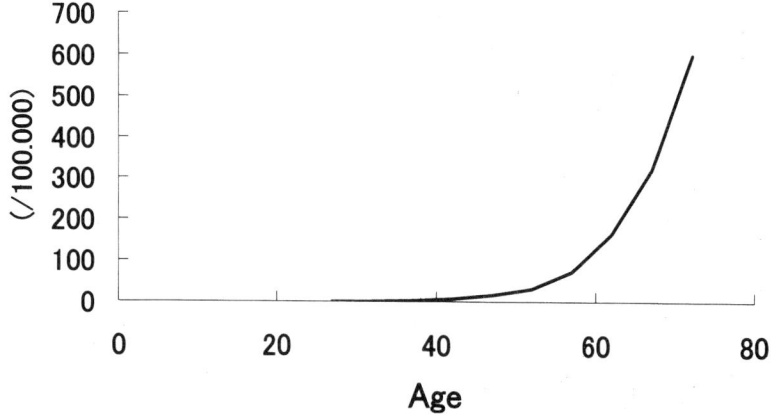

FIGURE 2. The lung cancer death rate among male smokers consuming 20 cigarettes a day since age 20, estimated from regression equations of five-year age specific death rates and cumulative cigarette consumption.

cumulative cigarette consumption, as illustrated in FIGURE 1 for the death rate of the 70–74 year age group.[3] From a mechanistic viewpoint, this linear increase suggests that cigarette smoking acts on a single event, possibly damage to DNA, in the process of carcinogenesis. The lifetime lung cancer mortality risk of a person with any history of cigarette smoking can be estimated by calculating lung cancer death rates of different five-year age categories using the regression equations obtained for each five-year age group (TABLE 1), and then combining them into cumulative risk using the actuarial method. For example, the curve in FIGURE 2 shows a hypothetical age-mortality curve for males who have continued to smoke 20 cigarettes a day since age 20. This estimate is found to be in good agreement with other reports of the quantitative relationship between cigarette smoking and lung cancer risk, such as the prospective cohort study by British physicians.[4]

UNCERTAINTY CAUSED BY RESIDUAL CONFOUNDING

A potential confounding factor is an independent risk or preventive factor for a disease of interest. When the distribution of the potential confounding factor is associated with the agent under investigation, the risk estimate for the agent could be biased because of the existence of the confounding factor (see FIGURE 3). In this situation, the factor is called an *actual* confounding factor, or *confounder*. The bias caused by confounding factors is usually eliminated by selecting a proper study design, such as matching; or by using proper analytical methods, such as stratified analysis or multivariate analysis. However, since there is no disease for which all the risk and preventive factors have been elucidated, the risk estimate could be biased by unknown confounding factors, these are called *residual* confounding factors. The magnitude of distortion by residual confounding factors cannot be visualized in an actual study, but it can be evaluated by examining the effect of a known confounding factor when it is not properly controlled.

In 1997, the International Agency for Research on Cancer (IARC) classified 2,3,7,8-tetrachlorodibenzo-*para*-dioxin (TCDD) as a human carcinogen, although epidemiologic studies were considered to provide only limited evidence on the car-

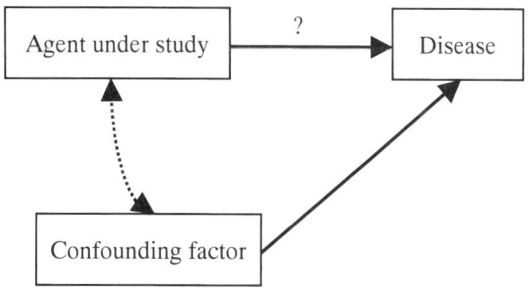

FIGURE 3. Schematic explanation of a confounding factor. *Solid lines* indicate causal relationships; *dotted line* indicates a noncausal association.

cinogenicity.[5] For the lung cancer risk, the standardized mortality ratio (SMR) was estimated at 1.4 with a 95% confidence interval of 1.1–1.7, obtained by pooling four retrospective cohort studies.[5–9] Among various epidemiologic methods, the retrospective cohort study is used most frequently for occupational cancer risks. One of the problems that could have distorted the results of these retrospective cohort studies is the confounding effect of cigarette smoking. If the smoking history of cohort members differs from that of the comparison group, which is usually the general population, the comparison of lung cancer mortality would be biased by the difference.

To provide a numerical example, consider a hypothetical retrospective cohort study of Japanese male workers, whose age is uniformly distributed between 40 and 64. According to the regression equations shown in TABLE 1, the expected annual lung cancer death rate in this cohort is 57.4 per 100,000, if none of them had smoked cigarettes, and 283.1 per 100,000 if they had smoked 20 cigarettes a day since the age of 20. Suppose, for simplicity, that the members of the cohort consist of lifetime non-smokers and current smokers who had smoked 20 cigarettes a day since the age of 20. The lung cancer death rate in the entire cohort is then an average of the two rates, non-smokers and 20-cigarette smokers, weighted by the smoking prevalence. Since the smoking prevalence in the general male population of Japan is estimated at 55%, the expected lung cancer death rate of the cohort is 181.5 per 100,000 ($= 0.55 \times 283.1 + 0.45 \times 57.4$). If the smoking prevalence of the cohort members is higher than the national average of 55%, the expected lung cancer mortality rate of the co-

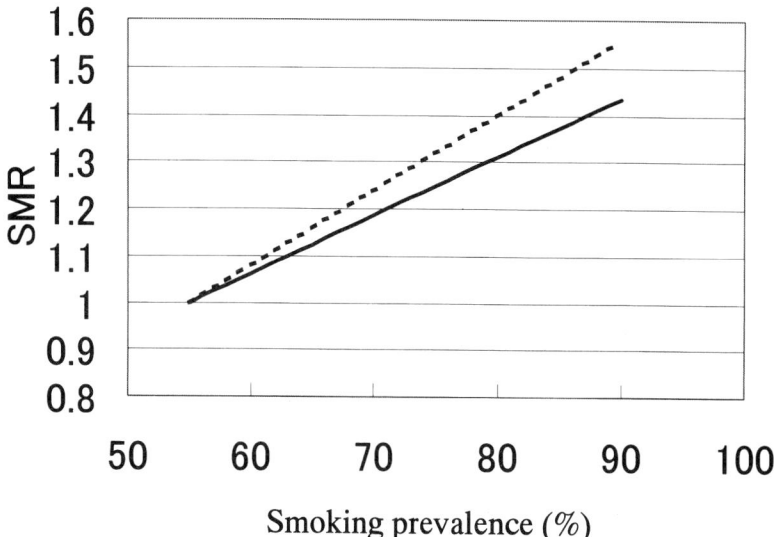

FIGURE 4. Increase in standardized mortality rate (SMR) of lung cancer, in proportion to the smoking prevalence, for hypothetical cohorts of Japanese males aged 40 to 64 (*solid line*) and 50 to 74 (*dotted line*). The smoking prevalence in the general population, with which the mortality experience of cohorts is compared, is assumed to be 55%.

hort would be larger than 181.5 per 100,000, due solely to the higher smoking prevalence. In FIGURE 4, the SMR is plotted against the smoking prevalence for two hypothetical cohort studies: the cohort mentioned above, and a similar cohort consisting of Japanese male workers whose age is uniformly distributed between 50 and 74. FIGURE 4 shows that the SMR increases in proportion to the smoking prevalence of the cohort, and that the increase is larger for the cohort of older subjects. The SMR of 1.4, as observed for 2,3,7,8-TCDD in the pooled analysis of four cohort studies by IARC, would be observed in the absence of carcinogenic risk, if the smoking prevalence was 87%, for the cohort aged 40–64; and 80% for the cohort aged 50–74. Since the smoking prevalence among blue collar workers is known to be higher than that of others, the SMR would overestimate the true risk to some extent, unless smoking is properly controlled in any retrospective cohort study of workers.

The above hypothetical examples indicate that cigarette smoking, unless appropriately controlled, might have biassed the results of lung cancer mortality to by as much as the SMR observed for 2,3,7,8-TCDD. It is also noteworthy that this bias cannot be reduced by increasing the number of subjects in the cohort. The best way to eliminate this bias is to control for the smoking by collecting smoking history data from all the cohort members as well as from the comparison group. However, this is not always possible, particularly when the cohort is compared with the general population as the external comparison group. As shown in FIGURE 4, the confounding effect of smoking increases as the cohort becomes older and the effect of smoking becomes stronger. Therefore, a cohort consisting of younger subjects might be better than older subjects, although the lower death rate in younger age groups necessitates a larger sample size to ensure adequate statistical significance.

EFFECT MODIFICATION AND UNCERTAINTY IN EPIDEMIOLOGIC INFERENCE

An effect modifier is a factor that modifies the effect of an agent on disease occurrence.[1] The effect modification depends on the effect measure that is used to quantify the relationship between agent and disease occurrence. Here we focus the discussion on ratio measures, such as the SMR, because these are used most frequently as effect measures in epidemiology of occupational and environmental cancers. In cancer epidemiology, synergistic or antagonistic interaction of two factors often occurs according to the modes of action of two factors in the carcinogenic processes. The simplest classification of modes of action widely used in animal carcinogenesis models is the distinction between initiation and promotion. For example, cigarette smoking is believed to act as an initiator, causing DNA damage to target cells. For an agent coacting with cigarette smoking, three different modes of action need to be considered, as shown schematically in FIGURE 5. In Case 1, both smoking and the agent of interest act as initiators. In Case 2, smoking acts as initiator, the agent acts as promoter, and the two factors act by different causal pathways. In Case 3, smoking acts as initiator, the agent acts as promoter, and the two factors act by the same causal pathway.

To examine how different modes of action influence the risk estimate, consider two hypothetical studies in which lung cancer risk is analyzed in relation to an agent.

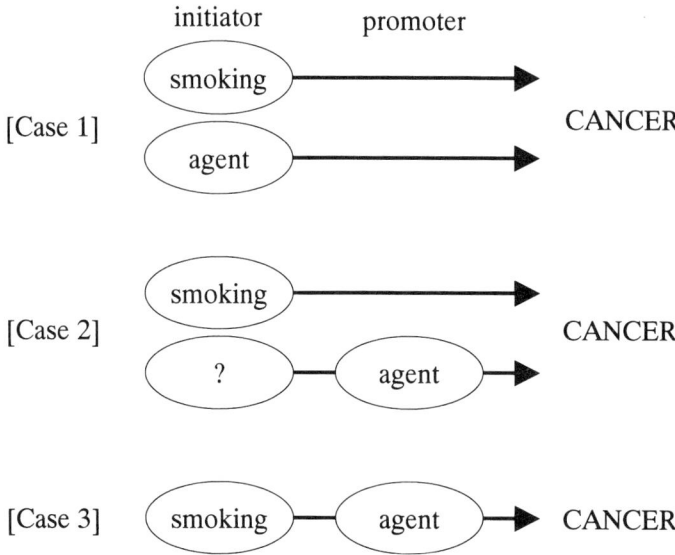

FIGURE 5. Three different relationships between the agent under study and smoking acting as an effect modifier. In *Case 1*, both agent and smoking act as initiators. In *Case 2*, smoking acts as an initiator and the agent acts as a promoter; smoking and agent act by different causal pathways. In *Case 3*, smoking acts as an initiator and the agent acts as a promoter; smoking and agent act by the same causal pathway.

The subjects of one study are all lifetime nonsmokers, whereas those of the other study are all regular smokers who have consumed 20 cigarettes a day since the age of 20. For simplicity, the cumulative lung cancer risk by age 75, more precisely the probability of dying from lung cancer by age 75 conditional on the absence of other causes of death, is used as the effect measure.

Suppose that the agent was found to increase the cumulative lung cancer risk 1.4-fold in the study of nonsmokers. As shown in FIGURE 6, the cumulative lung cancer risk by age 75 can be estimated, by using the regression equations in Table 1, at 0.456% for a lifetime nonsmoker and at 0.729% for a male regular smoker who consumed one cigarette a day since age 20. Therefore, the 1.4-fold increase in risk, which corresponds to the cumulative risk of 0.638%, is comparable to the increase in risk caused by consuming one cigarette a day. If this agent acts as initiator (as is shown in Case 1 of FIG. 5), the exposure of a smoker to this agent is to add one cigarette to the number of cigarettes smoked daily. For example, for a 20-cigarette regular smoker, the effect of exposure to the agent is equal to smoking 21 cigarettes a day. The cumulative lung cancer risk by age 75 is 5.77% and 6.03% for a regular smoker consuming 20 and 21 cigarettes a day, respectively, according to the regression equations in TABLE 1. This indicates that the effect of the agent for 20-cigarette regular smoker is 1.04-fold (= 6.03/5.77)—much smaller than the effect for nonsmokers (see FIGURE 7). For cases in which the agent acts as a promoter on a causal

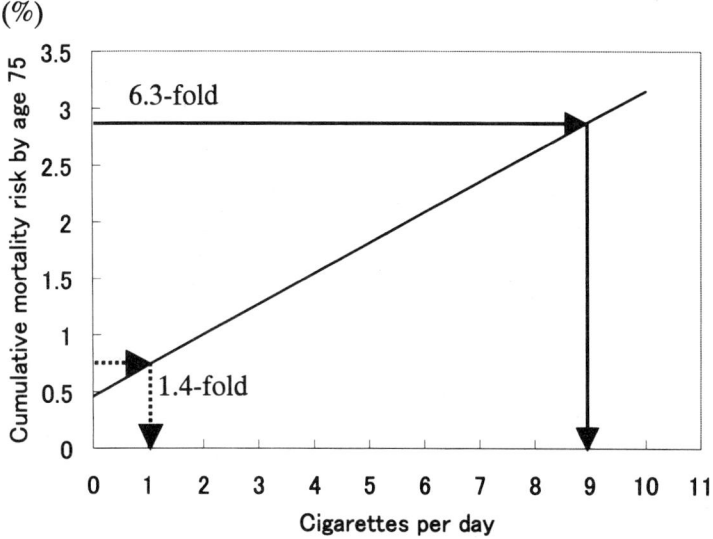

FIGURE 6. The cumulative lung cancer mortality risk by age 75 in relation to the number of cigarettes consumed per day, ranging from 0 to 10.

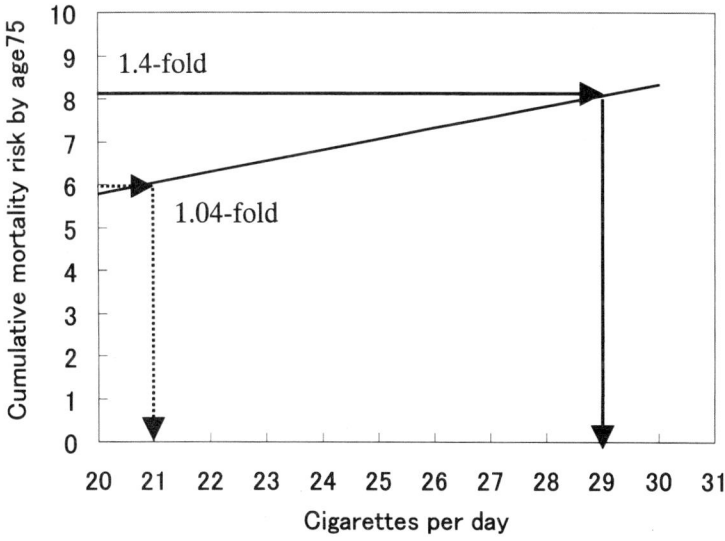

FIGURE 7. The cumulative lung cancer mortality risk by age 75 in relation to the number of cigarettes consumed per day, ranging from 20 to 30.

pathway different from that of smoking (Case 2 of FIG. 5), the effect of the agent is again to add one cigarette a day. No distinction can be made between Cases 1 and 2 of FIGURE 5 as far as effect modification is concerned. Only in cases where smoking acts as initiator, the agent acts as promoter, and both act on the same causal pathway (as in Case 3 of Fig. 5), can exposure to the agent be expected to multiply the risk by 1.4 regardless of the smoking status. For example, for a regular smoker consuming 20 cigarettes a day, the cumulative risk by age 75 will increase from 5.77% to 8.08% (= 5.77 × 1.4), which corresponds to adding nine cigarettes a day, as shown in FIGURE 7.

Now consider an agent that has been shown to increase, by 1.4-fold, the cumulative lung cancer mortality risk by age 75 of regular smokers consuming 20 cigarettes a day. The 1.4-fold increase among smokers consuming 20 cigarettes per day corresponds to the addition of nine more cigarettes, as shown by solid arrows in FIGURE 7. Therefore, if this agent acts as an initiator (Case 1 of FIG. 5) or as a promoter independent of the causal pathway of smoking (Case 2 of FIG. 5), the exposure of nonsmokers to this agent will increase the cumulative risk from 0.456% to 2.89%—a 6.3-fold increase—corresponding to a consumption of nine cigarettes a day. If the agent acts as promoter using the same causal pathway as smoking, the increase in cumulative risk among nonsmokers is the same as for smokers, a 1.4-fold increase.

These two hypothetical studies of nonsmokers and smokers indicate that the risk ratio can be influenced by coexisting risk factors, such as cigarette smoking. Such factors are called effect modifiers. It is also suggested that the effect modification depends on the mode of action in the carcinogenic pathways. The results seem to have several implications for the risk assessment of weak carcinogens. First, they indicate that an initiator with weak potency is difficult to identify in a situation where stronger initiators such as cigarettes smoking coexist. An agent that has been shown to be carcinogenic in animal experiments without concurrent exposures to other agents, might sometimes be very difficult to identify by an epidemiologic study, because of coexisting carcinogens. Second, an agent that has been shown to be a weak carcinogen in an epidemiologic study of subjects with concurrent exposure to carcinogens such as cigarettes smoking, might exert a stronger effect in people without concurrent exposure. In actual epidemiologic studies there are always smokers among the study subjects, and this means that the effect on nonsmokers could be stronger than the observed risk estimate if the agent acts as initiator or as promoter independent of the causal pathway of smoking.

DISCUSSION

In this paper, the effects of coexisting factors on risk estimation were discussed from two different aspects, confounding and effect modification. The results for the confounding effect of smoking indicate that the slight increase in cancer risk observed in an epidemiologic study should be interpreted with caution. At least a part of the increase might be attributable to residual confounding factors. An external comparison with national death rates always suffers from the confounding effect of cigarette smoking, because of the lack of reliable data on national death rates that are specific to smoking status. If smoking status data were available for cohort members, analysis within each cohort could be performed to assess the separate, as well as the combined, effects of smoking and exposure to the agent under study. This type of multivariate analysis also enables us to investigate the degree of effect modification by examining the improvement in model fit when interaction terms are incorporated.

The results for effect modification by smoking indicate that the magnitude of increased risk should be interpreted with caution, because it might change when the prevalence of effect modifier in the target population is different from that of the study subjects. It is particularly noteworthy that the relative risk of 1.4, when identified for smokers, is not applicable to nonsmokers if the agent acts as an initiator. Even if the effect on nonsmokers is as high as 6.3-fold, as shown in our hypothetical study, it is often difficult to identify the increased risk among nonsmokers because of high smoking prevalence, as well as lack of smoking data.

What are the implications of the present discussions for cancers other than lung cancer? In other cancer sites that could possibly be involved in occupational and environmental cancers, we have much less (and unreliable) information on confounders and effect modifiers. The effect of genotoxic agents could be diluted in epidemiologic studies, and for such cases, long-term rodent bioassays and other laboratory tests would be useful for hazard identification. Nonetheless, epidemiology should continue to play its role in identifying occupational and environmental cancer risks by exploring unusual occurrence of cancer in workers and general populations, because further studies, including laboratory experiments, will not be initiated unless possible hazardous effect is perceived by a scientific society or regulatory agency. Even though the risk estimate expressed by epidemiologic risk measures, such as SMR, is subject to uncertainty, an increased risk observed in epidemiologic studies provides a good starting point to explore hazards that might otherwise remain undetected.

REFERENCES

1. KLEINBAUM, D.G., L.L. KUPPER & H. MORGENSTERN. 1982. Epidemiologic research. Wadsworth, Belmont.
2. YAMAGUCHI, N. 1998. Role of epidemiology in cancer risk assessment. Rev. Toxicol. **2:** 53–58.
3. YAMAGUCHI, N., Y. MOCHIZUKI-KOBAYASHI & S. WATANABE. 1998. Tobacco in Japan. Proc. 10th World Conference on Tobacco or Health. In press.
4. DOLL, R. & PETO, R. 1978. Cigarette smoking and bronchial carcinoma: dose and time relationships among regular smokers and lifelong non-smokers. J. Epidemiol. Community Health **32:** 303–313.
5. INTERNATIONAL AGENCY FOR RESEARCH ON CANCER. 1997. Polychlorinated dibenzo-*para*-dioxins and polychlorinated dibenzofurans. IARC Monograph. **69:** 335–343.
6. OTT, M.G. & A. ZOBER. 1996. Cause specific mortality and cancer incidence among employees exposed to 2,3,7,8-TCDD after a 1953 reactor accident. Occup. Environ. Med. **53:** 606–612.
7. HOOIVELD, M., D. HEEDERIK & H.B. BUENO DE MESQUITA. 1996. Preliminary results of the second follow-up of a Dutch cohort of workers occupationally exposed to phenoxy herbicides, chlorophenols and contaminants. Organohalogen Compounds **30:** 185–189.
8. FINGERHUT, M.A., W.E. HALPERIN, D.A. MARLOW, L.A. PIACITELLI, P.A. HONCHAR, M.H. SWEENEY, A.L. GREIFE, P.A. DILL, K. STEENLAND & A.J. SURUDA. 1991. Cancer mortality in workers exposed to 2,3,7,8-tetrachlorodibenzo-*para*-dioxin. N. Engl. J. Med. **324:** 212–218.
9. BECHER, H., D. FLESCH-JANYS, T. KAUPPINEN, M. KOGEVINAS, K. STEINDORF, A. MANZ & J. WAHRENDORF. 1996. Cancer mortality in German male workers exposed to phenoxy herbicides and dioxins. Cancer Causes & Control **7:** 312–321.

Reducing Uncertainty in the Derivation and Application of Health Guidance Values in Public Health Practice

Dioxin as a Case Study

CHRISTOPHER T. DE ROSA,[a,b] HANA R. POHL,[b] HUGH HANSEN,[b] ROBIN C. LEONARD,[c] JAMES HOLLER,[b] AND DENNIS JONES[b]

[b]*Agency for Toxic Substances and Disease Registry Public Health Service, U.S. Department of Health and Human Services, Atlanta, Georgia 30333, USA*

[c]*Haskell Laboratory for Toxicology and Industrial Medicine, Newark, Delaware 19714, USA*

ABSTRACT: We were requested by the U.S. Environmental Protection Agency (EPA) to clarify the relationships among the minimal risk level (MRL), action level, and environmental media evaluation guide (EMEG) for dioxin established by the Agency for Toxic Substances and Disease Registry (ATSDR). In response we developed a document entitled "Dioxin and Dioxin-Like Compounds in Soil, Part I: ATSDR Interim Policy Guideline"; and a supporting document entitled "Dioxin and Dioxin-Like Compounds in Soil, Part II: Technical Support Document". In these documents, we evaluated the key assumptions underlying the development and use of the ATSDR action level, MRL, and EMEG for dioxin. We described the chronology of events outlining these different health guidance values for dioxin and identified the areas of uncertainty surrounding these values. Four scientific assumptions were found to have had a great impact on this process; these were: (1) the specific uncertainty factors used, (2) the toxicity equivalent (TEQ) approach, (3) the fractional exposure from different pathways, and (4) the use of body burdens in the absence of exposure data. This information was subsequently used to develop a framework for reducing the uncertainties in public health risk assessment associated with exposure to other chemical contaminants in the environment. Within this framework are a number of future directions for reducing uncertainty, including physiologically based pharmacokinetic modeling (PBPK), benchmark dose modeling (BMD), functional toxicology, and the assessment of chemical mixture interactions.

INTRODUCTION

The mission of the Agency for Toxic Substances and Disease Registry (ATSDR) is to prevent, or mitigate, adverse human health effects and diminished quality of life resulting from exposure to hazardous substances from waste sites, unplanned releas-

[a]Address for correspondence: C.T. De Rosa, ATSDR, Division of Toxicology, E-29, 1600 Clifton Road, Atlanta, Georgia 30333, USA. 404-639-6300 (voice); 404-639-6315 (fax).
e-mail: cyd0@cdc.com

es, and other sources of pollution present in the environment. ATSDR evaluates information from hazardous waste sites and uses this information to prepare site-specific public health assessments and consultations. Health assessors must have a knowledge of many site-related issues, including site description and history, land use, community concerns, health outcome data, environmental contaminants of concern, and completed exposure pathways. Health-based guidance values, specifically the ATSDR minimal risk levels (MRLs) and environmental media evaluation guides (EMEGs), play an important role in assessing the public health implications of low-level exposures to substances found at hazardous waste sites. By staying abreast of the latest research relating to toxicity, toxicokinetics, and toxicodynamics of hazardous chemicals, ATSDR continually refines the judgment that is used in developing these values.[1,2] Nevertheless, the health assessment process involves many assumptions, limitations, and uncertainties that must be dealt with. This paper outlines some of the uncertainties encountered during development of an ATSDR interim policy guideline for dioxin and dioxin-like compounds in soil[3,4] and describes the approach taken by ATSDR to further address uncertainty in health guidance values, in consultation with its Board of Scientific Councillors.

BACKGROUND ON THE ATSDR INTERIM POLICY GUIDELINE FOR DIOXIN AND DIOXIN-LIKE COMPOUNDS IN SOIL

The ATSDR interim policy guideline for dioxin and dioxin-like compounds in soil addressed several issues.[3,4] The three primary issues evaluated were: (1) the relationship between the ATSDR action level of 1 ppb dioxin and dioxin-like compounds in residential soil and the ATSDR EMEGs, (2) concern that current analytic and sampling techniques employed for soil contaminated with dioxin and dioxin-like compounds may not be sufficiently sensitive, and (3) concern that the ATSDR action level of 1 ppb dioxin and dioxin-like compounds in residential soil may be too high.

ATSDR outlined three steps to evaluate human exposure from soil contaminated with hazardous chemicals: (1) screening for contaminants of concern, (2) evaluating potential exposure pathways, and (3) defining public health implications and actions. This approach was also used to evaluate dioxin exposure from soil. ATSDR outlined a framework that can be used by health assessors to evaluate dioxin-contaminated soil (TABLE 1). The ATSDR decisions were based on an extensive review of current literature pertaining to dioxin and dioxin-like compounds that was presented in an ATSDR draft "Toxicological Profile for Chlorinated Dibenzo-p-dioxins",[5] with more recent data cited and discussed in the policy paper itself.

With reference to the specific issues listed previously, the ATSDR interim policy concluded that:

1. The ATSDR action level of 1 ppb of dioxin and dioxin-like compounds expressed in toxicity equivalents (TEQs) in residential soil is consistent with the ATSDR EMEG. These values are used for distinctly different purposes in evaluating dioxin-contaminated sites (TABLE 1).

2. Currently used soil analytic methods may not be sufficiently sensitive. Determination of an appropriate analytic method should be made on a site-specific basis. Specific knowledge of different dioxin-like compounds at a given site is required in order to evaluate the adequacy of a soil-sampling protocol.
3. The ATSDR action level of 1 ppb for dioxin and dioxin-like compounds (TEQs) in residential soil is not too high. Use of the 1 ppb action level should be decided on a site-specific basis in which residential soil levels greater than 50 ppt and less than 1 ppb are further evaluated in the context of site-specific parameters.

While developing the interim policy guideline, ATSDR dealt with assumptions, limitations, and uncertainties pertaining to both health assessments in general, and to some dioxin-specific issues. Dealing with these topics was a complex and evolving experience. Because dioxin exposure is associated with effects at very low levels and a wide range of considerations was taken into account, the approach used by ATSDR in addressing these issues can serve as an example that may provide a framework for health assessment of other toxic chemicals.

TABLE 1. ATSDR decision framework for sites contaminated with dioxin and dioxin-like compounds

Screening Level	Evaluation Levels	Action Level[a]
≤ 50 ppt TEQs[b]	> 50 ppt but < 1 ppb TEQs	≥ 1 ppb TEQs
•The EMEG for TCDD is 50 ppt	Evaluation of site-specific factors, such as	Potential public health actions considered, such as
• This is based on an MRL of 1 pg/kg/day for TCDD.	• Bioavailability	• Surveillance
• For screening purposes 50 ppt TCDD is assumed to be equivalent to 50 ppt TEQs	• Ingestion rates	• Research
	• Pathway analysis	• Health studies
	• Soil cover	• Community education
	• Climate	• Physician education
	• Other contaminants	• Exposure investigations
	• Community concerns	
	• Demographics	
	• Background exposures	

[a]A concentration of chemicals at which consideration of action to interdict/prevent exposure occurs, such as surveillance, research, health studies, community education, physician education, or exposure investigations. Alternatively, based on the evaluation by the health assessor, none of these actions may be necessary.

[b]The toxicity equivalent (TEQ) of 2,3,7,8-tetrachlorodibenzo-p-dioxin (TCDD) is calculated by multiplying the exposure level of a particular dioxin-like compound by its toxicity equivalency factor (TEF). TEFs are based on congener-specific data and the assumption that Ah receptor-mediated toxicity of dioxin-like chemicals is additive. The TEF scheme compares the relative toxicity of individual dioxin-like compounds to that of TCDD.

UNCERTAINTIES ASSOCIATED WITH THE DERIVATION OF MRLS

Areas of Uncertainty

Data Used in Various Risk Assessment Methods Are Incomplete

An incomplete database is the first source of uncertainty introduced into the risk assessment process. We may, for example, know that a certain effect occurs following oral exposure to a chemical, but can we infer from this observation that there are other routes of exposure? Similarly, extrapolation among exposure-duration categories may be difficult. Often information is available from laboratory studies in animals but relevant studies in humans are lacking. Interspecies anatomical differences (e.g., nasal turbinate in rodents, forestomach in rodents, Zymbal glands in rats, stomach in herbivores) may obviously contribute to differences in the chemical toxicity mechanism. Interspecies differences in pathophysiological responses and in pathogenesis of diseases must be also considered. For example, chronic progressive nephropathy is an age-related spontaneous disorder of rats that is more severe in males than in females and that affects certain strains more than others.[6] Chronic exposure of male rats to $\alpha_2\mu$-globulin-inducing agents results in the aggravation of chronic progressive nephropathy, characterized by increased severity and earlier onset of the disease. It has been postulated that this pathophysiology of renal disease may not be applicable to humans.

Scientific uncertainty on validity of the endpoint was also considered in the derivation of chronic oral MRL for 2,3,7,8-tetrachlorodibenzo-*p*-dioxin (2,3,7,8-TCDD). The chronic oral MRL was based on the neurobehavioral endpoint from teratology studies in monkeys (mothers exposed to dietary concentration of 5 ppt 2,3,7,8-TCDD). No significant alterations in reflex development, visual exploration, locomotor activity, or fine motor control were found.[7] In tests of cognitive function, object learning was significantly impaired, but no effect on spatial learning was observed.[8] When the monkeys were placed in social groups, altered social behavior was observed.[7,9] This lowest-observed-adverse-effect level (LOAEL) was classified as minimal—an uncertainty factor of 90 was used for MRL derivation (see TABLE 2).

Rier *et al.*[10] identified a less serious LOAEL of 5 ppt (0.00012 µg/kg/day) for moderate endometriosis. However, monkeys appear to be more susceptible to endometriosis, based on a background incidence of endometriosis (in monkeys) of 30%[10] compared with a background incidence of 10% in humans.[11] Thus, derivation of a chronic oral MRL based on endometriosis would necessitate using an uncertainty factor of at most 1 to account for the increased sensitivity of monkeys to endometriosis as compared with humans. ATSDR considered using the Rier *et al.*[10] study to calculate an oral MRL, based on the LOAEL of 0.00012 µg/kg/day divided by an uncertainty factor of 100 (10 to extrapolate from a LOAEL, 10 for human variability, and 1 for interspecies differences). This would have resulted in a computed MRL that was essentially the same as the chronic oral MRL of 1 pg/kg/day based on developmental toxicity, as described in the preceding paragraph. Moreover, (1) the clinical history for these rhesus monkeys during the 10-year period between the Schantz *et al.*[9] study and examination by Rier *et al.*[10] is unknown (not reported); (2) Boyd *et al.*[12] did not find an association between exposure to chlorinated dibenzo-*p*-dioxins (CDDs), chlorinated dibenzofurans (CDFs), or polychlorinated biphenyls

TABLE 2. Comparison of MRLs for 2,3,7,8-TCDD derived in 1989 and 1997

Year	Exposure duration	MRL in pg/kg/d	UF LOAEL/NOAEL	UF interspecies	UF sensitivity	Endpoint	See reference
1989	acute	1000	10	10	10	LOAEL for hepatic focal necrosis and hypertrophy	25
1997	acute	200	1	3	10	NOAEL for immunological effects	26
1989	intermediate adopted also as chronic	1	10	10	10	LOAEL for reproductive, abortions and developmental effects	22, 23
1997	chronic	1	3	3	10	LOAEL for neurobehavioral developmental effects	9

NOTE: The MRL is calculated as MRL = (NOAEL or LOAEL)/(UF × MF), where MRL is the minimal risk level (mg/kg/day), NOAEL is the no-observed-adverse-effect level (mg/kg/day), LOAEL is the lowest-observed-adverse-effect level (mg/kg/day), UF is the uncertainty factor (dimensionless), and MF is the modifying factor (dimensionless).

(PCBs) and endometriosis in a clinical study in women; and (3) the U.S. Environmental Protection Agency (EPA)[13] concluded that "the evidence for supporting the hypothesis that CDDs and PCBs are causally related to human endometriosis via an endocrine-disruption mechanism is very weak." Thus, even though there is information to indicate that endometriosis may also be a sensitive toxicological endpoint for 2,3,7,8-TCDD exposure, the developmental endpoint (altered social behavior) reported in the Schantz et al.[9] study was determined to be the most appropriate endpoint for derivation of an MRL for chronic oral 2,3,7,8-TCDD exposure.

Approach to Calculation of MRLs Is Based on Incomplete Knowledge

By definition, a minimal risk level (MRL) is an estimate of the daily human exposure to a hazardous substance that is likely to be without an appreciable risk of adverse noncancer health effects over a specified route and duration of exposure.[2,14] The formula for derivation of an oral MRL is:

$$MRL = \frac{NOAEL\ (LOAEL)}{UF \times MF},$$

where MRL is the minimal risk level (mg/kg/day), NOAEL is the no-observed-adverse-effect level (mg/kg/day), LOAEL is the lowest-observed-adverse-effect level (mg/kg/day), UF is the uncertainty factor (dimensionless), and MF is the modifying factor (dimensionless).

Traditionally, the operational approach to lack of data has been the use of analytic steps to address the scientific uncertainty. UFs are used to account for uncertainties associated with extrapolation from a LOAEL to a NOAEL and from animal to human data, and to provide adjustments for intraspecies variability. UFs with default values of ten are usually used for all three of the previously cited categories of extrapolation. A factor of ten is used for a LOAEL, if a NOAEL was not identified, for the purposes of low dose extrapolation (i.e., to identify a biologically plausible NOAEL). This adjustment is supported by analyses of several chemicals for which at least one experimental NOAEL and LOAEL were available. These analyses indicate that dividing the lowest LOAEL by a factor of ten usually yields a value that is less than the experimental NOAEL in 95% of cases.[15,16]

Although humans are qualitatively similar to other animals with respect to health outcomes following exposures, interspecies differences do exist. Significant variations may arise from toxicokinetic and toxicodynamic differences in interactions between organisms and toxic chemicals that are species-specific. UFs of 10 have been used to offset the uncertainties surrounding these differences. Dourson and Stara[15] support the use and selection of this uncertainty factor. That support is based on empirical evidence in the literature suggesting that the tenfold reduction in animal dose is sufficient to encompass the variability between animals and humans 95% of time.

Conditions that may enhance susceptibility to adverse health effects include age, sex, genetic make-up, nutritional status, and preexisting disease conditions. UFs of 10 are usually used to derive MRLs that are protective of these sensitive subpopulations. Following an extensive literature review, Calabrese[17] concluded that the commonly used UF of 10 seems to provide protection for 80% to 95% of the human population. Recently, however, some policy makers, in order to be protective of children's health, suggest applying an additional margin of safety for exposure to infants and children so as to account for potential toxicity and incompleteness of the database.

Combining UFs without further evaluation can lead to overestimation of the actual risk. For example, if two factors of 10 are multiplied and each factor encompasses an extrapolation at the 95% level, the product will result in an estimate that is more conservative than the 95% level (i.e., in the direction of the 99% level or greater).

Under current ATSDR methodology, default UFs of 10 are applied to extrapolate from a LOAEL to a NOAEL, for interspecies extrapolation, and for intraspecies variability. However, chemical-specific toxicity and toxicokinetic information have sometimes made it necessary and appropriate to deviate from using the standard UF of 10.[1,2] Once again, MRLs for 2,3,7,8-TCDD can be used to provide examples for decreasing uncertainty based on the available data.

A UF of 3 instead of 10 was used in computing the chronic oral MRL for 2,3,7,8-TCDD for the extrapolation from a LOAEL to a NOAEL No overt signs of toxicity were observed in the mothers or offspring, and birth weights and growth were not adversely affected by 2,3,7,8-TCDD exposure. Significant alterations were observed in play behavior, displacement, and self-directed behavior in the 2,3,7,8-TCDD-exposed offspring. 2,3,7,8-TCDD-exposed monkeys tended to initiate more rough-and-tumble play bouts and retreated less from play bouts than controls; they were less often displaced from preferred positions in the playroom than the controls; and they engaged in more self-directed behavior than controls. No other significant alterations in behavior or alterations in reflex development, visual exploration, locomotor activity, or fine motor control were noted.[7] In tests of cognitive function, object learning was significantly impaired, but no effect on spatial learning was observed.[8] In summary, only some of the results from a battery of tests showed significant changes. Therefore, the overall evaluation of seriousness of these effects was reduced.

A UF of 3 instead of 10 was used to extrapolate from animals to humans in deriving the chronic oral MRL for 2,3,7,8-TCDD. A comparison of species sensitivity suggests that even though there are wide ranges of sensitivity for some 2,3,7,8-TCDD-induced health effects, for most health effects the LOAELs for the majority of animal species cluster within an order of magnitude. Based on the weight of evidence of animal species comparisons, and human and animal mechanistic data, it is reasonable to assume that human sensitivity would fall within the range of animal sensitivity. This causes the uncertainty to be lowered. On the other hand, neurobehavioral toxicity is a recently developed discipline; not enough data are yet available to develop animal models that parallel or convincingly simulate known effects in humans. Evidence of similarities may often be concealed by inadequate testing or interpretation of data, interspecies differences in developmental maturity of the central nervous system (CNS), and differences in behavioral patterns. A UF of 3 for interspecies extrapolation acknowledges these differences and the reservations associated with them.

In contrast, a UF of 10 for human variability was not changed. A UF for intraspecies differences was introduced to account for differences in response to toxic chemicals and to protect sensitive individuals. Age, sex, genetic composition, nutritional status, and preexisting diseases may all alter susceptibility to hazardous chemicals.

The MRL was based on studies in very young animals. It is reasonable to assume that young children with developing neurological systems would be protected. However, uncertainties in the genetic make-up (e.g., differences in Ah receptors) would preclude decreasing the UF.

The level of uncertainty has also been addressed by modifying factors. For example, in the derivation of an acute oral MRL for 2,3,7,8-TCDD, a modifying factor of 0.7 was applied to adjust for the differences in higher bioavailability of 2,3,7,8-TCDD from gavage with an oil vehicle than from food. Support for this modifying factor comes from toxicokinetic studies in Sprague Dawley rats. In rats fed 0.35 or 1 µg/kg/day 2,3,7,8-TCDD in the diet for 42 days, approximately 60% of the administered dose was absorbed.[18] In contrast, 70%–84% of a single or repeated gavage dose of 0.01–50 µg/kg/day 2,3,7,8-TCDD in corn oil was absorbed in rats.[19,20] Thus, the ratio of 2,3,7,8-TCDD absorption from the diet to gavage with an oil vehicle is 0.71–0.85.

Sources of Concern

Uncertainty Factors That Are Based on Incomplete Knowledge of Substance-Specific Chemistry or Toxicology

Dioxin and dioxin-like compounds have been studied more than any other type of chemical during the last decade. Although our knowledge has increased greatly, significant scientific uncertainty remains. Increased knowledge about 2,3,7,8-TCDD toxicity was reflected in changes that MRLs underwent over the decade (TABLE 2). For example, the acute oral MRL of 1000 pg 2,3,7,8-TCDD/kg/day was based on a LOAEL of 0.1 µg/kg/day in 1989.[21] Later studies showed the toxicity of 2,3,7,8-TCDD at even lower levels, and the 1997 MRL was based on a NOAEL of 0.005 µg/kg/day (the LOAEL in this study was 0.01 µg/kg/day).[5] This would have resulted in deriving an MRL of 50 pg/kg/day, using the UF of 10 each for interspecies extrapolation and intraspecies variability. However, greater knowledge about 2,3,7,8-TCDD toxicity enabled ATSDR to lower the uncertainty and to use an MF that resulted in an MRL of 200 pg/kg/day. In summary, as an outcome the new MRL is protective but not overly conservative.

In 1989, the LOAEL of 0.001 µg/kg/day was used in deriving the intermediate-duration oral MRL of 1 pg/kg/day. At this exposure level, dilated pelvises and changes in gestational index were observed in rats,[22] and abortions were reported in monkeys.[23] A UF of 10 was used to extrapolate from animals to humans, a factor of 10 for human variability, and a factor of 10 for the use of a LOAEL. The intermediate-duration exposure MRL was adopted for chronic exposure. No UF was used to extrapolate across durations. In 1997, the chronic MRL of 1 pg/kg/day was based on a LOAEL of 0.12 ng/kg/day in monkeys administered in a diet for a total exposure of 16.2 ± 0.4 months.[9] An uncertainty factor of three was used for extrapolation from animals to humans, a factor of 10 for human variability, and a factor of three for the use of a LOAEL. In summary, although based on a lower LOAEL, the final value is the same because of the decreased uncertainty. From that, results our greater confidence in the new value.

Recognition That the Larger the Uncertainty, the Higher the Cost to Society

Discernment of real threats to public health is harder when uncertainty is high. A preeminent feature of the ATSDR mission statement is the concept of prevention. This concept extends not only to the prevention of exposure and disease, but also to diminished quality of life. Pollution and the attendant health risk potentially arising from pollution can directly impact quality of life—not only in terms of direct health effects but also in terms of lost resources.

Dioxin and other pollutants such as mercury and PCBs make significant contributions to pollutant body burdens in human populations. The primary pathway of exposure is via the diet, with fish accounting for approximately 95% of total exposure.[24] In public health practice, the precautionary principle dictates that in the face of uncertainty, larger margins of safety (sometimes referred to as margins of exposure) are invoked in the interest of public health. If potential risk is overestimated due to data limitations or gaps, natural resources may be perceived as unsafe.

Furthermore, "[t]he identification of a threshold body burden/blood serum level, below which adverse health effects are not anticipated, would help to better define potential health risks at sites contaminated with dioxin and dioxin-like compounds. However, since significant uncertainties remain regarding such levels, especially for at-risk populations by virtue of exposure or physiologic sensitivity, a threshold level cannot be identified at present".[3,4]

High social and financial cost when we try to solve every perceived problem. The same is true of hazardous waste sites and abandoned industrial sites (*brown fields*). In practice, there is a big difference in cost when cleaning up a hazardous waste site so that the final residue of dioxins is at the 10 ppb, 1 ppb, or 0.1 ppb level. Such levels may be driven by, or considered to be, artifacts of the application of uncertainty factors. Because of the limited budget for environmental clean-up, overprotection at one site may result in lack of funds for another site where the resources are needed.

UNCERTAINTIES ASSOCIATED WITH THE DERIVATION OF EMEGs

Assumptions Used in the Derivation of EMEGs

By definition, an environmental media evaluation guide (EMEG) is a media-specific comparison value that is used to select contaminants of concern at hazardous waste sites.[27] ATSDR uses EMEGs for air, water, and soil. EMEGs for water and soil are calculated from the following formula:

$$\text{EMEG} = \frac{\text{MRL} \times \text{BW}}{\text{IR}}$$

where EMEG is the environmental media evaluation guide (mg/kg), BW is the body weight (kg), and IR is the soil ingestion rate (mg/day).

The assumptions used to develop EMEGs include: (1) exposure occurs 24 hours a day for each day of the exposure period; (2) body weight is 10 kilograms (22 pounds) for a child, and 70 kilograms (154 pounds) for an adult; (3) the ingestion rate for drinking water is two liters per day for adults, and one liter for children; and (4) the ingestion rate for soil is 100 milligrams per day for adults, 200 milligrams per day for children, and 5 grams per day for a geophagic child.

These assumptions bring further inaccuracies into the process. Special attention was given to soil ingestion rates in several studies. Soil ingestion rates are assumptions that are included in the derivation of EMEGs. ATSDR uses assumptions based on a consumption of 100 mg/day for adults and 200 mg/day for children. The soil ingestion for children is based on studies[28,29] that estimated the average soil ingestion in populations of normal children. In their calculations, Kimbrough et al.[30] assumed that children between 1.5 and 3.5 years of age ingest about 10 g of soil daily, and their risk assessment was based on "extreme total daily dose estimates". This estimate was later disputed, and several studies were conducted to evaluate the daily intake of soil by children. One of the reports suggested that an average child ingests only about 25–40 mg of soil daily.[31] However, about 1%–2% of children are geophagic and ingest from 5 to 10 g of soil daily.[32] Uncertainties associated with this issue are acknowledged, but ATSDR[27] views ingestion rates of 100 mg/day and 200 mg/day for adults and children, respectively, to be reasonable. In the event that geophagic children are at risk, ATSDR considers this issue further in the public health assessment.

Other Limitations and Uncertainties Encountered in Developing the ATSDR Policy Guideline for Dioxin and Dioxin-like Compounds

Dioxin and dioxin-like compounds serve as good examples of the multiple uncertainties that have to be considered in deliberations on health-based guidance values. As excerpted from the De Rosa et al. papers,[3,4] additional limitations and uncertainties were considered in outlining the ATSDR policy guideline.

Bioavailability

Bioavailability is an integral factor in the estimation of the internal dose (or dose at target-tissue) of the chemical. The gastrointestinal absorption of 2,3,7,8-TCDD and related compounds is variable, incomplete, and is congener- and vehicle-specific. More lipid-soluble congeners, such as 2,3,7,8-tetrachlorodibenzofuran, are almost completely absorbed, however, the extremely insoluble, octachlorodibenzodioxin is less well absorbed depending on the dose regimen; high doses may be absorbed at a lower rate, whereas low repetitive doses may be absorbed at a greater rate. The only study of 2,3,7,8-TCDD bioavailability in humans was reported by Poiger and Schlatter[33] and was based on a single male in which the gastrointestinal absorption exceeded 87% when 2,3,7,8-TCDD was administered in corn oil.

Laboratory data suggest that there are no major interspecies differences in the gastrointestinal absorption of CDDs and CDFs. However, absorption of 2,3,7,8-TCDD depends on conditions and characteristics of the soil medium; in animals, absorption of 2,3,7,8-TCDD from different soils ranged from 0.5%[34,35] to 50%.[35] Absorption from a diet was 50%–60% in rats.[18] Therefore, exposure, with food as a vehicle rather than oil, relates more closely to exposure from soil. Bioavailability has to be considered when calculating the hypothetical ingestion dose.

If it is assumed that 100% of 2,3,7,8-TCDD is bioavailable, the risk may be overestimated. The health assessor should recognize that other assessors may have used different assumptions in their calculations. Kimbrough et al.[30] assumed 30% bioavailability from ingestion of soil, but pointed out that animal studies with contaminated Missouri soil indicated absorption up to 30%–50%.[37] Pohl et al.[38] assumed

40% bioavailability from soil. In contrast, Paustenbach et al.[39] estimated bioavailability at 10%–30%. Unless toxicokinetic studies that use soil samples from the specific site are available, it is difficult to speculate about the quantity of 2,3,7,8-TCDD and related compounds that will be absorbed. Therefore, the estimate of the actual intake has limitations.

The chronic MRL is based on studies where food was the vehicle. Results from animal studies indicate that bioavailability of 2,3,7,8-TCDD from soil varies between sites because dioxin and dioxin-like compounds bind tightly to soil— increasingly so with the passage of time and clay content of soil.[31] Therefore, 2,3,7,8-TCDD content alone may not be indicative of the potential for human health hazard from contaminated environmental materials Again, site-specific evaluation is essential.

Background Exposure

EMEGs represent an estimate of exposure dose from one source only. All relevant sources of exposure from the hazardous waste site and all possible background exposures should be included in the final evaluation of actual exposure.

Dioxin and dioxin-like compounds are known to readily enter the food chain. It has been estimated that about 98% of exposure occurs through food. It should be noted that the average background intake of TCDD and of total TEQs of dioxin and dioxin-like compounds for adults in the general population were estimated as 0.35 pg/kg/day and 1.9 pg/kg/day, respectively.[40] Furthermore, it is important to consider the background level of dioxin and dioxin-like compounds in contaminated soil. The U.S. background 2,3,7,8-TCDD soil levels ranged from undetected to 10 ppt in industrialized areas of groups of midwestern and mid-Atlantic states.[41]

Exposure from Soil by Different Routes

Kimbrough et al.[30] estimated that the lifetime uptake of 2,3,7,8-TCDD from soil consists of 95% from soil ingestion, 3% from soil dermal exposure (assuming 1% dermal absorption), and 2% from inhalation. Paustenbach et al.[39] indicated that the 1% dermal absorption proposed for 2,3,7,8-TCDD–contaminated soil may be too high. Similarly, he further lowered the estimates of inhalation intake, speculating that 2% from inhalation may be too high.

Unless indicated otherwise by the specific on-site circumstances, exposure by routes other than oral can be considered to be insignificant.

Exposure to Dioxin-like Compounds

Dioxin-like compounds, or related chemicals, are other compounds containing chlorine or bromine whose molecules are similar on shape to 2,3,7,8-TCDD and that produce similar toxic effects. These include some other dioxin congeners, some furan compounds, some PCBs, and some polybrominated biphenyls (PBBs).[42] TEQs are used to estimate toxicity of dioxin-like compounds (see TABLE 3).

Some of the assumptions for using the TEQ approach cover a well-defined group of chemicals, a broad database of information, consistency across endpoints, additivity of effects, and a common mechanism of action.[43] According to EPA guidelines for risk assessment of complex mixtures, potency-weighted additivity is assumed for mixtures in the absence of information to the contrary.[44]

TABLE 3. World Health Organization TEFs for humans, mammals, fish, and birds

Congener	Humans/mammals	Fish[a]	Birds[a]
2,3,7,8-TCDD	1	1	1
1,2,3,7,8-PeCDD	1	1	1[f]
1,2,3,4,7,8-HxCDD	0.1[a]	0.5	0.05[f]
1,2,3,6,7,8-HxCDD	0.1[a]	0.01	0.01[f]
1,2,3,7,8,9-HxCDD	0.1[a]	0.01[e]	0.1[f]
1,2,3,4,6,7,8-HpCDD	0.1	0.001	<0.001[f]
OCDD	0.0001[a]	—	—
2,3,7,8-TCDF	0.1	0.05	1[f]
1,2,3,7,8-PeCDF	0.05	0.05	0.1[f]
2,3,4,7,8-PeCDF	0.5	0.5	1[f]
1,2,3,4,7,8-HxCDF	0.1	0.1	0.1[c,f]
1,2,3,6,7,8-HxCDF	0.1	0.1[c]	0.1[c,f]
1,2,3,7,8,9-HxCDF	0.1[a]	0.1[c,e]	0.1[c]
2,3,4,6,7,8-HxCDF	0.1[a]	0.1[c]	0.1[c]
1,2,3,4,6,7,8-HpCDF	0.01[a]	0.01[b]	0.01[b]
1,2,3,4,7,8,9-HpCDF	0.01[a]	0.01[b,e]	0.01[b]
OCDF	0.0001[a]	0.0001[b,e]	0.0001[b]
3,4,4′,5-TCB (81)	0.0001[a,b,c,e]	0.0005	0.1[e]
3,3′,4,4′-TCB (77)	0.0001	0.0001	0.05
3,3′,4,4′,5-PeCB (126)	0.1	0.005	0.5
3,3′,4,4′,5,5′-HxCB (169)	0.01	0.00005	0.001
2,3,3′,4,4′-PeCB (105)	0.0001	<0.000005	0.0001
2,3,4,4′,5-PeCB (114)	0.0005[a,b,c,d]	<0.000005[b]	0.0001[g]
2,3′,4,4′,5-PeCB (118)	0.0001	<0.000005	<0.00001
2′,3,4,4′,5-PeCB (123)	0.0001[a,c,d]	<0.000005[b]	0.00001[g]
2,3,3′,4,4′,5-HxCB (156)	0.0005[b,c]	<0.000005	0.0001
2,3,4,4′,5′-HxCB (157)	0.0005[b,c,d]	<0.000005[b,c]	0.0001
2,3′,4,4′,5,5′-HxCB (167)	0.00001[a,d]	<0.000005[b]	0.00001[g]
2,3,3′,4,4′,5,5′-HpCB (189)	0.0001[a,c]	<0.000005	0.00001[g]

[a]Limited data set.
[b]Structural similarity.
[c]Quantitative structure activity relationships (QSAR) modeling prediction from CYP1A induction (monkey, pig, chicken, or fish).
[d]No new data from 1993 WHO review.
[e]*In vitro* CYP1A induction.
[f]*In vivo* CYP1A induction after *in ovo* exposure.
[g]QSAR modeling prediction from class-specific TEFs.
SOURCE: Table derived from Van den Berg, *et al.*[45]

Limitations associated with the use of TEQs must be considered in developing health guidance values. TEQs are derived using toxicity equivalency factors (TEFs) that are constants determined from experimental studies for each congener. Although TEFs are considered to be constants, they are dependent on the specific study (endpoint, dose, and duration of exposure).

As defined, TEQs are assumed to be additive and neither synergistic nor antagonistic. In actual mixtures of dioxin and dioxin-like compounds, competitive inhibition may occur at sufficiently high doses. As with MRLs and EMEGs, biomedical judgment must be used in considering site-specific conditions that would reasonably modify the estimates to be applicable to an individual site.

CONCLUSIONS

Defining the Status Quo

In summary, this paper illustrates the use of dioxin and dioxin-like compounds to illustrate that the methodology for deriving health guidance values encompasses two kinds of uncertainty issues, both of which comprise less than certain science. The upper portion of the box in FIGURE 1, represents the area of the basic toxicology practice and endpoints used in risk assessment. This portion of the box contains the assumptions that underlies the use of traditional toxicology and, less often, epidemiology data as the starting point for estimating health guidance levels. The lower half of the box represents the traditionally applied uncertainty factors, including default values, used in the calculations.

Identifying a New Approach

To date, efforts to think "out of the box" have been almost exclusively confined to the lower half of the box (see FIGURE 2). These efforts have led to the development of analytic methodologies that refine the uncertainty factors. Although these methods have not removed all the uncertainty in health guidance values, in many cases they have increased confidence in these estimates or increased the biological plausibility of a significant effect level. Continuous decrease of factors of ten, based on greater scientific knowledge, may be one approach, as demonstrated in this paper. However, there are other methods that decrease the reliance on default values. Scientists and health assessors should be encouraged to use these methods more often.

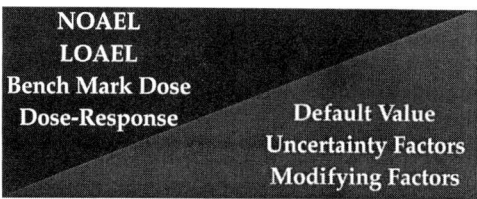

FIGURE 1. Recommendations/framework. Defining the status quo.

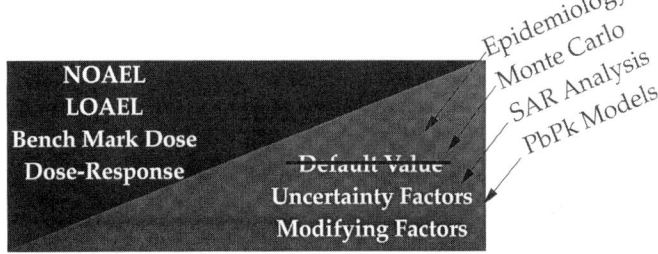

FIGURE 2. Identifying a new approach.

Two broad issues surrounding the use of these methodology refinements have been identified. The first is that complex methods have the potential to obscure the degree of uncertainty that remains after their use. The complexity of the analysis provides an artificial sense of precision. The second issue is that the refinements do not meet the criteria for a paradigm shift in scientific thinking. ATSDR envisions this exercise of refining uncertainty factors as a step out of the box for a better tool, which is then used in an essentially unchanged process. The basis of the ATSDR approach is to provide the highest level of protection for the most people in the population, recognizing that every individual in the population may not experience the same level of protection. Inherent in public health approaches is the variability of the means related to individual genotypes and variability in environmental exposures. The unchanged process, which is based on fundamental principles of toxicology, is anchored solidly in the concept of risk assessment held by the scientific community. Identifying new scientific approaches, difficult enough in itself, is probably not nearly so difficult as effecting a genuine paradigm shift among scientists and policy makers.

ACKNOWLEDGMENT

This policy guideline and evaluation of uncertainty was developed in consultation with and endorsed by the ATSDR Board of Scientific Counselors: E. Bingham, C. Xintaras, L. Claudio, M.D. Collins, J.W. Hoffbuhr, R.C. Leonard, M.T. Morandi, M.A. Roberts, J.M. Roseman, A.D. Stark, and L.E. White.

REFERENCES

1. DE ROSA, C.T., H. POHL, M. WILLIAMS, A. ADEMOYERO, S. CHOU & D. JONES. 1998. Public health implications of environmental exposures. Environ. Health Perspect. **106** (Suppl.1): 369–378.
2. POHL, H.R. & H.G. ABADIN. 1995. Utilizing uncertainty factors in minimal risk levels derivation. Regulat. Toxicol. Pharmacol. **22:** 180–188.

3. DE ROSA, C.T., D. BROWN, R. DHARA, W. GARRETT, H. HANSEN, J. HOLLER, D. JONES, D. JORDAN-IZAGUIRRE, R. O'CONNOR, H. POHL & C. XINTARAS. 1997. Dioxin and dioxin-like compounds in soil, part I: ATSDR interim policy guideline. Toxicol. Ind. Health **13**(6): 759–768.
4. DE ROSA, C.T., D. BROWN, R. DHARA, W. GARRETT, H. HANSEN, J. HOLLER, D. JONES, D. JORDAN-IZAGUIRRE, R. O'CONNOR, H. POHL, C. XINTARAS. 1997. Dioxin and dioxin-like compounds in soil, part II: Technical support document for ATSDR interim policy guideline.Toxicol. Ind. Health **13**(6): 769–804.
5. AGENCY FOR TOXIC SUBSTANCES AND DISEASE REGISTRY (ATSDR). 1997. Toxicological profile for chlorinated dibenzo-p-dioxins. U.S. Department of Health and Human Services, Agency for Toxic Substances and Disease Registry, Atlanta.
6. AGENCY FOR TOXIC SUBSTANCES AND DISEASE REGISTRY (ATSDR). 1995. Guidance for developing toxicological profiles. U.S. Department of Health and Human Services, Agency for Toxic Substances and Disease Registry, Atlanta.
7. BOWMAN, R.E., S.L. SCHANTZ, M.L. GROSS *et al.* 1989. Behavioral effects in monkeys exposed to 2,3,7,8-TCDD transmitted maternally during gestation and for four months of nursing. Chemosphere **18**: 235–242.
8. SCHANTZ, S.L. & R.E. BOWMAN. 1989. Learning in monkeys exposed perinatally to 2,3,7,8-tetrachlorodibenzo-p-dioxin (2,3,7,8-TCDD). Neurotoxicol. Teratol. **11**: 13–19.
9. SCHANTZ, S.L., S.A. FERGUSON & RE. BOWMAN 1992. Effects of 2,3,7,8-tetrachlorodibenzo-p-dioxin on behavior of monkey in peer groups. Neurotoxicol. Teratol. **14**: 433–446.
10. RIER, S.E., D.C. MARTIN & RE. BOWMAN *et al.* 1993. Endometriosis in Rhesus monkeys following chronic exposure to 2,3,7,8-tetrachlorodibenzo-p-dioxin. Fund. Appl. Toxicol. **21**: 433–441.
11. WHEELER, J.M. 1992. Epidemiology and prevalences of endometriosis. Infertil. Reprod. Med. Clin. N.A. **3**: 545–549.
12. BOYD, J.A., G.C. CLARK, D.K. WALMER *et al.* 1995. Endometriosis and the environment biomarkers of toxin exposure. Abstract of Endometriosis 2000 Workshop, May 15–17.
13. U.S. ENVIRONMENTAL PROTECTION AGENCY (EPA). 1997. Special report on environmental endocrine disruption: An effects assessment and analysis. Risk Assessment Forum. U.S. Environmental Protection Agency, Washington DC. EPA/630/R-96/012.
14. AGENCY FOR TOXIC SUBSTANCES AND DISEASE REGISTRY (ATSDR). 1996. Minimal risk levels for priority substances and guidance for derivation. Federal Register **61**(101): 25873–25882.
15. DOURSON, M.L. & J.F. STARA. 1983. Regulatory history and experimental support of uncertainty (safety) factors. Regul. Toxicol. Pharmacol. **3**: 224–238.
16. U.S. ENVIRONMENTAL PROTECTION AGENCY (EPA). 1989. General quantitative risk assessment guidelines for noncancer health effects (draft). U.S. Environmental Protection Agency, Washington DC. ECAO-CIN-538.
17. CALABRESE, E.J. 1985. Uncertainty factors and interindividual variation Regul. Toxicol. Pharmacol. **5**: 190–196.
18. FRIES, G.F. & G.S. MARROW. 1975. Retention and excretion of 2,3,7,8-tetrachlorodibenzo-p-dioxin by rats. J. Agric. Food Chem. **23**: 265–269.
19. PIPER, W.N., R.Q. ROSE & P.J. GEHRING 1973. Excretion and tissue distribution of 2,3,7,8-tetrachlorodibenzo-p-dioxin in the rat. Environ. Health Perspect. **5**: 241–244.
20. ROSE, J.Q., J.C. RAMSEY, T.H. WENTZLER *et al.* 1976. The fate of 2,3,7,8-tetrachlorodibenzo-p-dioxin following single and repeated oral doses to the rat. Toxicol. Appl. Pharmacol. **36**: 209–226.

21. AGENCY FOR TOXIC SUBSTANCES AND DISEASE REGISTRY (ATSDR). 1989. Toxicological profile for 2,3,7,8-tetrachlorodibenzo-*p*-dioxin. U.S. Department of Health and Human Services, Agency for Toxic Substances and Disease Registry, Atlanta.
22. MURRAY, F.J., F.A. SMITH, K.D. NITSCHKE, C.G. HUMISTON, R.J. KOCIBA & B.A. SCHWETZ. 1979. Three-generation reproduction study of rats given 2,3,7,8-tetrachlorodibenzo-*p*-dioxin isomers using a polymeric liquid crystal capillary column. J. Chromatogr. **369**(1): 203–207.
23. ALLEN, J.R., D.A. BARSOTTI, L.K. LAMBRECHT et al. 1979. Reproductive effects of halogenated aromatic hydrocarbons on nonhuman primates. Ann. N.Y. Acad. Sci. **320**: 419–425.
24. JOHNSON, B.L., H.E. HICKS, D.E. JONES, W. CIBULAS, A. WARGO & C.T. DE ROSA. 1998. Public health implications of persistent toxic substances in the Great Lakes and St. Lawrence Basins. J. Great Lakes Research. **24**(2): 698–722.
25. TURNER, J.N. & D.N. COLLINS. 1983. Liver morphology in guinea pigs administered either pyrolysis products of a polychlorinated biphenyl transformer fluid or 2,3,7,8-tetrachlorodibenzo-*p*-dioxin. Toxicol. Appl. Pharmacol. **67**: 417–429.
26. BURLESON, G.R., H. LEBREC, Y.G. YANG et al. 1996. Effects of 2,3,7,8-tetrachlorodibenzo-p-dioxin (TCDD) on influenza virus host resistance in mice. Fund. Appl. Toxicol. **29**: 40–47.
27. AGENCY FOR TOXIC SUBSTANCES AND DISEASE REGISTRY (ATSDR). 1992. Public health assessment guidance manual. U.S. Department of Health and Human Services, Agency for Toxic Substances and Disease Registry, Atlanta. NTIS PB92-147164.
28. BINDER, S., D. SOKAL & D. MAUGHN. 1986. The use of tracer elements in estimating the amount of soil ingested by young children. Arch. Environ. Health **41**: 341–345.
29. CLAUSING, P., B. BRUNEKREFF & J.H. VAN WIJEN. 1987. A method for estimating soil ingestion by children. Int. Arch. Occup. Environ. Health **59**: 73–82.
30. KIMBROUGH, R.D., H. FALK, P. STEHR et al. 1984. Health implications of 2,3,7,8-tetrachlorodibenzo-*p*-dioxin (2,3,7,8-TCDD) contamination of residential soil. J. Toxicol. Environ. Health **14**. 47–93.
31. GOUGH, M. 1991. Human exposures from dioxin in soil—a meeting report. J. Toxicol. Environ. Health **32**: 205–245.
32. U.S. ENVIRONMENTAL PROTECTION AGENCY (EPA). 1989. Exposure Factors Handbook. U.S. Environmental Protection Agency, Office of Health and Environmental Assessment, Washington, DC. EPA/600/8-89/043. July 1989.
33. POIGER, H. & C. SCHLATTER. 1986. Pharmacokinetics of 2,3,7,8-TCDD in man. Chemosphere **15**: 1489–1494.
34. UMBREIT, T.H., E.J. HESSE & M.A. GALLO. 1986. Bioavailability of dioxin in soil from a 2,4,5-T manufacturing site. Science **232**: 497–499.
35. UMBREIT, T.H., E.J. HESSE & M.A. GALLO. 1986. Comparative toxicity of 2,3,7,8-TCDD contaminated soil from Times Beach, Missouri, and Newark, New Jersey. Chemosphere **15**: 2121–2124.
36. LUCIER, G.W., R.C. RUMBAUGH, Z. MCCOY et al. 1986. Ingestion of soil contaminated with 2,3,7,8-tetrachlorodibenzo-*p*-dioxin (2,3,7,8-TCDD) alters hepatic enzyme activities in rats. Fundam. Appl. Toxicol. **6**: 364–371.
37. MCCONNELL, E.E., G.W. LUCIER, R.C. RUMBAUGH et al. 1984. Dioxin in soil: bioavailability after ingestion by rats and guinea pigs. Science **223**: 1077–1079.
38. POHL, H., C.T. DE ROSA & J. HOLLER. 1995. Public health assessment for dioxins exposure from soil. Chemosphere **31**(1): 2437–2454.
39. PAUSTENBACH, D.J., H.P. SHU & F.J. MURRAY. 1986. A critical examination of assumptions used in risk assessments of dioxin contaminated soil. Regul. Toxicol. Pharmacol. **6**: 284–307.

40. WORLD HEALTH ORGANIZATION (WHO). 1991. Consultation on tolerable daily intake from food of PCDDs and PCDFs. Summary Report. World Health Organization, Bilthoven, the Netherlands.
41. NESTRICK, T.J., L.L. LAMPARSKI, M.N. FRAWLEY *et al.* 1986. Perspectives of a large scale environmental survey for chlorinated dioxins: overview and soil data. Chemosphere **15:** 1453–1460.
42. SCHIEROW, L.J. 1995. Dioxin: reassessing the risk. CRS Report to Congress. Environment and Natural Resources Policy Division.
43. U.S. ENVIRONMENTAL PROTECTION AGENCY (EPA). 1989. Interim procedures for estimating risks associated with exposure to mixtures of chlorinated dibenzo-p-dioxins and dibenzofurans (CDDs and CDFs) and 1989 update. U.S. Environmental Protection Agency, Risk Assessment Forum. EPA 625/3-89/016. NTIS PB90-145756.
44. U.S. ENVIRONMENTAL PROTECTION AGENCY (EPA). 1987. The risk assessment guidelines of 1986. U.S. Environmental Protection Agency, Office of Health and Environmental Assessment. EPA/600/8-87/045.
45. VAN DEN BERG, M., L. BIRNBAUM & A.T.C. BOSVELD. 1998. Toxic equivalency factors (TEFs) for PCBs, PCDDs, PCDFs for humans and wildlife. Environ. Health Perspect. **106**(12): 775–792.

Uncertainty in Risk Characterization and Communication

Discussion

ALISTAIR WOODWARD[a]

*Department of Public Health, Wellington School of Medicine,
University of Otago, New Zealand*

It is widely appreciated that variability in individual susceptibility to toxic effects is an important element of uncertainty in risk assessment. Models to explore the nature and magnitude of this variability, such as that presented by Dale Hattis, have generally been based on the effects of single exposures. However, in practice, chemicals are seldom experienced as single exposures. One would expect the variability between individuals in susceptibility to multiple, concurrent exposures to be greater than that predicted from a single exposure model. This is a difficult area to work in, given the very large number of possible combinations of exposures that might occur, but there are obvious and important implications for standard setting.

Risk assessments are powerfully shaped by preconceptions. John Bailar demonstrates in his paper how important are differences between scientific disciplines in the interpretation of data—*interaction* may mean something quite different to an epidemiologist than to her toxicological colleague. In a broader sense, culture is a significant but underrated cause of disagreement and uncertainty. The gaps between different cultural views of risk are not the kind that can be bridged with quantitative methods. An example is the question of how water quality standards should be set. In New Zealand there is a tension between the traditional approach to characterizing health risks from drinking water (using measures such as coliform counts) and Maori concepts of environmental integrity, that forbid altogether the discharge of human waste into waterways. In the past, issues such as this may have been regarded as a headache for the risk manager, but scarcely an issue for scientists involved in risk assessment. However public perceptions of risk should and do impinge directly on the work of the scientist. (Applicants for research grants in New Zealand, for example, must explain the implications of their work for Maori health.) Discussion of risk characterization and communication should include reflection on what we mean by risk and hazard.

As a consequence of its history, risk assessment is primarily focussed on chemical exposures in the environment. Without detracting from the importance of chemical hazards, it is important to recognize that there are other threats to health, that may have similar or even greater impacts. Examples include economic disruption and poverty, social policies leading to mass unemployment, and global environmen-

---

[a]Address for correspondence: Alistair Woodward, Department of Public Health, University of Otago, PoBox7343 Wellington South, New Zealand.
e-mail: woodward@wnmeds.ac.nz

tal changes such as climate change. Can the risk assessment approach be applied to *big picture* risks of this kind? Can we learn from other disciplines, outside the health sciences, such as ecology and economics, that are familiar with large-scale assessments? It is always most comfortable to stay within a disciplinary framework, but sometimes the most important advances are made by extending and redefining boundaries. Models of integrated risk assessment that are being tested in the climate-change area may offer a useful example.

Uncertainty in Risk Assessment
Current Efforts and Future Hopes

A. JOHN BAILER[a]

Department of Mathematics and Statistics, Miami University, Oxford, Ohio 45056-1641, USA

Education and Information Division, National Institute for Occupational, Safety and Health, Cincinnati, Ohio 45226-1998, USA

> ABSTRACT: The incorporation of sampling variability in estimates of excess risk has been part of risk assessment practice for decades. Currently, there is a strong desire to incorporate understanding of biological mechanisms into the models used for exposure assessment and exposure-response modeling. In addition, representing population heterogeneity in the assessment of risks and the identification of sensitive subpopulations is of great concern. Finally, the communication of uncertainty and variability remains a challenge to risk assessors. Based upon the presentations of workshop faculty, a summary of current practice when addressing uncertainty together with conjectures concerning future challenges for addressing uncertainty, are presented.

It is my pleasure, and my challenge, to provide a quick reaction and summary to the presentations made at the Workshop on Uncertainty in the Risk Assessment of Environmental and Occupational Hazards. This workshop brought together an international collection of scientists from government, academia, and industry. As an organizing principle, the presentations were grouped into four categories based upon the National Academy of Sciences risk assessment model.[1] These categories included hazard identification, exposure assessment, exposure-response modeling, and risk characterization. Regardless of the category to which a presenter was assigned, all were asked to consider how we can improve understanding of the sources and magnitude of uncertainty in the risk assessment process. Speakers were also asked to explore how uncertainty in this process can be reduced and how uncertainty should be described, characterized, and expressed with a particular view towards policy implications. My summary follows the order in which presentations were made. As a caveat, before I begin, these observations represent what I heard in these presentations and should be read as one perspective of the meeting.

In his opening remarks, Dr. P. Landrigan introduced the concept of sensitive subpopulations. He focused on the risk assessment of children and warned against a simple treatment of children as "little adults". The exposure routes and patterns for children along with metabolism and developmental differences may place them at

---

[a]Address for correspondence: Department of Mathematics & Statistics, Miami University, 123 Bachelor Hall, Oxford, Ohio 45056-1641, USA. 513/529-3538 (voice); 513/529-1493 (fax).
e-mail: ajbailer@muohio.edu

much higher risk of adverse health outcomes when exposed to an environmental hazard. After he addressed the uncertainty inherent in the risk assessment for sensitive subpopulations, Dr. Landrigan described how variability in food consumption distributions and pesticide residue distributions were convoluted to obtain a distribution of pesticides in children. This type of calculation, in which the distribution of an outcome attribute is constructed from distributions of input variables, proved to be a common theme of this workshop.

In the hazard identification session, Dr. C. Maltoni challenged us to consider the concordance of animal and human studies. In particular, he reminded us that if a lack of agreement is observed between human and animal studies, then careful consideration of the adequacy of each study type is needed. In addition, Dr. Maltoni strongly argued for the utility of animal studies in identifying human hazards. His presentation argued that the uncertainty associated with extrapolating to human risks from mammalian models may not be as large as many have claimed. The second presentation of this session was given by Dr. A. Ahlbom. He provided a summary of the vexing case of evaluating the potential risks associated with exposure to electromagnetic fields (EMF). The fundamental question underlying this presentation was what provides sufficient evidence of a hazard? Dr. Ahlbom suggested a structure for hazard identification that represents mechanistic belief as a prior distribution potentially modified by data. Implicit in this Bayesian formulation was the potential for controversy in defining the prior distribution. In this example, should the prior distribution for EMF effects be a distribution about zero (no effect) or about some positive value (suggesting an *a priori* belief in positive risk associated with exposure). One possible strategy is to start with a different prior distributions and then examine the posterior distributions. If the posterior distribution does not vary much with specification of prior probability distributions, then this eliminates this concern. Dr. M. Soffritti provided examples of other hazards that were difficult to evaluate. These examples included EMF and gamma radiation exposure. In particular, evaluating hazards associated with low carcinogenic risks is a special challenge. This evaluation requires large studies with low level exposures and lifetime follow-up of exposed individuals. The next speaker of this session, Dr. C. Portier, summarized recent activities in the United States for assessing the risks associated with EMF exposures. Noteworthy in his presentation was a description of a national sample that was conducted in order to generate a picture of current EMF exposure. This appeared to me to be an important general message for risk assessment: better assessment of the distribution of the exposures leads to stronger, and more valid, variability analyses. Dr. Portier also noted the challenge of risk communication. Labeling of EMF as a *possible carcinogen* was described as being too fuzzy, and potentially confusing. Finally, he discussed risk characterization issues for which the integration of the exposure-distributions and dose-response models was needed. The final speaker of the session, Dr. J. Huff, reviewed issues concerning the use of animal studies to predict human cancer risks. Since cancer is a very complicated disease that is multi-causal and multi-step involving multiple genes and mechanisms, perfect concordance between animal models and human responses is unreasonable. The concordance of effects between mammals but not necessarily between sites should be viewed as encouraging. In addition, he noted that data sets generated for screening purposes, that is, qualitative cancer assessments, are often called upon to provide the foundation for quantitative dose-response projections.

Kinetic models are often employed in exposure assessment as a means to extrapolate across routes of exposure, or across species. In the first presentation of the session devoted to uncertainty and variability in exposure assessment, Dr. L. Edler looked at how uncertainty could be incorporated into these models. His particular interests were in physiologically-based pharmacokinetic (PBPK) models. He commented that the basic formulation of these models involved a fundamental uncertainty issue—how many compartments should be included in the model? (As an aside, this may not be as important as the kinetic description of the compartments.) This was a structural uncertainty question. A related question addressed which parameter was most influential. He also raised the question of how uncertainty should be incorporated in a PBPK model—as a parameter distribution? Range of values? Can we consider correlation between model parameters? An uncertainty raised by Dr. Edler that may be overlooked was the differing laboratory analytics. This lab-to-lab variability in estimating PBPK model traits should also be considered in any uncertainty analysis. Finally, what factors influence the choice of error structure, for example, additive or multiplicative errors? Dr. P. Schulte then provided an overview of molecular epidemiology and how this might give us better understanding of the mechanism of the pathway from exposure to disease. He noted the importance of validation of biomarkers, both in terms of laboratory reproducibility and in terms of epidemiology utility. Finally, he challenged the audience to consider that more information does not necessarily reduce variability in the system. The more details we appreciate about exposure, susceptibility, and disease, the more we may appreciate our ignorance of other important issues. Dr. ten Berge addressed the definition of cumulative exposure metrics for safe dose assignment and stressed the importance of considering survival-adjusted analysis methods. Dr. A. Salvan took up the theme of toxicokinetic models again. He contrasted statistical models with PBPK and minimal physiologic toxicokinetic models in the context of dioxin risk assessment. In essence, the models range from completely empirical to extensive mechanistic models. Some compromise between these extremes is required. Dr. Salvan also noted that different estimation methods may inject yet another source of uncertainty in an analysis. Since human studies often include observations with incomplete data records, another source of uncertainty arises from whether such observations are omitted from an analysis or whether imputed values are supplied for the missing variables. Dr. H. Kromhout and Dr. D. Loomis presented an analysis of a large study of workers occupationally exposed to EMF. They identified numerous potential uncertainties in the assessment of EMF effects. Exposure assessment was a difficult exercise with concerns about the definition of job exposure matrices, the effects of duration and the effects of exposure intensity present. The effects of employing the wrong exposure measure are haunted with concerns about imprecision, and attenuation in the dose-response model is of greatest concern. Drs. Kromhout and Loomis used simulation studies to explore measurement error issues and presented dose-response with *bands of uncertainty* associated with different exposure patterns and window/lag assumptions. Dr. A. Woodward raised exposure assessment issues in the context of evaluating environmental tobacco smoke (ETS) exposure. He commented that the proper choice of an exposure measurement method depends upon its intended use, and that biomarkers and questionnaires possessed similar predictive validity for ETS. Dr. Woodward raised the important issue of uncertainty induced by different values and expectations. For example, risk tolerant and risk sensitive individuals, in a risk assessment based upon the same data, will be influenced by their very different frames of reference. The final session in the exposure assessment section was presented by Dr. A. Zavatti. Dr. Zavatti described the development of monitoring and prevention strategies. He argued that a network of specialists was required to manage resources for sustainable development and use of environmental resources.

The third session that focused on uncertainty in dose-response modeling was the home of many statistical talks. In the first presentation, Dr. R. Kodell provided a probabilistic structure for uncertainty factors that are commonly employed in noncancer risk assessments. By characterizing the distribution of uncertainty factors with a log-normal distribution, he illustrated that the current defaults may correspond to an approximate 99th percentile for combined uncertainty factors. Dr. L. Ryan gave an overview of issues in developmental toxicology. She highlighted the challenges that arise when multiple endpoints are considered. If multiple responses might be considered for dose-response modeling and quantitative risk estimation, should the most sensitive site be considered or should we model the likelihood of at least one adverse response? The former may not be as protective as is widely believed. In addition, Dr. Ryan noted that the default omission of non-responders (nonpregnant in the context of teratology studies) may seriously bias the results. Dr. L. Stayner reviewed sources of uncertainty when employing human data from epidemiology studies for risk estimation. Included in this uncertainty list was the choice of best data set that might be addressed by multiple analyses, misspecification of the dose-response model which might be addressed by presenting multiple model projections, and all of the uncertainty inherent in observational study designs (causality, confounders, etc.). For retrospective cohort studies, the reconstruction of historical exposure patterns necessitates an analysis of uncertainty and variability. Dr. Stayner illustrated the use of Monte Carlo techniques to generate a distribution of parameter estimates for use in evaluating lung cancer responses in railroad workers exposed to diesel. He advocated reporting ranges of risk estimates for risk communication. Dr. K. Ulm introduced an alternative dose-response that accommodated thresholds in dose-response levels. Thresholds can be viewed as an estimated alternative to the no-adverse-effect level. With new German cancer guidelines including categories for nongenotoxic thresholds and genotoxic, low potency carcinogens, threshold ideas have become more important. Both of the talks by Drs. Stayner and Ulm described the uncertainty of the shape and form of the dose-response models that are used in risk estimation. Dr. K. Crump described a statistical meta-analysis based upon the distribution of p-values over different studies. This presentation predicted a larger number of liver carcinogens than have been observed by the United States National Toxicology Program. Dr. D. Krewski closed this session with a discussion of residential radon cancer risks. He presented the interesting idea of decomposing total variability/uncertainty into constituent parts. He described a characterization of model uncertainty and variability in a multiplicative model. He defined variability as the distribution of a component, and uncertainty as the distribution of a parameter that is a characteristic of the variability distribution. This definition led to discussion and debate, with some feeling that the definition was overly restrictive. Developing a shared definition and understanding of uncertainty and variability is an important step. Risk assessment researchers must reach an understanding of these issues before we can effectively communicate uncertainty and variability to risk managers and to the public.

The fourth and final session addressed uncertainty in risk characterization and communication. Dr. J. Bailar raised the issue that perspectives on uncertainty are discipline dependent. This was initially illustrated with an example of perspectives on synergy, where the same pattern of data led to different interpretations of the presence and direction of interaction. Dr. D. Hattis reported on his work to develop a database of human variability in parameters of PBPK models. He employed a lognormal probability model that he justified on the grounds of a multiplicative effects model. A major message to take away from this presentation was that highly variable traits may not be covered by tenfold safety factors. Dr. F. Bois described a detailed analyses of PBPK models. He suggested an approach in which PBPK model fitting fed into cancer data fitting, followed by the establishment of human risk. Variability would be appropriately incorporated at each of these three phases of analysis. Dr. Bois argued for the need for better model validation and modification of model parameters by data based on a Bayesian framework. In addition, identifiability of population parameters and interspecies and interpopulation uncertainty factors were noted to be not well established. Extensions of this work may ultimately include integration with transport and effect models. Dr. N. Yamaguchi raised issues of external and internal validity when characterizing hazards. He continued the earlier theme of Dr. Stayner and others by discussing uncertainty in epidemiology studies, mentioning unrecognized confounding and effect modification. He also noted that the perception of risks and hazards among the public was an important component that may determine support for risk assessment activities. The closing speaker of this session, Dr. C. De Rosa, commented on data gaps in risk characterization and emphasized the need to conduct the research necessary to address ignorance and uncertainty. He advocated an open model of risk assessment with full involvement of all stakeholders in the process. The need to assess and articulate uncertainty in the risk assessment process, to risk managers and to the public in general, was another conclusion in his presentation.

As can be inferred from the preceding paragraphs, we had a rich collection of presentations that generated much discussion. Dr. J. Bailar commented during one discussion period that "we never know as much as we think we know" to which Dr. L. Stayner added "there is more uncertainty than we capture in our uncertainty analysis". Appreciation of these observations will sober even the boldest of risk assessors and will serve to keep us all focused on the need to view the analysis of uncertainty and variability in risk assessment as an evolving exercise. We are not yet close to any established formal paradigm for this analysis. Perhaps the establishment of guidelines for sensitivity analyses of varying types might be an objective for future deliberations. Even if we agree on sensitivity/uncertainty assessment guidelines, will we be able to communicate these concerns to risk managers and to the public? Perhaps one of our communication headaches is associated with the linguistic difficulties that remain—uncertainty versus variability; sensitivity versus uncertainty analyses (not *versus* but tools to analyze sensitivity and uncertainty simultaneously?). As noted in many of the presentations at this meeting, addressing *data gaps* to mitigate uncertainty should be a goal we all share. Even if we can adequately address these concerns, the expansion of this debate to consider humans as part of the larger ecosystem looms on the horizon. My intention is not to close on a depressing note. I am excited about the innovation and development of tools to incorporate uncertainty and variability in risk assessments. I believe this workshop addressed the goal of understanding the sources and magnitude of uncertainty in the risk assessment process. Furthermore, I believe the workshop also addressed the objective of describing, characterizing and expressing uncertainty and variability. I believe that more effort can and should be spent addressing the policy implications of uncertainty and the communication of uncertainty to the public.

ACKNOWLEDGMENTS

Drs. Eileen Kuempel and Leslie Stayner provided suggestions and comments on a previous draft of this manuscript that improved the presentation contained herein.

REFERENCE

1. NATIONAL ACADEMY OF SCIENCES. 1983. Risk Assessment in the Federal Government: Managing the Process. National Academy Press, Washington, D.C.

Common Themes at the Workshop on Uncertainty in the Risk Assessment of Environmental and Occupational Hazards

JOHN C. BAILAR III[a] AND A. JOHN BAILER[b,c]

[a]*Department of Health Studies and Harris School of Public Policy, University of Chicago, 5841 South Maryland Avenue, MC 2007, Chicago, Illinois 60637, USA*

[b]*Department of Mathematics and Statistics, Miami University, Oxford, Ohio 45056, USA*

[c]*National Institute for Occupational Safety and Health, Education and Information Division, Risk Evaluation Branch, 4676 Columbia Parkway, Cincinnati, Ohio 45226, USA*

The workshop entitled "Uncertainty in the Risk Assessment of Environmental and Occupational Hazards", which was held during September 21–26, 1998 in Bologna, Italy in the historic council chamber of the Bologna Town Hall, was a collaborative effort of the European Ramazzini Foundation and the International Statistical Institute. The workshop had three objectives: (1) to improve understanding of the sources and magnitude of uncertainty in the risk assessment process; (2) to discuss and disseminate means for reducing such uncertainty; and (3) to describe, characterize, and express uncertainty in risk assessment, with a particular view towards its implications on policy. The workshop sessions revolved around the themes of uncertainty and variability in the four components of a common model of the risk assessment process. The presentations were grouped into sessions that considered uncertainty in hazard identification, exposure assessment, exposure-response modeling, and risk characterization. The workshop was designed to be highly practical. The uncertainties associated with the assessment of health risks of electromagnetic fields and of dioxin were the focus of more than one presentation. The perspectives of participants from academia, industry, and government enriched discussions about the evaluation and communication of uncertainty and variability throughout the risk assessment process.

The municipal council chamber in Bologna played host to a three-day workshop devoted to uncertainty in the risk assessment of environmental and occupational hazards. The sessions were organized into four components reflecting hazard identification, exposure assessment, concentration-response modeling and risk characterization. These four sessions were based on a common risk assessment paradigm suggested by the National Academy of Sciences in 1983.[1] After three days of deliberations, we noted ten general issues that appeared in more than one presentation and discussion. Here is what we heard and saw, or thought we did.

Addresses for correspondence:
[a]John C. Bailar, 773-834-1242 (voice); 773-702-1979 (fax). e-mail: jcbailar@midway.uchicago.edu
[b]John Bailer, 513-529-3538 (voice); 513-529-1493 (fax). e-mail: ajbailer@muohio.edu

1. Heterogeneity in responses should not be treated as just another source of uncertainty. Imagine a population for which several human studies indicate that some compound C is carcinogenic, but that quantitative assessments derived by similar methods range from 5 to 45 cases per thousand exposed—a ninefold difference. (This would be very small uncertainty in many risk assessment contexts.) Imagine now that you discover that the adverse effect is limited to persons who lack a detoxifying enzyme, and that a nonrandom segment of the population is so affected. The true risk is zero for some and 50 for others, with risks in the study populations determined by enzyme status, although we do not know the status of the next person we will encounter. This seems to be fundamentally different from the situation in which there are serious measurement problems, or errors in default assumptions, or other kinds of uncertainty.

There is a problem with this. Whether we call something heterogeneity or uncertainty depends on our state of knowledge. In an extreme *clockwork* universe every person has probability zero or unity of some dread outcome under any fixed set of circumstances—but we still do not know individual risks because we cannot tell what is going on cell by cell, molecule by molecule. Both variability (from unknown causes), as is reflected by this heterogeneity, and other uncertainties, are measures of our ignorance.

Some speakers highlighted special kinds of heterogeneity in risk, including:

- children are not little adults;
- sensitive subpopulations;
- synergies with prior, concurrent, or later exposures to other agents.

Some of these variations can be removed by appropriate scaling (e.g., by body weight) or other transformation (e.g., to a power of body weight as a surrogate for metabolic differences) but analytic methods that reduce the range or impact of variation (e.g., logarithmic transformation)—especially at the high end of risk—may run directly contrary to what is needed in protecting the public health.

2. Laboratory animal and human observational studies may lead to quite different risk estimates, but data often agree that a risk exists despite variations in specific outcomes or magnitudes of risk. Thus, there was a strong sense that animal studies offer a valid and important tool for identifying human hazards. In general, moves toward biologically-based models, and away from the familiar *default assumptions,* may simply replace a few large uncertainties with many small ones and offer no guarantee of any improvement in the product. However, this may provide a more honest depiction of our state of knowledge about potential hazards. Possible explanations of differences include substantial laboratory-to-laboratory variation in estimates of parameters that are critical in PBPK models.

3. What is sufficient evidence to justify what kind of risk management response? Intervention may be based on levels of evidence ranging from a faint suspicion, to an equivocal laboratory finding, or to conclusive epidemiologic studies, with many steps between. Similarly, the level of interven-

tion can range from a little private worry, to voluntary personal avoidance, to public warnings, to strict labeling, to controlled use, or to outright prohibition, again with many intermediate steps. Somehow these two continuous scales, strength of evidence and risk management steps, should be linked. There appears to be little or no research on this topic, either theoretical or applied, although opinions are rife.

4. Each new study should be interpreted in a context of what is already known. This implies a Bayesian approach to each step of risk assessment. This is a fairly new and evolving approach in risk assessment. Interesting questions concerning the nature of a prior distribution may be related to risk management ideas. For example, should a prior distribution reflect a belief that a potential hazard has no adverse effect—perhaps as reflected in the distribution of an associated regression coefficient, with the hazard being centered at zero? Alternatively, should we start with a prior distribution that reflects a belief that the substance is hazardous? Answers to these specific questions are necessarily political and philosophical as much as they are scientific.

5. The more that a particular risk is concentrated on a small, identifiable subpopulation, the easier it is to identify and measure the risk, but the greatest population-wide hazards may be from very low exposures of millions of people. In the limit, if every person is affected by some exposure, the risk will merge into the background rate and be undetectable, or even unsuspected. The challenges to evaluating the risks associated with such small exposures are very great and these need to be addressed in well-designed and extensive animal and human studies.

6. Toxic hazards are complex. Cancer has multiple causes, with multiple steps, and a likelihood of response heterogeneity, as well as multiple biologic mechanisms of causation. Laboratory observations suggesting that risk has a threshold or sublinear form may not carry over to humans who live in a sea of toxic agents and may already be well along some biologic pathway before they encounter the new hazard, which could then create linear or supralinear risks. Reproductive responses are even more complex—aspermia, failure to ovulate or implant, birth defects, failure of nursing, and many others.

These complexities are well-understood by workers in the field, but not always by risk managers or by the public, who want sharp lines between what is risky and what is safe. Communicating this complexity to risk managers and to the public remains one of our great challenges in risk assessment.

7. All critical assumptions underlying the risk assessment process must be identified and, to the extent possible, validated. For example, the shape of concentration-response models, mechanism of toxicity, and questions of species extrapolation haunt most or all risk assessments. However, even the identification of assumptions may be difficult and incomplete. Sensitivity analysis can help to define the range of uncertainty, but this approach

depends on knowing all of the critical inputs and reasonable ranges for their values.

8. It has become a truism that the greatest uncertainties in risk assessment are likely to come from poor understanding of exposures. In addition to uncertainties about levels of exposure, we often do not know how to summarize the exposure captured by the risk. For example, for some reproductive hazard, should we use the cumulative exposure at low levels over a lifetime, or the maximum eight-hour time-weighted average during the third month of pregnancy, or something else? Choices of metrics for exposure are seldom justified or formally evaluated. This was stated or implied in several presentations, but not addressed in a direct way by any speaker.

9. Completion of a risk assessment document is not the end of the road. Contrary to the recommendations of the National Academy of Sciences in their 1983 *Red Book*, risk assessors must be involved in all later stages of risk management and risk communication, with special attention to uncertainty, however unpopular that may be.

10. There are many critical gaps in the data for specific toxic agents, but there are also gaps in matters that lie beyond concerns about toxic hazards taken one-by-one. Examples include the parameters needed in PBPK modeling, critical aspects of transport, general responses to very low exposures or background levels of risk, and many other things. Building databases may be less exciting scientifically and less appealing politically than the carcinogen-of-the-week approach, but it is essential for improvements in risk assessment, including reduction of uncertainty. Sensitivity analyses based on solid data will have more credibility than those based on a series of convenient *ad hoc* distributional assumptions.

Given these impressions, what is next? We believe that uncertainty and variability will always be a part of the risk assessment process. This implies a need to continue to develop the tools to appropriately accommodate these concerns in risk assessment. However, this activity will not be enough. A closer collaboration between risk assessment scientists and social scientists specializing in risk communication is needed. We must communicate uncertainty and variability to risk managers and to the public in order to be effective risk assessors.

REFERENCE

1. NATIONAL ACADEMY OF SCIENCES. 1983. Risk Assessment in the Federal Government: Managing the Process. National Academy Press, Washington, DC.

Index of Contributors

Ahlbom, A., 27–33
Al-Delaimy, W., 156–172

Bailar, III, J.C., ix, 273–285, 373–376
Bailer, A.J., 212–222, 273–285, 367–372, 373–376
Banati, P., 286–316
Belpoggi, F., 10–26, 34–55
Bois, F.Y., 317–337
Bortot, P., 125–140
Bua, L., 34–55

Crump, K.S., 232–244

De Rosa, C.T., 348–364

Edler, L., 80–100

Feychting, M., 27–33

Gaylor, D.W., 188–195
Gilbert, S., 212–222
Goble, R., 286–316

Hansen, H., 348–364
Hattis, D., 286–316
Holler, J., 348–364
Hopke, P.K., 245–272
Huff, J., 56–79

Jones, D., 348–364

Kleckner, R.C., 141–155
Kodell, R.L., 188–195
Krewski, D., 232–244, 245–272
Kromhout, H., 141–155
Kuempel, E., 212–222

Landrigan, P.J., 1–9
Lauriola, P., 173–187
Leonard, R.C., 348–364
Loomis, D.P., 141–155

Maltoni, C., x–xi, 10–26, 34–55
Minardi, F., 34–55
Molenberghs, G., 196–211

Pohl, H.R., 348–364

Rai, S.N., 245–272
Rice, F., 212–222
Ryan, L., 196–211

Salvan, A., 125–140
Sartori, N., 125–140
Schulte, P.A., 101–111
Smith, R., 212–222
Soffritti, M., 10–26, 34–55
Stayner, L., 212–222

Ten Berge, W.F., 112–124
Thomaseth, K., 125–140

Ulm, K., 223–231

Van den Broecke, M., xii
Van Landingham, C., 232–244

Waters, M., 101–111
Woodward, A., 156–172, 365–366

Yamaguchi, N., 338–347

Zavatti, A., 173–187
Zielinski, J.M., 245–272